Madness and Literature

LANGUAGE, DISCOURSE AND MENTAL HEALTH

Series Editors:

Laura Cariola, Lecturer in Applied Psychology at the University of Edinburgh

Billy Lee, Lecturer in Psychology at the University of Edinburgh

Lisa Mikesell, Associate Professor of Communication at Rutgers University, USA

Michael Birch, Professor of English & Communications at Massachusetts College of Liberal Arts, USA

Mental Health Ontologies
How We Talk About Mental Health, and Why it Matters in the Digital Age
Janna Hastings, 2020

Madness and Literature
What Fiction Can Do for the Understanding of Mental Illness
ed. Lasse R. Gammelgaard, 2022

Eating Disorders in Public Discourse
Using Language-Based Approaches to Explore Media and Lived Experiences
ed. Laura Cariola, 2022

MADNESS AND LITERATURE

What Fiction Can Do for the Understanding of Mental Illness

Edited by
Lasse Raaby Gammelgaard

UNIVERSITY
of
EXETER
PRESS

First published in 2022 by
University of Exeter Press
Reed Hall, Streatham Drive
Exeter EX4 4QR, UK

www.exeterpress.co.uk

Copyright © Lasse Raaby Gammelgaard and the contributors 2022

The right of Lasse Raaby Gammelgaard and the contributors to be identified as authors of this work has been asserted by them in accordance with the Copyright, Designs and Patents Act 1988.

Language, Discourse and Mental Health

The publishers gratefully acknowledge the assistance of the Independent Research Fund Denmark in the publication of this volume.

British Library Cataloguing in Publication Data
A catalogue record for this book is available from the British Library.

https://doi.org/10.47788/PMMG3806

ISBN 978-1-90581-637-8 Hardback
ISBN 978-1-90581-638-5 ePub
ISBN 978-1-90581-639-2 PDF

Cover image: iStock.com/enjoynz

Every effort has been made to trace copyright holders and obtain permission to reproduce the material included in this book. Please get in touch with any enquiries or information relating to an image or the rights holder.

Typeset in Caslon and Myriad by Deanta Global Publishing Services, Chennai, India

Contents

Contibutors   viii

    Introduction: Madness and Literature and the Health Humanities   1
    Lasse Raaby Gammelgaard (Aarhus University, Denmark)

Part I: Literary History and Socio-Political Perspectives   21

1. *Layla and Majnun* in Historical and Contemporary Conceptions of Madness in Islamic Psychology   23
   Alan Weber (Weill Cornell Medical College, Qatar)

2. The Anti-Psychiatry Ethos in Samuel Beckett's *Murphy*   41
   Shoshana Benjamin (Ben-Gurion University of the Negev, Israel)

3. Apartheid's Garden: Dismantling Madness in J.M. Coetzee's *Life & Times of Michael K*   58
   Sebastian C. Galbo (University of Buffalo—SUNY, USA)

4. Sniffs and Dribblers: *Poppy Shakespeare* and the Identities of Madness   75
   Clare Allan (novelist)

Part II: Literary Theory and Experiencing Mental Illness   91

5. Reading Shattering Minds and Extended Selves in Virginia Woolf's *Mrs Dalloway*   93
   Anna Ovaska (Tampere University, Finland)

CONTENTS

6   Spill the Words: Speechlessness and Creativity in the
    Writing of Janet Frame   111
    Mary Elene Wood (University of Oregon, USA)

7   Pronominal Shifts and the Confusion of Self with
    Not-Self   128
    Alice Hervé (writer and independent scholar)

8   Rethinking Clinical and Critical Perspectives on Psychosis
    in Kathy Acker's Writing   143
    Charley Baker (University of Nottingham, UK)

9   Countering the DSM in Poetry about Bipolar
    Disorder   164
    Lasse Raaby Gammelgaard (Aarhus University, Denmark)

10 Seeing Feeling: Dissociation and Post-Traumatic Memory
    in the Graphic Novel *Perfect Hair*   180
    Penni Russon (University of Technology Sydney)

Part III: Literary Instrumentality and Clinical Psychopathology   199

11 Writing Therapy, Writing Data: Therapeutic Writing as
    a Methodological and Ethical Approach in Researching
    Digital Sexual Assault   201
    Signe Uldbjerg (University of Southern Denmark)

12 A Question of Context: Sites for Cultural Negotiation in
    Narratives of Manic Depression   220
    Megan Milota (University Medical Center Utrecht, Netherlands)

13 Conscripting Dante: History, Anachronism, and the Uses
    of Literary Precedents in the 'New' Diagnosis of Hoarding
    Disorder   239
    David Orr (University of Sussex, UK)

14 Opening Up the Discourse of Male Eating Disorders: Personal Experience in German and English Narratives 259
Heike Bartel (University of Nottingham, UK)

Afterword 281
Lasse Raaby Gammelgaard (Aarhus University, Denmark)

Index 285

Contibutors

Clare Allan is a novelist, author of *Poppy Shakespeare* and of the forthcoming *Everything is Full of Dogs*. From 2006 to 2018 she wrote a column for *The Guardian* newspaper on matters relating to mental health, and for many years lectured in novel writing at City, University of London.

Dr Charley Baker is an Associate Professor of Mental Health at the University of Nottingham. She has broad expertise across a range of mental health and illness, with a particular interest in 'psychosis', self harm, suicidality, anxiety and obsessive compulsive disorder. She is known internationally for her work in the Health Humanities, particularly in the subfields of literature and mental health, and heavy metal music and self harm. She has worked with a broad range of organizations including the NHS, BBC and different publishers.

Heike Bartel is Professor of German Studies and Health Humanities at the University of Nottingham, UK. Her key publications include *Men Writing Eating Disorders*: *Autobiographical Writing and Illness Experience in English and German Narratives* (2020).

Shoshana Benjamin, retired Senior Lecturer from Ben-Gurion University of the Negev and Beit Rivka Teachers' College, Kfar Chabad, Israel, specializes in the study of cryptic literature. Her publications include 'On the Distinctiveness of Poetic Language' (2012) and 'Is There a Single Right Interpretation for Cryptic Texts?' (2013).

Sebastian C. Galbo is a PhD student in the English Department at the State University of New York–Buffalo. He holds an MS in information and library science and works as a graduate assistant in the University at Buffalo's Robert L. Brown History of Medicine Collection. He has been a contributing editor to New York University's Literature, Arts, & Medicine Database for the last five years. His research interests are interdisciplinary and include the medical humanities, history of medicine and nineteenth-century American literature.

Lasse Raaby Gammelgaard is Associate Professor at the Department of Communication and Culture at Aarhus University, Denmark. He has published articles and book chapters on the depiction of madness in Danish and English literature. He co-directs the research group Health, Media and Narrative at Aarhus University.

Alice Hervé was awarded a Master of Arts in Literature and a PhD in Creative Writing. She writes poetry and prose as well as non-fiction. Post-doctorate, she worked as an Associate Lecturer at Bath Spa University. She has been a full-time writer since 2019.

Megan Milota is an Assistant Professor in Medical Humanities at the University Medical Center Utrecht in the Netherlands. She has published on a variety of topics, including end-of-life conversations in *Supportive Care in Cancer* (2021) and narrative medicine in the medical school classroom in *Medical Teacher* (2019) and *Medical Education* (2021).

David Orr is Senior Lecturer in Social Work at the University of Sussex. He is co-editor of the *Palgrave Handbook of Sociocultural Perspectives on Global Mental Health* (2017) and sits on the Editorial Board of the international journal *Anthropology in Action*.

Anna Ovaska is a postdoctoral scholar at Narrare (Centre for Interdisciplinary Narrative Studies) at Tampere University, Finland. Her monograph *Shattering Minds: Reading Experiences of Mental Distress in Modernist Finnish Literature* (Finnish Literature Society, forthcoming) explores the interaction between a reader and a text in first-person narratives of mental illness.

Penni Russon is a Senior Lecturer in Writing and Publishing at University of Technology Sydney. She is a widely published, critically acclaimed author for

CONTIBUTORS

young people. Her research concerns the intersections between creative reading and writing and youth mental health.

Signe Uldbjerg is a postdoctoral scholar at the University of Southern Denmark. Other publications on the project presented in this book include 'Writing victimhood: a methodological manifesto for researching digital sexual assault' (2021) in *Women, Gender and Research*, and 'The rhythms of shame in digital sexual assault' (2021) in *First Monday*.

Alan S. Weber has taught the medical and health humanities for the last 15 years at Weill Cornell Medicine–Qatar in Doha, Qatar. He has held previous appointments at Cornell University and Pennsylvania State University.

Mary Elene Wood is a Professor of English at the University of Oregon. She is author of *The Writing on the Wall: Women's Autobiography and the Asylum* (1994) and *Life Writing and Schizophrenia: Encounters at the Edge of Meaning* (2013).

Introduction: Madness and Literature and the Health Humanities

Lasse Raaby Gammelgaard

Although madness (a term that is often reappropriated by scholars working on mental illness in literature) does not exist as 'an aesthetic category like the grotesque, the sublime or the uncanny' (Bernaerts, Herman, and Vervaeck 285), the relation of madness to literature has been examined as far back as in Plato's *Ion*. Furthermore, psychiatry and the arts have always been reciprocally interested and influenced. They share the endeavour to explain the human mind and human behaviour (cf. Rieger; Oyebode; Baker et al.; Gammelgaard and Boström). To take just two examples, it was the psychologist William James who first coined the term 'stream of consciousness' that would become important to the modernist novel, and Karl Jaspers, founder of modern psychiatry, states that we need to study authors like Shakespeare and Dostoevsky to gain a sufficient store of images and symbols and exercise the necessary understanding (Clarke ii).

In spite of the diversity of theory, methodology, literary examples under scrutiny, and national and cultural background of the contributors, this book fits under the umbrella term of the health humanities and literature and medicine. The authors explore mental illness (as a cultural, historical, phenomenological concept) through interpretations of salient literary examples. Hence, literature and psychopathology are put into dialogue by mounting research questions concerning the representation of mental illness in literature. The output of any representation is informed by the affordances and limitations of the chosen medium, and different types of literature are suited to advancing different purposes. This book offers academic engagements with madness literature from a wide diachronic, cultural, and generic spectrum (from medieval Islamic narrative poetry about love and melancholia to contemporary comics about trauma and abuse). The authors engage critically with a range of theories, examining the interplay between medical knowledge of and the humanities' discourses about mental illness. The individual chapters may hold relevance for a wide group of audiences such as humanities scholars, practitioners (psychologists, doctors, nurses, social workers), patients, their next of kin, and those members of the public who might be interested in the topic.

In *Poetic Madness and the Romantic Imagination*, Frederick Burwick makes reference to Michel Foucault's rationality paradox, according to which 'every attempt to examine irrationality reveals only the rigorous categories of reason' (Burwick 8–9). However, representing mental illnesses through literature entails conveying fragments, silences, abnormal thinking, strange voices, and more. So the question is whether irrationality might not be examined more freely through imaginative literature than other modes of discourse. The chapters in this volume address how historical and socio-political implications of mental illness have been explored through literature, how literature can help us to better understand the subjectivity of mental illness experiences, and how literature can be instrumentalized—that is, put to use in order to help inform clinical praxis.

This book is titled *Madness and Literature: What Fiction Can Do for the Understanding of Mental Illness*. At a surface level, two concepts seem to be doubled in the main title and the subtitle—namely, madness/mental illness and literature/fiction. This calls for explanation, if not justification. 'Madness' and 'mental illness' arguably try to cover roughly the same phenomenon. 'Madness', though, is loose, colloquial, and decidedly not politically correct, whereas 'mental illness' resonates more with medicalized language use. The term 'madness' connotes a distance to a biomedical discourse. It can even—but does not have to—be used to implicate anti-psychiatric sentiments (cf. Rapley, Moncrieff, and Dillon). Individual contributors to this book vary in terms of how critical or endorsing they are of the system in place. 'Madness' is used in the title to state that madness literature is not subservient to the discourse of clinical psychiatry in terms of providing insights into mental illness. Additionally, this move places the book in line with academic publications on

INTRODUCTION: MADNESS AND LITERATURE AND THE HEALTH HUMANITIES

madness literature that use both 'madness' and, for instance, 'mental illness' in their titles. More recent publications on the topic, however, often opt for 'mental illness' instead. In her entry on 'Mental Disorder (Illness)' in the *Stanford Encyclopedia of Philosophy*, Jennifer Radden states that '[f]requently the term "*illness*" in "mental illness" has been replaced by "*disorder*," apparently without a consistent rationale beyond avoiding explicitly medical language' (Radden 2019; italics in the original). This seems strange, though, since 'disorder' is at least as medicalizing as 'illness'. In the title for this book, I use both 'madness' and 'mental illness'. This is not to suggest that they are identical or interchangeable, but rather to suggest that they are in reciprocally interdependent dialogue with one another.

The other two terms that operate within the same domain of meaning are 'literature' and 'fiction'. Again, the purpose of this book is not to suggest that they are interchangeable. Literature can be both fictional and non-fictional, and in many of the cases analysed here the lines between the fictional and the non-fictional are blurred or mixed. Fiction, in its turn, is not limited to literature, but exists in movies and television among other things. While this book is limited to literature (with one chapter about comics as a multimodal example, combining text with visual material), it is not limited to strictly speaking fictional literature. However, many of the cases analysed are fictional, and 'fiction' in the title also draws attention to the aim of the book to use fictional (i.e. made-up) stories in a wider theoretical and cultural context.

Critical Tendencies within the Study of Madness and Literature

Madness and literature has been approached via different theoretical perspectives and with various purposes in mind. In this brief overview, I want to demarcate five different approaches to researching interrelations between literature and mental illness: politically oriented studies, psychoanalytic approaches, narrative research, history of medicine, and studies on creativity and madness. Of course, these five cannot always be separated completely from one another, as there are many potential overlaps. The authors of this volume tap into several of the five approaches, often combining one or more of them.

Madness in literature is more often than not in some way tied with political sentiments. Given that mental illness and the treatment of psychiatry patients involve precarious ethical issues such as confinement, forced medication, and other means of coercion and losses of essential liberties, both authors of literature and of academic works are disposed to form an opinion on such aspects. The anti-psychiatry movement emerged because of large-scale anti-humanistic experiments around the treatment of people suffering from mental illness in the twentieth century, such as lobotomy and insulin-induced seizure. The anti-psychiatry movement is associated with the works of Thomas Szasz, R.D. Laing, Michel Foucault, and Erving Goffman (cf. the references for each scholar's most important work in this regard). In *Post-Capitalist Subjectivity in Literature and Anti-Psychiatry* from 2021, Hans A. Skott-Myhre revisits Marxist and post-Marxist theories and literary examples to argue that the portrayal of institutions and families therein contains the potential to imagine a new social organization in which subjectivity is freed from capitalist structures.

More recently, a movement labelled 'mad studies' has emerged. Peter Beresford, who is a co-editor of *The Routledge International Handbook of Mad Studies* (2021), states that '[mad studies] rejects a bio-medical approach to the domain widely known as "mental illness" or "mental health" and substitutes instead a framework of "madness"' (Beresford 2020: 1337). Instead of describing human conditions as illnesses or disorders, as is the case within a biomedical framework, mad studies prefers designations like 'distress' (Beresford) or 'misery' (Rapley, Moncrieff, and Dillon). Depictions of madness as something that goes counter to the established system can be observed in a large number of works of fiction.

Another salient approach to madness and literature is found in psychoanalytic literary criticism. This is inherent in much of Sigmund Freud's own work, in that he often employed literary examples as illustrations of his psychoanalysis. Perhaps the most prominent example of this is his study *The Uncanny*, which is partially a reading of E.T.A. Hoffmann's short story entitled 'The Sandman'. Shoshana Felman's book *Writing and Madness* (first published in French in 1978) mixes anti-psychiatry and psychoanalysis in its conceptual framework. She makes the following claim:

> In the nineteenth century, the age of the establishment of the clinician's power, literature interrogates and challenges this power, gives refuge and expression to what is socially or medically repressed, objectified, unauthorized, denied and silenced. Literature becomes the only recourse for the self-expression and the self-representation of the mad. (Felman 4)

INTRODUCTION: MADNESS AND LITERATURE AND THE HEALTH HUMANITIES

As such, the author takes up the position as anti-psychiatrist. Felman argues that the discourse of the madman can be reclaimed through literature. With reference to Lacanian psychoanalysis, she explains a theory of misprision as a 'theory of the *rhetoric* of the unconscious' (Felman 123; italics in the original), because psychoanalytic defense mechanisms employ 'all kinds of "tropes" and "figures of speech"' (Felman 122). Psychoanalysis is an approach taken up frequently, but it can take the literary analysis in different directions—which is also acknowledged by Branimir Rieger in the introduction to the anthology *Dionysus in Literature: Essays on Literary Madness* from 1994, in which he writes that the contributions reflect 'pluralism in psychological or psychoanalytic criticism' (Rieger 12; in addition, cf. Wiesenthal).

Psychoanalytic approaches to madness narratives have affinities with some of the approaches from narrative theory. The literary category of the fantastic, proposed by Tzvetan Todorov, is frequently exemplified by texts in which madness plays a role, where readers oscillate between supernatural and naturalistic, scientific explanations of an irrational element in a story. Though not the main focus of this book, madness is a powerful resource for constructing a suspenseful plot in general. In *Reading for the Plot*, Peter Brooks explicitly sets out to employ psychoanalysis to explain various phenomena in fictional narrative. In chapter four on 'Freud's Masterplot: A Model for Narrative', he employs Freud's notion of the death drive from *Beyond the Pleasure Principle* to speculate on narrative desire as a readerly interest. Much of narrative theory's engagement with madness has to do with understanding authors' various styles when trying to depict madness. This, of course, has a diachronic dimension. As narrative innovations develop over time, so do authors' ways of representing mad characters. In *Transparent Minds: Narrative Modes for Presenting Consciousness in Fiction*, the structuralist narratologist Dorrit Cohn invokes the distinction between showing and telling and states that authors of the nineteenth century 'choose to tell rather than show those psychic happenings that their characters cannot plausibly verbalize, employing analyses, analogies, and other authorial indirections to penetrate the speechless nether realm' (Cohn 88). This, however, is not the case with surrealism or the beat writers (for instance William S. Burroughs) of the twentieth century.

Narrative theory has a long-standing interest in mad narrators, who are often analysed as being unreliable. The anthology *Les narrateurs fous / Mad Narrators* from 2014 (edited by Jaëck et al.) is devoted to the examination of mad narrators in fiction. The contribution by Lars Bernaerts is about the rhetoric of first-person narrators who are mad, and in it he makes a useful distinction between '*fou raisonnant*' (referring to clinical-pathological discourse) and '*fou imaginant*' (referring to the existential-phenomenological delirium) to help navigate the madness discourse. *Fou imaginant* proposes a more positive and engaging assessment of a narrative delirium. Instead of merely labelling the narrator as mad and hence unreliable in what they narrate, the category of the *fou imaginant* shows how literature can present the experience of madness as meaningful and mind-expanding, something that Virginia Woolf also advocates in her essay entitled *On Being Ill*. The narration of madness does not, of course, only take place with first-person narrators. Sometimes fiction uses shifts in the personal pronoun to mark madness. This is the move that William Faulkner employs when Darl goes mad in *As I Lay Dying*.

Another aspect of narrative theory engaging with madness literature is research into illness narratives. This genre has proliferated since the 1990s, both in terms of publications and of research into the topic. Several advances have been made in the genre of the pathography, where one can distinguish between different illness narratives. For instance, Arthur Frank has described three illness narratives: the restitution narrative, the chaos narrative, and the quest narrative. This raises questions of fiction versus non-fiction, and, in this regard, pathographies about mental illness can challenge autobiography's 'preference for the literal and verifiable' as well as 'its anxiety about invention' (Gilmore 129).

Arguably, all approaches to madness and literature have—at least to some extent—a historical dimension. Some publications explicitly mix literary criticism with the history of medicine. And, indeed, publications on the history of medicine frequently use literary examples. This is, for instance, the case with Roy Porter's book *Madness: A Brief History*, which provides a concise overview of the history of madness. Two of the seminal books combining madness literature with a history of medicine approach are Lillian Feder's *Madness in Literature* from 1980 and Allen Thiher's *Revels in Madness* from 1999. Feder's book draws on literary depictions of madness from ancient Greece to the twentieth century. She foregrounds the discoveries made in fictive texts and how the works reflect contemporary philosophical, medical, social, religious, and political issues. Thiher's book is in two parts. The first part is on madness from Hippocrates to Hölderlin, whereas the second part is about 'The Modernity of Madness' (Thiher 159)—i.e. from madness in romanticism up to the end of the twentieth century. Hence, Thiher's book has a historically progressing structure, tracing developments in medicine alongside examples taken from literature.

Historical approaches that cite literature in conjunction with medical advances have also led to comparison between symptoms of mental illnesses and textual features from the imaginative world of literature. Two important books that were published just one year apart epitomize this approach—namely Louis A. Sass's *Madness and Modernism: Insanity in the Light of Modern Art, Literature, and Thought* from 1992; and Kay Redfield Jamison's *Touched with Fire: Manic-Depressive Illness and the Artistic Temperament* from 1993. Both books examine creativity, more generally, in relation to literature. Jamison's book is inscribed in a long tradition of seeing relations between what is today labelled 'bipolar disorder' and creativity. *Touched with Fire*, she states, is about 'manic-depressive illness—a disease of perturbed gaieties, melancholy, and tumultuous temperaments—and its relationship to the artistic temperament and imagination' (Jamison 2). This line of thought can be dated back at least to Aristotle's Problemata 30 on the relationship between melancholy and greatness in human beings (and, of course, the topos of *furor poeticus* dates further back to Plato's *Ion* and *Phaedrus*). However, as Jennifer Radden has argued, it is not unproblematic to align past melancholia with present-day depression—among other reasons, because melancholia covered more symptoms than accounted for in present-day depression (Radden 2003).

Positing relations between creativity and mental illness is often presented as a notion rooted in romanticism, where madness is viewed as individualistic and liberating (cf. Burwick; James; and Whitehead). The view of madness as creative is, in its turn, often associated with manic depression or bipolar disorder. Louis A. Sass challenges this in *Madness and Modernism*, in which the interpretive strategy 'is to view the poorly understood schizophrenic-type illnesses in the light of the sensibility and structures of consciousness found in [...] the epoch of modernism' (Sass 1992, 8). He argues that modernist art forms 'are characterized not so much by unreflectiveness and spontaneity as by acute self-consciousness and self-reference, and by alienation from action and experience—qualities we might refer to as "hyperreflexivity"' (Sass 1992, 8). The question of whether creativity is more associated with schizophrenia-type illnesses or affective illnesses (like bipolar disorder and variations thereof) resulted in a special issue of the *Creativity Research Journal* in 2000–2001, about creativity and the schizophrenia spectrum. In his article in the special issue, Sass states the following:

> there seems to be a fairly sharp difference between romantic yearnings for unity with the world, heightened emotional arousal, and intense personal engagement and the modernist preference for isolation, coolness, and detachment. (Sass 2000–2001, 60)

Sass wants to emphasize that schizophrenia is not a dementing illness, but rather one characterized by alienation and hyperreflexivity; that is, whereas the romantic notion of creativity and affective illnesses highlight impulsivity and natural processes, schizophrenic creativity underscores deliberation and rational processes.

Regardless of whether the question of creativity in relation to madness and literature—from a psychological and philosophical perspective—is better aligned with romanticism and aspects of the affective disorders, or with modernism and the schizophrenic spectrum, literary scholars would foreground the creative potential inherent in composing literature about mad characters. Nathalie Jaëck has drawn attention to the notion 'that mad narrators may provide some writers with an experimental poetical matrix, a metaphor for an ideal literary form, a literary temptation—delirium as the horizon for literature, what Deleuze called "*le devenir-fou de la structure*"' (Jaëck 15).

The Health Humanities

The 'illness' in mental illness differs from somatic illnesses. To put it crudely, it is easier to give a diagnosis of, say, bone fracture or high blood pressure, while relying on empirical, objective science, than to diagnose someone with schizophrenia, schizoaffective disorder or bipolar disorder. Additionally, the causes of a mental illness rely on different scientific paradigms. From a medical perspective, one may highlight, for instance, neurological implications or genetic dispositions, but it is difficult to disregard social causes such as one's upbringing and traumatic experiences. Hence, inputs from the human sciences are indispensable. Jennifer Radden describes some intersecting issues related to foundational assumptions behind one's understanding of mental illness:

> Thus, objectivist (or naturalist) accounts, hold that mental disorders are empirically discoverable items that can be provided value-free description, while evaluativist (or normative) analyses deny the possibility of such value-free description […] And finally, the nature of mental disorder will be sought either through *a posteriori* scientific research based in cognitive science, or through conceptual analysis derived in part or whole from social and cultural norms. (Radden 2019; italics in the original)

Whether one believes mental illness is caused by traumatic experiences, by genetic predisposition or has neurological implications, and to what degree one wants to take these into account, or whether one predominantly wants to look at particular symptoms and clusters of symptoms, there is a shared assumption across the chapters in this volume that literature has the potential to play a role in understanding mental illness, and in negotiating values associated with mental illness.

In his seminal article from 2018 entitled 'What Does It Mean to Be Mad? Diagnosis, Narrative, Science, and the DSM', Porter Abbott takes issue with diagnostic typology and advances the following argument:

> [Diagnostic typologies are] acts of scientific domestication applied to individuals who nonetheless have, in Savarese's apt phrase, 'Irreducible particularity' (Savarese 2015: 395). This particularity, which not only separates every one of us but lies beyond reach of the finest scientific instruments, is one of the things that make even the most seemingly settled psychiatric classifications necessarily unstable—as witness the constant definitional tinkering in successive editions of the *Diagnostic and Statistical Manual of Mental Disorders* (DSM). (Abbott 20)

Abbott furthermore argues that the DSM-III from 1980 'consolidated a revolution in a field that had been up to then dominated by psychoanalytic theory and practice, and ushered in an era of biomedical dominance' (Abbott 23). One consequence of this was that the individual case history, which had been 'the primary instrument in a narrative-based psychology' would almost cease to be employed as a scientific resource (Abbott 23). Abbott makes reference to a study by Carol Berkenkotter that shows how articles using a case history to support their argument gradually disappeared from contributions to *The American Journal of Psychiatry* from 1980 to 1991.

However, the subsequent dominance of empirical and biomedical research has created a gap in our human endeavours to grasp what mental illness is, why it exists, and what types of meanings it can maintain. In his article, Abbott contends that madness disables one's 'mind-reading capability', which has an impact on the beholders that 'registers as an urgent need for a diagnosis that will sufficiently explain the frightening combination of unpredictability and obscurity of intention that signifies madness' (Abbott 18). Hence, the ascription of madness becomes a necessary 'placeholder' when one encounters behaviour that is difficult to understand (Abbott 18). Due to the irreducible particularity of individuals, this placeholder is not sufficient, and the decline of the case history has created a void. Abbott suggests that narrative fiction can to some extent fill that void, since it can 'let us actually know, without a doubt, what a character is thinking' (Abbott 24).

The notion that narratives (within fiction as well as non-fiction) can supplement the empirical, positivistic vantage point of medicine resonates well with the field of narrative medicine and more broadly the proliferating interdisciplinary field of the health humanities. For instance, Rita Charon writes that 'bedrock aspects of narrative practice' such as 'temporality, singularity, causality/contingency, intersubjectivity, and ethicality' are also indispensable narrative features of medicine (Charon 39).

In *Health Humanities*, a book from 2015 co-written by Paul Crawford, Brian Brown, Charley Baker, Victoria Tischler, and Brian Abrams, the authors contend that 'in the health humanities, the arts and humanities are used to provide insight into the human condition, and issues such as suffering, personhood and our responsibility to each other' (Crawford et al. 18). The idea of the health humanities entails a privileged position for literature and the arts in general, for understanding what it means to be in ill health and to be treated by the healthcare system. *Health Humanities* devotes a significant amount of text space to mental illness in particular, and mental illness does seem to pose a particular challenge for a biomedical discourse (as is evident from the main ideas in Abbott's article). Crawford et al. write:

> Unlike a physical illness, the most extreme test of personal integrity and identity comes in the form of challenges to mental well-being, from depression and anxiety through to psychotic disorders which challenge not only the 'regular' experience of emotional health but the sense of secure and reliable perceptions and beliefs. (Crawford et al. 43)

INTRODUCTION: MADNESS AND LITERATURE AND THE HEALTH HUMANITIES

In mental illness representation, for example proprioceptive dysfunctions might be accompanied by disturbances of what phenomenology terms 'the minimal self', resulting in an altered sense of bodily demarcation (Brice et al.; Sass, Parnas, and Zahavi). Part of the project of this book is to engage critically with literature that emphasizes and tries to depict the experience of mental illness. It may be that someone experiencing a psychosis makes reference to an object that is actually not there in the world for other people to confirm (say, the dagger in Shakespeare's *Macbeth*), and, hence, this could be interpreted as a visual hallucination—yet it truly is something that the person experiencing the psychosis sees. The middle section of this book is thus devoted to the experience of mental illness—for which literary examples can be a great auxiliary resource to aid understanding. Literature has a definite advantage over the case study that one finds in textbooks designed for the education of doctors and healthcare workers specializing in psychiatry, in that literature has more space at its disposal—which enables it to add more context and complexity to psychological descriptions and to conveying human relations. The authors of *Health Humanities* write the following in this regard:

> Whereas the vignette or case study, under the guise of presenting a narrative of a unique experience, portrays a madness experience under a homogenizing diagnostic framework, the literary text instead presents the individual human specificity of cognition, emotion and internality in imaginative and unique form. This in turn reminds us that there is no 'typical' experience of madness, despite the homogenizing tendency of the common diagnostic systems. Nosology denies the elements of human agency and autonomy that the literary text epitomizes. (Crawford et al. 44)

Literature can nurture the imagination of both patients and practitioners, so they perceive of individuals *'outside* and *beyond* the biomedical gaze' (Crawford et al. 59; italics in the original). However, to get the full output from literature about mental illness, readers must avoid the trap of merely treating it thematically. Literary form or composition is indispensable to the meaning authors create. The authors of this book aim to show how stylistic choices are integral to advancing thematic points and hence, conveying—among other purposes—the thematic meaning of a particular piece of literature. Conversely, the attention to the formal experiments in selected examples of madness literature feed back into the theory employed, causing the authors to modify and rethink central theoretical concepts.

The Structure and Individual Contributions

In spite of multiple theoretical overlaps as well as overlaps in terms of the overall purpose of the individual contributions, this book is divided into three separate sections. The first section is about 'Literary History and Socio-Political Perspectives' on the topic of madness and literature. This feeds into a health humanities programme, in which it is stressed that 'it is not only *personal* madness that is told through literary narratives, but also forms of societal or cultural *otherness*, that which is "excluded" or "decreed abnormal"' (Crawford et al. 44; italics in the original). The second section is about 'Literary Theory and Experiencing Mental Illness'. Contributions in this part examine how authors try to give aesthetic, literary form to mad experiences. The third section is about 'Literary Instrumentality and Clinical Psychopathology'. The contributions here exemplify how knowledge gained from literary texts informs and interacts with knowledge gained via clinical psychopathological approaches. Additionally, this section accounts for the instrumental use of literature within health-related contexts. It should be emphasized that even though each chapter of this book is placed in one of these sections, one could argue that literary history, theory, and instrumentality (or, at least, the potential to be instrumentalized)—as well as the socio-political, the experience of mental illness, and clinical psychopathology—are to some degree inherent in all the contributions.

In 'Layla and Majnun in Historical and Contemporary Conceptions of Madness in Islamic Psychology', Alan Weber examines the medieval love story of Layla and Majnun predominantly through the version by the poet Nizami Ganjavi. He explains how Nizami provides interpretations of abnormal behaviours in the poem, which are explained with reference to physiology, psychology, and magical/religious beliefs. Weber then argues that pre-Islamic conceptions of madness as can be found in the story of *Layla and Majnun* persist in the modern-day Muslim world, and that the story therefore provides a modern view on madness in Islam.

In 'The Anti-Psychiatry Ethos in Samuel Beckett's *Murphy*', Shoshana Benjamin compares anti-psychiatric sentiments expressed in Samuel Beckett's 1938 novel *Murphy* to the positions on the matter championed by the proponents of the anti-psychiatry movement that emerged in the subsequent decades. In particular, Benjamin compares Beckett's and R.D. Laing's shared interests in the conditions of the asylums, and in the mental disorder labelled schizophrenia.

INTRODUCTION: MADNESS AND LITERATURE AND THE HEALTH HUMANITIES

Continuing the discussion of power struggles but within a postcolonial framework, Sebastian Charles Galbo employs Édouard Glissant's understanding of madness as a tactic of resistance in his chapter on 'Apartheid's Garden: Dismantling Madness in J.M. Coetzee's *Life & Times of Michael K*'. In an interpretation of Coetzee's novel, Galbo argues that Coetzee finds a way to both criticize Apartheid's use of madness as a method of codifying otherness, justifying extrajudicial incarceration, and controlling populations, and to present madness as a tactic of resistance and a mode of counter-discourse.

In 'Sniffs and Dribblers: *Poppy Shakespeare* and the Identities of Madness', Clare Allan discusses issues of identity in relation to experiences of mental distress. Allan explored these in her novel *Poppy Shakespeare*, and in this chapter, she demonstrates how fictional narratives about mental distress might contribute to conversations about the validity of the psychiatric diagnosis system in place. Furthermore, she argues that engaging with fiction about madness might enable readers to gain an understanding of experiences of mental distress and by extension help to break down barriers between sanity and insanity. Hence, Allan's chapter is unique in this volume in that it is personal, essayistic, and adds a dimension of praxis.

The first chapter in the second part of the book, which is about 'Literary Theory and Experiencing Mental Illness', is Anna Ovaska's 'Reading Shattering Minds and Extended Selves in Virginia Woolf's *Mrs Dalloway*'. Ovaska argues that Virginia Woolf managed to show—through her 'tunnelling' technique—the interconnectedness of people, as well as to depict how they are shaped by their surroundings. Ovaska explains how Woolf's fictional, narrative experiments anticipated what the 4E theories account for today—namely the embodied, enactive, embedded, and extended nature of the mind. The 4E theory, in its turn, can shed light on key passages in Woolf's fictional texts. In *Mrs Dalloway*, Woolf attempts to portray sanity and insanity side by side, which enables readers to understand and sympathize with experiences of mental illness.

In 'Spill the Words: Speechlessness and Creativity in the Writing of Janet Frame', Mary Elene Wood compares how the novelist Janet Frame and the psychoanalyst and memoirist Annie G. Rogers deal with trauma, psychosis, and schizophrenia. Speech in schizophrenia is altered, and Wood argues that Lacanian psychoanalysis provides a theoretical framework for understanding seemingly indecipherable uses of language in severe mental illness. Combining

Lacan's psychoanalysis with Jane Bennett's concept of vibrant matter, Wood argues that creativity and its connection with artistic expression can help shape the material world for people with schizophrenia, and that putting their creativity to use can help them to assume agency over their imaginative products, enabling them to re-enter the social world.

In her chapter entitled 'Pronominal Shifts and the Confusion of Self with Not-Self', Alice Hervé investigates pronominal shifts as a strategy that authors use to find a compromise and balance between clarity and plausibility when constructing mad characters. Hervé defines pronominal shifts as the substitution of one pronoun for another in a way that is inappropriate or bizarre. Examining works by Margaret Atwood, Samuel Richardson, Günter Grass, Charlotte Perkins Gilman, Patrick McGrath, and Jay McInerney, Hervé shows how a variety of authors writing in different time periods have employed a shift from the first-person singular pronoun to other pronouns without changing the focalization, to foreground and signpost alienation and what the phenomenologically oriented psychiatrist Louis A. Sass has labelled an 'ipseity disturbance'.

In 'Rethinking Clinical and Critical Perspectives on Psychosis in Kathy Acker's Writing', Charley Baker focuses on the portrayal and implications of psychosis as represented in the writings of Kathy Acker. Baker argues that Acker's contextual, textual, and experiential representations offer a version of what might be referred to clinically as 'psychosis' that is personally meaningful and understandable. Acker's writing details the context and content of strange or unusual mental experiences and distress, while often simultaneously structurally mirroring the form of expressions of psychosis. Baker additionally argues that Acker's writings offer insights relevant for clinical practice in working with and supporting people who are experiencing psychosis.

In 'Countering the DSM in Poetry about Bipolar Disorder', Lasse Raaby Gammelgaard probes how authors can depict experiences associated with bipolar disorder in a way that supplements clinical psychiatry. Engaging with Mark Rapley, Joanna Moncrieff, and Jacqui Dillon's theory of de-medicalizing misery, he argues that literature can fill a gap left by clinical psychiatry in which mental illness is decontextualized to make it generalizable. He uses Virginia Woolf's essay *On Being Ill* to draw attention to similarities between the ill and the aesthetic mind. Selecting three poems about bipolar disorder, he demonstrates how poetry can counter the DSM by directly or indirectly

INTRODUCTION: MADNESS AND LITERATURE AND THE HEALTH HUMANITIES

playing off its discourse. The poets employ the unique affordances of poetry to different ends, but all three poems display an alternative approach to making sense of bipolar disorder.

In 'Seeing Feeling: Dissociation and Post-Traumatic Memory in the Graphic Novel *Perfect Hair*', Penni Russon argues that the graphic novel is a genre well equipped to represent trauma and dissociation. In a reading of Tommi Parrish's *Perfect Hair*, she employs Jill Bennett's theory of empathy to argue that Parrish creates an affective dynamic of putting insides into contact with outsides. Additionally, Russon introduces Bennett's notion of the art of sense memory to make the case that readerly engagements with the sequences of images must pay attention to the sensorial body and the gaps or spaces in the narrative, rather than the narrative itself, to feel the truth. The body of the character 'Figure' is foregrounded and represents the traumatized self that stores the affective memory within the body rather than within the mind.

Signe Uldbjerg's contribution, entitled 'Writing Therapy, Writing Data: Therapeutic Writing as a Methodological and Ethical Approach in Researching Digital Sexual Assault', is the first chapter in part three of this book, about 'Literary Instrumentality and Clinical Psychopathology'. Uldbjerg describes and reflects on her research design for her project on victim survivors of digital sexual assault (DSA), which is defined as the sharing of intimate images on digital media without the consent of the people displayed in the images. DSA can have severe psychological consequences (among them anxiety, depression, and PTSD). Drawing on theories and methodologies promoted by Kathleen McNichol, James W. Pennebaker, and Gillie Bolton, Uldbjerg uses writing to help facilitate conscious self-reflection and to help the participants reshape their narratives of themselves. Engaging with literature as an intervention and from the vantage point of producing texts, the chapter also reflects on the ethical aspects of using writing to gain knowledge about the affective consequences of DSA.

In her chapter 'A Question of Context: Sites for Cultural Negotiation in Narratives of Manic Depression', Megan Milota sees fictional and biographical stories of bipolar disorder as being enmeshed in cultural negotiations about illness. Employing theoretical concepts from Pierre Bourdieu, Jerome Bruner, Judith Butler, Janet Wolff, Luc Herman and Bart Vervaeck, and Miranda Fricker, she aims to understand the habitus of readers as well as the contexts in which such illness narratives are produced and consumed. Milota analyses texts from two databases of patient narratives—the Story Bank for Psychiatry, and PsychoseNet—which are meant to be instrumental in helping tellers and readers move towards understanding and recovery. Additionally, she analyses the novel *Karkas* by Femke Schavemaker. Although supportive of the aims of the narratives, Milota also reflects on the risk that the cases being contained within the cultural sites they inhabit may contribute to two types of epistemic injustice related to pathographies: testimonial injustice and hermeneutical injustice.

In 'Conscripting Dante: History, Anachronism, and the Uses of Literary Precedents in the "New" Diagnosis of Hoarding Disorder', David Orr explains that the sociology of diagnosis has shown how new diagnostic categories in psychiatry are the result of extensive social, cultural, and political work by multiple parties to stabilize their claims and maximize their persuasive power so that they gain official acceptance. Orr contends that historical accounts of the proposed condition in earlier times play a role in establishing legitimacy for it. The diagnostic classification of 'Hoarding Disorder' was officially recognized by the American Psychiatric Association only in 2013, but Dante's *Divine Comedy* is commonly adduced as evidence for the significance of hoarding as far back as the fourteenth century. In this chapter, Orr contextualizes Dante's discussion in order to question the equivalence drawn between hoarders in Dante and in the DSM, and considers the uses to which the claim of connection across the centuries is put in legitimizing new diagnostic developments.

In the final chapter, 'Opening up the Discourse of Male Eating Disorders: Personal Experience in German and English Narratives', Heike Bartel sheds light on the overlooked issue of eating disorders in men. Analysing three cases of autobiographical writing about men with eating disorders—Michael Krasnow's *My Life as a Male Anorexic*, Dave Chawner's *Weight Expectations: One Man's Recovery from Anorexia*, and Benjamin von Stuckrad-Barre's *Panikherz*—Bartel argues that there is a need for a comprehensive socio-cultural approach towards understanding men and boys' experience of eating disorders, since this illness has a strong association with females, which can be detrimental to recovery when applied to men with eating disorders. Bartel explains how these autobiographic illness narratives by men straddle the divide between narratives of illness/recovery and self-help books, and suggests that these types of literature might beneficially be used to inform and influence clinical treatment of male eating disorder.

INTRODUCTION: MADNESS AND LITERATURE AND THE HEALTH HUMANITIES

In sum, the chapters in this book contribute to debates about what constitutes normalcy, and give voice to difficult, ineffable experiences and to patient views that tend to be cancelled out in a purely biomedical discourse. In a society where mental disturbances gain considerable media attention and public interest, just as they affect patients, relatives, and the healthcare system, finding ways of understanding different experiences is an urgent project—and literature about mental illness has the potential to play a vital role in comprehending and negotiating this understanding. We hope to have made a contribution, however small, to the limited but constantly expanding knowledge of the field.

References

Abbott, Porter, 'What Does It Mean to Be Mad? Diagnosis, Narrative, Science, and the DSM' in Zara Dinnen and Robyn Warhol (eds), *The Edinburgh Companion to Contemporary Narrative Theories* (Edinburgh: Edinburgh University Press, 2018), 17–29. https://doi.org/10.1515/9781474424752-005

Aristotle, *Problems II: Books XXII–XXXVIII. Rhetorica ad Alexandrum*, trans. by W.S. Hett (Cambridge, MA: Harvard University Press, 1939).

Baker, Charlotte, Paul Crawford, B.J. Brown, Maurice Lipsedge, and Ronald Carter, *Madness in Post-1945 British and American Fiction* (London: Palgrave Macmillan, 2010). https://doi.org/10.1057/9780230290440

Beresford, Peter, '"Mad", Mad Studies and Advancing Inclusive Resistance', *Disability & Society* 35.8 (2020): 1337–42. https://doi.org/10.1080/09687599.2019.1692168

Bernaerts, Lars, 'Tell-Tale Minds: The Rhetoric of Mad First-Person Narration' in Nathalie Jaëck, Clara Mallier, Arnaud Schmitt, and Romain Girard (eds), *Les narrateurs Fous / Mad Narrators* (Pessac: Maison des sciences de l'homme d'aquitaine, 2014), 185–206.

Bernaerts, Lars, Luc Herman, and Bart Vervaeck, 'Narrative Threads of Madness', *Style* 43.3 (2009): 283–90.

Brice, Martin, Marc Wittmann, Nicolas Franck, Michel Cermolacce, Fabrice Berna, and Anne Giersch, 'Temporal Structure of Consciousness and Minimal Self in Schizophrenia', *Frontiers in Psychology* 5 (2014): 1–12. https://doi.org/10.3389/fpsyg.2014.01175

Brooks, Peter, *Reading for the Plot: Design and Intention in Narrative* (New York: A.A. Knopf, 1984).

Burwick, Frederik, *Poetic Madness and the Romantic Imagination* (Pennsylvania: The Pennsylvania State University Press, 1996).

Charon, Rita, *Narrative Medicine: Honoring the Stories of Illness* (Oxford: Oxford University Press, 2006).

Clarke, Liam, *Fiction's Madness* (Exeter: PCCS Books, 2009).

Cohn, Dorrit, *Transparent Minds: Narrative Modes for Presenting Consciousness in Fiction* (Princeton: Princeton University Press, 1980).

Crawford, Paul, Brian Brown, Charley Baker, Victoria Tischler, and Brian Abrams, *Health Humanities* (London: Palgrave Macmillan, 2015). https://doi.org/10.1057/9781137282613

Feder, Lillian, *Madness in Literature* (Princeton, NJ: Princeton University Press, 1980).

Felman, Shoshana, *Writing and Madness (Literature/Philosophy/Psychoanalysis)* (Palo Alto, CA: Stanford University Press, 2003). https://doi.org/10.1515/9781503620001

Foucault, Michel, *Madness and Civilization: A History of Insanity in the Age of Reason* (New York: Vintage Books, 1988).

Frank, Arthur, *The Wounded Storyteller: Body, Illness, and Ethics* (Chicago: Chicago University Press, 1995). https://doi.org/10.7208/chicago/9780226260037.001.0001

Freud, Sigmund, *The Uncanny: Essays* (New York: Penguin Classics, 2003).

Gammelgaard, Lasse, and Thomas Boström, *Galskab i litteraturen* (Aarhus: Systime, 2019).

Gilmore, Leigh, 'Limit-Cases: Trauma, Self-Representations, and the Jurisdictions of Identity', *Biography: An Interdisciplinary Quarterly* 24.1 (2001): 128–39. https://doi.org/10.1353/bio.2001.0011

Goffman, Erving, *Asylums: Essays on the Social Situation of Mental Patients and Other Inmates* (Somerset: Routledge, 2007).

Jaëck, Nathalie, '"Mad Narrators": Oxymoron or Pleonasm?' in Nathalie Jaëck, Clara Mallier, Arnaud Schmitt, and Romain Girard (eds), *Les narrateurs Fous / Mad Narrators* (Pessac: Maison des sciences de l'homme d'aquitaine, 2014), 13–19.

James, Tony, *Dream, Creativity, and Madness in Nineteenth-Century France* (Oxford: Clarendon Press, 1995). https://doi.org/10.1093/acprof:oso/9780198151883.001.0001

Jamison, Kay Redfield, *Touched with Fire: Manic-Depressive Illness and the Artistic Temperament* (New York: Free Press Paperback, 1993).

Laing, Ronald David, *The Divided Self: An Existential Study in Sanity and Madness* (London: Penguin Books, 1965).

Oyebode, Femi, *Mindreadings: Literature and Psychiatry* (London: RCPsych P, 2009). https://doi.org/10.1192/bjp.194.2.122

Porter, Roy, *Madness: A Brief History* (Oxford: Oxford University Press, 2002).

Radden, Jennifer, 'Is This Dame Melancholy? Equating Today's Depression and Past Melancholia', *Philosophy, Psychiatry, and Psychology* 10.1 (2003): 37–52. https://doi.org/10.1353/ppp.2003.0081

INTRODUCTION: MADNESS AND LITERATURE AND THE HEALTH HUMANITIES

Radden, Jennifer, 'Mental Disorder (Illness)', *Stanford Encyclopedia of Philosophy*, 2019, https://plato.stanford.edu/entries/mental-disorder/, accessed 25 September 2021.

Rapley, Mark, Joanna Moncrieff, and Jacqui Dillon (eds), *De-Medicalizing Misery: Psychiatry, Psychology and the Human Condition* (New York: Palgrave Macmillan, 2011). https://doi.org/10.1057/9780230342507

Rieger, Branimir M. (ed.), *Dionysus in Literature: Essays on Literary Madness* (Bowling Green, OH: Bowling Green State University Popular Press, 1994).

Sass, Louis A., *Madness and Modernism: Insanity in the Light of Modern Art, Literature, and Thought* (New York: BasicBooks, 1992).

Sass, Louis A., 'Schizophrenia, Modernism, and the "Creative Imagination": On Creativity and Psychopathology', *Creativity Research Journal* 13.1 (2000–2001): 55–74. https://doi.org/10.1207/S15326934CRJ1301_7

Sass, Louis A., Josef Parnas, and Dan Zahavi, 'Phenomenological Psychopathology and Schizophrenia: Contemporary Approaches and Misunderstandings', *Philosophy, Psychiatry & Psychology* 18.1 (2011), 1–23. https://doi.org/10.1353/ppp.2011.0008

Skott-Myhre, Hans A., *Post-Capitalist Subjectivity in Literature and Anti-Psychiatry: Reconceptualizing the Self Beyond Capitalism* (Milton: Taylor & Francis Group, 2021). https://doi.org/10.4324/9781003110545

Szasz, Thomas S., *The Myth of Mental Illness: Foundations of a Theory of Personal Conduct* (New York: Harper & Row, 1974). https://doi.org/10.1016/B978-0-08-017738-0.50007-7

Thiher, Allen, *Revels in Madness: Insanity in Medicine and Literature* (Michigan: Michigan University Press, 1999). https://doi.org/10.3998/mpub.16078

Todorov, Tzvetan, *The Fantastic: A Structural Approach to a Literary Genre* (Ithaca, NY: Cornell University Press, 1987).

Whitehead, James, *Madness and the Romantic Poet: A Critical History* (Oxford: Oxford University Press, 2017). https://doi.org/10.1093/oso/9780198733706.001.0001

Wiesenthal, Chris, *Figuring Madness in Nineteenth-Century Fiction* (London: Macmillan Press Ltd, 1997). https://doi.org/10.1057/9780230371316

Woolf, Virginia, *On Being Ill* (Ashfield, Massachusetts: Paris Press, 2002).

Part I
Literary History and Socio-Political Perspectives

1 *Layla and Majnun* in Historical and Contemporary Conceptions of Madness in Islamic Psychology

Alan Weber

'As for madness, it will remain silent, the pure object of an amused gaze.'
(Foucault 13)

The Persian/Arabic romance of *Leili o Majnun* (Persian) or *Majnun Layli* (Arabic) has not only provided generations of poetry aficionados with a popular story of the suffering of two lovers, but also stands as essential documentary evidence for both the medieval and modern Islamic conceptions of madness. The version of Azerbaijani poet Nizami Ganjavi (1141–1209 CE) composed in Persian in 1188 is the best-known and most imitated of the Layla and Majnun tales. Nizami provides multiple interpretations for the abnormal behaviors presented in the poem—spanning the physiological, psychological, magical, and religious—through his imagery, the character dialogue, and his own direct commentary.

Due to the persistence of pre-Islamic conceptions of madness in the Muslim world into the modern day (which have been enshrined in language, sharia law, literature, folk wisdom, and traditional religious-based therapeutic approaches to mental illness), the poem additionally provides a window on modern views of madness in Islam. Medieval Islamic philosopher-physicians interpreted the story within Islamicized paradigms of Galenic–Hippocratic obsessive love-melancholy or excessive passion (*al-'ishq* in Arabic). These physicians worked primarily within rationalist and materialist paradigms and sought the origins of mental disturbances in physiological fluids (humors; χυμόι) or material spirits derived from humors (πνεύματα or *spiritus*). Other poets transformed the myth into a spiritual allegory about divine madness as a pathway to enlightenment.

Nizami was fully aware of the myriad ways in which his contemporaries interpreted abnormal behavior, and when both the narrator and the characters in his poem struggle to frame Majnun's madness, Nizami presents us with a comprehensive catalogue of contemporary views on the causes and manifestations of mental illness. As a close observer of nature as well, Nizami depicted behaviors that we could categorize today as obsessive, delusional, bipolar, and depressive according to DSM-5 categories.

In contrast to Islamic physicians trained in Greek rationalist medicine (*unani tibb*), traditions more aligned with prophetic medicine, or *tibb al-nabawi*, attributed the lovers' extreme behaviors in *Layla and Majnun* to demonic possession by *djinn* or *qareen*. Nizami's great poetic achievement was, through the characters and his own direct narration, to examine all of the possible explanations for Majnun's mad behavior while creating an enduring poem of considerable psychological depth, as well as establishing empathy for two believable lovers. Meanwhile he was working within the conventionalized narrative and symbolic framework of the *ghazal* verse form and 'Udhrī poetry. Many of the possible root causes of mental illness presented in Nizami's work, such as demonic possession, intoxication, immoderate lifestyle (sin), or the inability to master excessive emotions (passionate love), are still believed by many Muslims to be central factors in antisocial and abnormal behavior in Muslim-majority societies in the present day.

Textual History and Love Madness in Arabic and Persian Literature

Krachkovskiĭ in a 1946 study determined that the Layla and Majnun story originated in Arabia, possibly during the early Umayyad period (Krachkovskiĭ 1–50). The legends may have a historical basis in the love of the Arab poet Qays ibn al-Mulawwah for Layla al-Amiriya. The earliest Arabic versions were in the *Kitab al-Aghani* and Ibn Qutaybah's *al-Shi'r wa al-shu'arā'*. These early works were undoubtedly based on orally circulating Bedouin folk tales and survive in only loosely structured episodic fragments, which Nizami skillfully wove into a compelling narrative structure. Nizami's poem is the third in a series of five poems called the *Panj Ganj* or *Khamsa* (Quintet).

The widespread cross-cultural popularity of the tale argues for the universality of its themes among Indo-Iranian cultures. Complete versions exist in Arabic, Persian, Turkish, Pashto, Urdu, and Kurdish. It is the most popular and imitated story in Persian literature with at least fifty-nine imitations recorded by Ḥasan Ḏulfaqāri, as compared to fifty-one versions of *Ḵosrow and Širin* (Seyed-Gohrab 2009). Dastgerdi, who prepared the Farsi edition of Nizami, believes that there may well be over a thousand versions of this story worldwide. Lord Byron in the notes to his poem 'The Bride of Abydos' called Nizami's work 'the Romeo and Juliet of the East' (Lord Byron 753; see also Clinton 15–27).

Much of the drama of Nizami's version is psychological in nature and follows the inner thoughts and interior lives of Majnun and Layla. The poem fits within the 'Udhrī genre of poetry dealing with unrequited or unrealizable love. Lovers in this tradition remain constant and idealized; the love is often nonphysical and they suffer from their separation. The recurrent themes of 'Udhrī poetry are enmeshed in what today we might recognize as delusional or obsessive disorders, as the poet and lovers both refuse to recognize the order of things (fate) and their passions become all-consuming; as Bürgel notes:

> the common features of 'Udhrite love are that Fate, or, rather, social conditions prohibit the physical or, at any rate, the constant matrimonial union of the loving couple, but they remain faithful to each other until death. 'Udhrite love is absolute love, love as idea, love as religion. Such love is almost of necessity tragic. And its tragedy is a symbol of the incompatibility of the absolute and the concrete, of the ideal and real life. (Bürgel 92)

Another important literary analogue was the poetic form called *ghazal* (sometimes termed *nassib* by Nizami). This widespread, originally Arabic verse form entered Persian poetry via the Rashidun Caliphate and later Umayyad dynasty and spread to Mughal India, North Africa and southern Europe (Al-Andalus). Elements of *ghazal* poetry depict the following psychological dimensions of love: 1) the focus on suffering; 2) the idealization of the beloved; 3) the overwhelming power of the passions experienced in love, often causing severe psychological anguish; 4) the sometimes cruel nature of the beloved, and the sense of isolation and despair that her rejections cause the poet. Nizami's challenge was, within these strictures, to create psychologically believable and non-stereotypical characters who suffer extreme emotion from love. As Aliyev points out, 'the ghazals of the overwhelming majority of Nizami's predecessors and contemporaries are somewhat of conventional nature and they rarely serve to express real feelings and emotions, as well as veritable reflections of human spirits and inner thrillings' (Aliyev 51). Additionally, Nizami was impacted by the ethical texts in the Adab tradition; for example, Naufal is depicted as an exemplar of nobility of spirit when he champions Majnun's cause against mortal enemies.

In secular Islamic literature as well as Qur'anic exegesis, 'martyrs of love' were celebrated as those rare souls who had died for love: Ibn Da'ud in the *Kitāb az-Zahra* relates, 'The Messenger of God—on him be blessing and peace—said: He who loves and remains chaste and conceals his secret and dies, dies a martyr' (Giffen 99). In al-Jauzi's *Dhamm al-Hawā*, Majnun is listed as 'the most famous of the famous' of the 'Passionate Lovers Who Became Proverbial for Their Love [chapter 41]' (Giffen 108–09).

Summary of the Poem

To summarize the plot briefly, Qays (later Majnun) falls in love with his cousin Layla at school. Due to his passion for Layla that inspires many poems as well as demonstrations of excessive love, the townsfolk begin to call him 'majnoon' or crazy. Layla's father rejects Majnun's offer of marriage due to his increasingly bizarre behavior and Layla is married to a rich merchant instead, but never consummates the marriage. Consequently, Majnun becomes further obsessed with Layla, abandoning all social conventions including clothing, and wanders in the desert alone. His sole occupation is writing love songs to Layla and he loses interest in food. His father and uncle are unable to return him to sanity. The nobleman Naufal takes pity on Majnun and launches a battle against Layla's tribe to avenge him. Majnun, however, tries to stop the battle, drawing the ire of Naufal's troops. In the desert, Majnun befriends wild animals who become his constant companions and protect him until his death. His relationship with animals is symbolic of his deep connection to nature and natural impulses, and his alienation from human society. Majnun and Layla meet briefly but stay at a distance. Although Layla's husband dies, Majnun cannot face achieving his desire and returns to the desert. Layla dies of grief and Majnun discovers her grave and dies of grief as well on her tomb. Layla and Majnun are buried side by side and reputedly become a king and queen in paradise.

Physiological Readings of the *Layla and Majnun* Mythos

Among Muslim scholars and jurists, excessive secular (profane) love was widely believed to be in and of itself a cause of madness. Erotic literature, impure thoughts, and intoxicants were therefore to be avoided to prevent both sin and mental instability. The topic inspired numerous lengthy treatments by both physicians and religious thinkers, such as Ibn Sina's *Risāla fī l-'ishq* (*Treatise on Love*). As Dols notes, 'love in the Qur'ān and romantic love in Arabic poetry, such as that of Majnun and the 'Udhrī poets generally, were strong incentives for the study of the subject by scholars in the early Islamic era. As a vital aspect of human life, love commanded the attention of philosophers and theologians, doctors and even astrologers' (Dols 313). Measurement of the pulse was frequently used in Islamic diagnosis, and Qatari cardiologist Hajar Ahmed Albinali, MD has analyzed Majnun's behavior in Nizami's poem as the somatic manifestations of extreme love, such as weight loss (cachexia), anemia, immune deficiency, palpitations, and syncope (Albinali 192–98). Ibn Sina pioneered sphygmology in his Persian treatise *Resaleye Ragshenasi* and he was reportedly able to tell through the pulse when the patient was suffering from love (Zarshenas et al.).

By the tenth century, Islamic writers were quoting classical Greek authors as well as Hellenistic texts on love-melancholy, such as pseudo-Aristotle's *Problemata*, with some frequency. Abū Bakr Muḥammad ibn Dāwūd al-Iṣbahānī quotes long passages from Plato, Ptolemy, and Galen on the topic in his late ninth-century book *Kitāb az-Zahra*. Nizami's other writings provide abundant evidence of his wide reading in the sciences of his day: he was knowledgeable about astronomy and astrology—although expressing skepticism that astrology determined man's fate—and he was familiar with the major medical doctrines and writings of Ishaq ibn Hunain, Galen, Al-Razi, and Ibn Sina (Aliyev 32).

Nizami's descriptions of Majnun throughout the poem parallel medieval medical descriptions of love-melancholy: isolation, lack of concern for personal appearance, loss of appetite, suicidal ideation, and obsessive behaviors. In a reciprocal feedback loop, Nizami's story and other analogues of the Majnun legend would later themselves serve as case histories of mental illness in subsequent medical writings.

Although not presented as the ultimate cause, Nizami offers one potential physiological explanation for Majnun's mental illness that fits firmly within the Greek humoral model: 'He endeavoured to conceal the secret of his heart, / to Struggle against the fire in his heart. / But the blood of his liver went up to his heart, / Passing the heart, it reached to his brain' (Nizami 38–39). In Galenic and pseudo-Aristotelian texts available to Muslim authors, mental illness could be attributed to the uncontrolled burning of humors (normally black bile or *melan cholia*; Arabic: *as-sauda*) in the heart or liver, or from vapors from excessive heat or combustion of humors that ascended to the brain. In Nizami's image, the heated blood itself overwhelms the brain. Excess black bile is also frequently cited as the direct cause of mental illness in medieval medical texts. The mechanism of action was often conceived in materialistic terms; the smoke or vapors produce darkness, obscurity, or a fog in the ventricles of the brain, interfering with or obscuring cognition, or excessive fluids swamp or drown the cognitive faculties.

Both Ibn Sina in his *Qanun fi al-tibb* and Ibn al-Jawzi report that "ishq or excessive love is a delusionary disease similar to melancholia; it possesses the reason and causes the person to act unwisely' (Dols 319). According to al-Jawzi, both gazing at the lover and exposure to love poetry can lead anyone to excessive passion or mental delusion (Dols 329). This physiological interpretation in the humoral model would account for the periods of brooding, suicidal ideation, and depression in Majnun's behavior, in addition to his manic periods. In Fuzuli's later retelling of the story, doctors attempt to cure Majnun unsuccessfully with cooling sherbets to restore his natural heat, an obvious reference to the humoral therapeutics of '*contraria contrariis curantur*', or 'opposites are cured by opposites' (Dols 338).

Fuzuli's sixteenth-century version *Dâstân-ı Leylî vü Mecnûn*, written in Azerbaijani (Turkic), however, reinterprets Nizami's tale in light of his deep studies in Sufism and appears to reject these medical interpretations of love-melancholy. Majnun's love, far from originating in an organic disturbance, serves instead as a stepping-stone to divine reunification with 'reality' (*al-haqq*)—that is, Allah. Nizami clearly stands as a transitional figure in the development of the Majnun–Layla mythos, from the early Arabic love poetry, to examinations of the underlying medical condition of Majnun, to later purely allegorical interpretations in which poetry serves as handmaiden to philosophy and religion.

By emphasizing Majnun's kindness to animals, Nizami along with Fuzuli may be critiquing the medical opinions of both Ibn Sina and Zayn al-Din Sayyed Isma'il ibn Husayn al-Jurjani (1040–1136 CE; a near-contemporary of Nizami) that love-melancholy bestializes the sufferer and manifests as a type of animal agitation. Jurjani defines 'ešq (Arabic: 'ishq) as exaggerated love and relates it to lycanthropy and animal rage: 'the cause [of 'ešq] is a too lively concupiscible faculty (šahwaniya). Delirious love thus possesses an animal quality' (des Epesse 116–17). But Majnun's continual calming of wild animals appears to be Nizami's refutation of the medical animality of Majnun's behavior. The protection and devotion that animals display towards Majnun in Nizami's version of the poem appear to signal Majnun's connection to all of nature, a suggestion that he may be existing in a divine state of universal peace and harmony, the underlying primary pillar of Islam (tawhid, or oneness).

Nizami's prologue is addressed to a *saqi* and the poet continually calls for cups of wine and praises the drink as the lubricant of genius. Two characters in Nizami's poem suggest a simple physiological cause for Majnun's illness: intoxication by wine. Nizami, in the same Sufi tradition as Rumi, playfully weaves the metaphors of intoxication throughout his work: 'a bearer had come and filled their cups to the brim. They drank what he poured out for them. They were children and did not realize what they were drinking; no wonder they became drunk. He who is drunk for the first time, becomes deeply drunk indeed' (Nizami 17). And Majnun's loss of sanity is later compared to a wine-drinking state: 'unconscious, he lay on the ground, motionless as the stones around him, like a man whom wine has driven to raving madness and then cut down, robbed of his senses' (Nizami 157). Thus, intoxication would have presented to a medieval Muslim audience an additional physiological explanation for Majnun's madness.

Madness and Demonic Possession in *Layla and Majnun*

Nizami continually flirts with the possibility that Majnun is demonically possessed: 'suddenly a demon seemed to seize his rigid figure. Like a raving madman he tore the rags from his body' (Nizami 157). Thus, he juxtaposes different potential meanings of Majnun's experience, and Nizami's noncommittal and ambiguous approach allows for more richness of interpretation and more reader participation in creating Majnun's story; Nizami, as a sceptical non-interventionist narrator, appears to be quite conscious of his own aims not to steer the reader's experience of the story in any one specific direction. This multiplicity of meanings has no doubt added to the popularity of Nizami's version—despite all of the elements leaning towards a mystical reading of the story, there is still 'an actual party, an actual beloved, real kisses, and a rose garden one can touch and smell' (Kalpaklı and Andrews 34). Thus Nizami, much like Shakespeare, can be enjoyed by a variety of readers of differing levels of education, understanding, and sophistication.

In both Semitic and Indo-Iranian languages, the words for madness are related to hidden worlds and demonic beings who inhabit them. In the Semitic consonantal root system, a series of letters denotes a constellation of related meanings. For example, k-t-b (kaf, ta, ba; ك – ت – ب) forms the basis of: *yaktubu*, he writes / *katib*, a writer / *maktab*, an office / *kutub*, books. The name '*majnun*' given to Qays is the most common word in Arabic for a 'mad', 'possessed', or 'obsessed' person, based on the triliteral root j-n-n (jim, nun, nun; ج – ن – ن) which in the form '*jann / junūn*' (جن / جنون) connotes hiddenness, secretness, to conceal, to veil, to go mad (Wehr 138). Thus '*al-junūn*' (الجنون) can mean 'possession, obsession, mania, madness, insanity, dementia, foolishness, folly, frenzy, rage, fury, ecstasy, rapture' and '*majnūn*' (مجنون) can mean 'possessed, obsessed, insane, mad, madman, maniac, lunatic, crazy, cracked, crackpot, foolish, fool' (Wehr 138). The rich range of meanings of the *jann* root reflects the diversity of opinions on the nature of madness in Arab and Persian culture, from simple and commonplace mental derangement and incapacity (i.e. senility or dementia), to potential spiritual dimensions (enraptured, carried off by divine powers), to the intercession of or possession by demonic forces. *Jann* also can mean to descend, fall, be or become dark (night), which is significant as '*lail*' (ليل) in Arabic means 'night'. Thus some potential meanings of the title of the poem are 'madness for night', 'darkness descending into night', or that Majnun literally descends into Layla—in other words, madness becomes darkness, possession becomes veiled and veils his identity. These etymologies will become more significant in the discussion below of possible Sufi elements in the poem.

J-n-n (*jann*) also forms the root for the Arabic words *djinni* and *djinn* (plural), cognate with English 'genie', due to their hidden nature as well as their reputation for frequenting dark, dingy, and hidden places such as toilets and graveyards. The Djinn are described in the Qur'an as a separate race of beings created by Allah, composed of 'scorching fire' or 'smokeless fire': 'And he created man from clay, like pottery / And He created Djinn from a smokeless flame of fire' (*Al-Qur'ān*, Sūrat l-raḥmān [The Most Gracious], 55.14–15). A djinni might fall in love with a human, or be jealous of them, and they have the ability to possess or cause harm to humans. In many Muslim-majority countries, djinn are widely believed to be the primary cause of mental illness (Weber 2012, 62).

Medieval muftis, hakims, and poets wrote extensively about the love relationships between djinn and men: djinn would take the form of a human or animal (most notably a deer, sacred to the pre-Islamic goddess al-'Uzza) called a *tabi'* (fem. *Tabi'ah*) or follower. Layla is compared to a gazelle or deer in Nizami ('eyes dark as a stag's'), a frequent incarnation of the *tabi'ah*. Although the *tabi'* often taught their beloved one skills such as sword-making and the healing arts, sharia law jurists passed laws against intermarriage with djinn, arguing that djinn and humans were different species (El-Zein 103–05).

In a field study of folk medicine in Oman in 2011, Weber found continued evidence of possession beliefs, as well as the use of *ruqya* or exorcism to cure deviant behavior by driving out demons (Weber 2011). In addition, in a scoping review of modern mental illness beliefs in the Gulf Cooperation Council (Persian Gulf), the authors reported that 'external stressors, particularly the supernatural (i.e. jinn, black magic, evil eye) were frequently seen as the root cause of mental illness by both patients and caregivers' (Hickey, Pryjmachuk, and Waterman 11). This finding may partially explain why allopathic mental health services based on psychopharmaceutical interventions are not available or underfunded in many Muslim-majority nations.

Thus the continuity of traditional practices for treating psychological stress has very real consequences for modern services provision: as Kronfol, Ghuloum and Weber point out, it is 'quite common for a patient suffering from a mental illness to be first seen by the motawwa who will do readings from the Koran and perform "special procedures" to neutralize the evil eye or get rid of the evil spirit' (Kronfol, Ghuloum, and Weber 276). Ironically, Nizami's near-contemporary Ibn Sina advanced rationalist and materialist approaches to psychology, including cognitive-behavioral therapies for delusional disorders, which closely foreshadowed Western methodologies (Weber 2016 and 2013).

Religious cures for mental illness, however, are currently the dominant paradigm in the non-urbanized areas of the Muslim world.

Majnun repeatedly denies, however, that he is possessed by demons, for example *ghuls*. Persian contains a similar derivation as Arabic for insanity—*diwanagi* (mad) is derived from *diw* or 'demon'. Majnun's own father asks him 'are you a ghoul, a demon of the desert in human shape?' (Nizami 124). Although Al-Qayyim among other medieval writers attributed mental conditions such as epilepsy to two causes—one physiological and the other due to evil spirits—many popular Islamic advice-givers on modern websites attribute the following mental states solely to attacks by Shaytan or djinn: 'intense fear [...] psychological and nervous diseases, insanity, depression, anxiety, tension, epilepsy, *Waswaas* (whispers from the *Shaytaan*), personality disorders [...] hallucinations' (Ameen 52–53). Many of the descriptions and epithets of Majnun could lead to an interpretation of him as some sort of pure spirit without a body: as his body wastes away, he appears evanescent, cloud-like, ethereal; and he is so seldom seen by those who seek him in the desert, that both his being and poetry achieve mythical status.

Djinn can also cast the evil eye (*al-ayn*) on a person, and Majnun uses the evil eye as one explanation for his misfortunes—he complains that the world itself has cast the evil eye on him. He laments:

> yes, I am a victim of the world's Evil Eye, which has stolen what was my own. Who would not be afraid of it? People try to protect their children with blue amulets; even the sun, afraid of its darkness, wears a veil of pure sky-blue. But I was not protected by amulets, no veil covered my secret, no ruins offered a hiding place for my treasure; that is why the world could rob me of it. (Nizami 27)

Majnun refers to the widespread folk belief that excessive praise, happiness, or good fortune can attract the destructive powers of the evil eye. Amulets and charms such as the *nazar* (blue concentric pattern) and *Hamsa* or Hand of Fatima are used throughout the Islamic world to counteract the evil eye. Among folk healers in the Kingdom of Saudi Arabia, Al-Habeeb found that traditional practitioners ascribed serious mental conditions such as psychotic disorders, altered consciousness, aphonia, etc. to either the Evil Eye, sorcery (*as-sihr*), or djinn possession (Al-Habeeb 35).

Spiritualist and Sufi Interpretations of *Layla and Majnun*

Modern scholars of Nizami's poem have advanced several widely divergent interpretations as to what Nizami was ultimately trying to say about Majnun's madness. According to readings by Khairallah and Seyed-Gohrab, the poem is deeply allegorical and they suggest that Majnun may be divinely inspired, and following ascetic or Sufi pathways to enlightenment. This was certainly Fuzuli's later interpretation. Seyed-Gohrab, for example, points out that many of the traits of Majnun—peripateticism, mortification, seclusion, abstinence, and devotion—are also the hallmarks of the ascetic (Seyed-Gohrab 2003, 144). Although the historian of medicine Michael Dols rejected the mystical reading of Nizami's poem, the later 1484 version of the legend by the Sufi author Nur ad-Dīn Abd ar-Rahmān Jāmī of Khorasan transformed Majnun allegorically into a saint, and Layla is symbolized as God. The suffering of the separated lovers became a symbol of the anguish of the Sufi mystic who remains divided from union with the divine.

There are repeated references to veils in Nizami's poem; veils are a common symbol in Sufism in that the soul and the world are coverings that make people forget God, thus they should be pulled back to reveal the true nature of the divine. Nizami at one point in the poem describes Majnun as a Sufi mystic, as 'a dervish dancing before [Layla]' (Nizami 29). And although Majnun's obsessive love—particularly in light of his inability to consummate his desire once the impediment of Layla's husband is removed by death—appears to be narcissistic and inwardly directed, Nizami remarks that Majnun's longing liberates him from himself, another central tenet of Sufi philosophy: 'he suffered because he could not find the treasure for which he was searching, yet his grief provided him with a free passage, liberating him from the fetters of selfishness' (Nizami 48).

Many of the Sufi traditions speak of a lower inner being, the *nafs*, that must be controlled or tamed in order to achieve spiritual purity; thus one common goal of Sufi practice is destruction of the ego or self (*nafs*); this process can be likened to the removing of a veil, revealing the divine inner spiritual dimensions or states of being called *ruh* (soul) and *qalb* (spirit or heart). Majnun indicates that he has become pure love by annihilating all feelings of selfish lust, as well as his own persona: 'my soul is purified from the darkness of lust, my longing purged of low desire, my mind freed from shame. Love is the essence of my being [...] I no longer exist. What you see is me' (Nizami 195).

Nizami remarks 'there was no veil which could hide his beloved from Majnun' (Nizami 59), possibly emphasizing again a spiritual allegory of Layla as Majnun's own soul, veiled by darkness or the material world. When Majnun finds a piece of paper with only the names 'Majnun and Layla' written on it, he tears off Layla's name leaving his own, which astonishes the bystanders who ask him why he left only his name. He replies: '"because one can see the shell, but not the kernel," said Majnun. "Do you understand? The name is only the outer shell and I am this shell, I am the veil. The face underneath is hers"' (Nizami 133). His words indicate his belief that he and Layla are part of one being, which he explicitly states later in the poem.

Layla is described as 'a pearl unpierced' in the same passage examined above. Nizami may have known the Christian Syriac poem *Hymn of the Pearl* (*Hymn of the Soul*, third century CE)—probably composed in Edessa in the region of his birthplace Ganja—which contains Manichean, Zoroastrian, gnostic, and Christian elements (Poirier). The world is depicted as a prison and the soul as a pearl. Additionally Layla describes her death as breaking the chain of the world, a Neoplatonic symbol (Nizami 204).

The Orientalist Sir William Jones believed Nizami's poem was an allegory of divine love:

> the beautiful poem on the loves of Laili and Majnun by the immortal Nizami (to say nothing of other poems on the same subject) is indisputably built on true history, yet avowedly allegorical and mysterious; for the introduction to it is a continued rapture on Divine Love; and the name of Laili seems to be used in the *Masnavi* and the *Odes* of Hafiz for the Omnipresent Spirit of God. (Jones, quoted in Atkinson vi)

Horace Hayman Wilson, Professor of Sanskrit at Oxford, likewise called the loves of Layla and Majnun 'the reciprocal affection of body and soul' (qtd in Atkinson vii)—a possible reference to the Aristotelian tradition of the soul as a principle of harmony.

According to Seyed-Gohrab:

> Majnun provided mystics with a palpable example of 'annihilation' (*fanā'*) in the Beloved. Majnun's famous saying, 'I am Leyli and Leyli is [I],' corresponded to Ḥallāj's mystical aphorism (*šaṭḥ*): 'I am he whom I love; whom

I love is [I].' Mystics had several other pairs of lovers such as Maḥmud and Ayāz, Farhād and Širin, Wāmeq and 'Aḏrā to explicate one aspect of love, but the story of Leyli and Majnun remained one of the most popular for mystic poets. (Seyed-Gohrab 2009)

The logic of Sufi mysticism is clear—the self (*nafs*) must be abandoned to achieve divine union; as Khairallah notes: 'if we accept the Sufi logic which conceives of the goal of perfect love as self-annihilation in the Beloved, then it will follow that the end of perfect gnosis is loss of reason, and the end of perfect expression is silence' (Khairallah 109). Thus, in this view, Majnun's loss of rationality and rational thought's traditional marker—language—is the gaining of eternal wisdom.

The poem also appears to have Christian or Neoplatonic elements. Majnun declares that 'He is a lamp, and she is the sun (soul)', a possible reference to Plato's allegory of the cave. Also, Nizami comments on Majnun's madness: 'the reins had slipped from the rider's hand [...] he had not only lost his beloved, but also himself' (Nizami 24). This passage may be an allusion to Plato's chariot allegory in the *Phaedrus*, in which reason or intellect (the charioteer) guides two horses, one representing our moral nature, the other the concupiscible desires (Plato 246a–54e). Plato was widely read in medieval Islamic intellectual circles and Socrates' dialogue investigates the same themes as Nizami: divine madness (θεία μανία).

Additionally, both Majnun and the narrator refer several times to the earth as a prison, or impure, with the self being chained to the body in metaphors that recall the Neoplatonic conception of the imprisonment of the soul within the body and the *contemptus mundi* philosophy of medieval Christianity. The most striking examples of Neoplatonic imagery—the world as a prison or cage, light metaphors, the rejection of the material world, and the insignificance of man—occur in Nizami's interpolation:

> What is human life after all? Whether it endures for a brief spell or longer—even if it could last a thousand years; take it as a breath of air merging into eternity [...] you yourself are the grain of sand; you are your own prisoner. Break your cage, break free from yourself, free from humanity; learn that what you thought was real is not so in reality. Follow Nizami: burn but your own treasure, like a candle—then the world, your sovereign, will become your slave. (Nizami 181)

Early and medieval Christianity share many mythic elements with Persian religions, such as light imagery, the dualism of Zoroastrianism, and the two spirits of Manichaeism, in which light/dark, good/evil, God/Satan spirits battle for supremacy—Spenta Mainyu and Angra Mainyu. Thus the possible Christian allusions and imagery of Nizami's poem may be Persian in origin, derived from the common cultural heritage of the Abrahamic religions. Also, all medieval Abrahamic theologians were influenced by the philosophies of Plato, Aristotle, and the Stoics. Nizami's 1177 poem 'The Depository of Mysteries' expounds a theory of love in the Neoplatonic tradition of the duality of spirit/world. Here Nizami notes about human love (*esgh*): 'man consists of the two sources—spiritual and corporal, hence [his] dual nature: "He is both clean and turbid, though in him Gold begins to shine"' (Aliyev 64).

For the literary critic As'ad Khairallah, Majnun represents a heroic figure battling against rationalism and social norms in order to achieve spiritual and poetic purity. By rejecting wealth, companions, and the cultural rules of courtship and marriage, and through his ascetic behaviour, he challenges the social order. According to Khairallah,

> if sanity is generally equated with conformity to established norms, then [...] the madman will represent the rebellion against the stifling laws of reasonable society and its common sense. His imagination is his reason, and where 'sane' people hesitate in front of social and intellectual norms, he simply asserts his mode of vision with the same innocence and force of prophetic utterance. This purity of vision, and the courage of expressing it make the madman an almost poetic ideal. (Khairallah 20)

Nizami's Poem and Modern Islamic Psychology

Several Islamic psychotherapeutic models have recently been advanced. The underlying theoretical principle is that Islam is a radically distinct habitus requiring a unique way of life, and unique educational, social, and political systems. These proposed models may be partially driven by postcolonial political rhetoric that strongly distinguishes Islam from Western modes of being. Abu-Raiya and Pergamant have reviewed the attempts to formulate an empirically based Islamic psychology, which in their opinion have not been successful (Abu-Raiya and Pergamant). Wahass and Kent have argued that it would be 'difficult to see, for example, how a therapist with a Western/Christian background could help deeply religious Muslim patients to apply religion-based strategies without developing knowledge and skills in this area' (Wahass and Kent 667). Any attempt to place an empirical Islamic psychology and psychotherapy on a useful basis that would be acceptable to adherents of Islam would obviously need to acknowledge current folk-medical views, and the metaphoric and literary analogues of madness found in the diverse and complex corpuses of fiction and poetry that are still alive today in the Muslim world. As discussed earlier, the common expressions for madness in Islam are linked etymologically to the spirit world, and the Qur'an, hadith, and the Islamicized Greek humoral model of medicine are still highly influential in modern Muslim thought. Thus Nizami is an obvious and rich source for exploring modern Muslim, Arabic, and Indo-Iranian views of mental illness.

Conclusion

Nizami's poem is clearly not a medical treatise (although it was later used as a case study for medical interpretations of love madness), nor can it be defined unambiguously as a religious text exploring divine madness in the Sufi tradition. Nizami is manifestly interested in the character of Majnun, his inner mental states, and how fate, his habits of mind, and his cultural milieu lead him to behavior that is labeled madness by his contemporaries. Although not explored in depth in this paper, Layla represents another complex character who also claims to be driven mad by the lovers' separation and Majnun's sufferings. Characters in the poem—as well as Nizami the narrator—attempt to solve the mystery of Majnun's mad behaviors in order to cure him and reintegrate him back into society, attributing his madness to humoral imbalance, demonic possession, intoxication, divine fate, the evil eye, or excessive passion.

Nizami's poem thus very thoroughly explores the medical, religious, folk traditional, and philosophical interpretations of madness in his culture; his work represents an important social documentary of popular conceptions of mental illness in medieval Islamic literature. The remarkable cultural continuity regarding conceptions of madness in modern Muslim-majority countries—whose healthcare professionals are striving to develop a paradigm of 'Islamic psychology'—argues for the continuing appreciation of Nizami's work as a sourcebook of insights into madness and love.

References

Abu-Raiya, Hisham, and Kenneth I. Pargament, 'Empirically-Based Psychology of Islam: Summary and Critique of the Literature', *Mental Health, Religion and Culture* 14 (2011): 93–115. https://doi.org/10.1080/13674670903426482

Albinali, Hajar A., *Majnoon Laila: Medical Analysis of an Arab Love Story*, trans. by Amer Chaikhouni, Janet King (Doha: Katara Publishing House, 2018).

Al-Habeeb, Ahmad, 'A Pilot Study of Faith Healers' Views on Evil Eye, Jinn Possession, and Magic in the Kingdom of Saudi Arabia', *Journal of Family and Community Medicine* 10.3 (2003): 31–38.

Aliyev, Rustam M., *Nizami Ganjavi* (Baku, Azerbaijan: Yazichi, 1991).

Al-Qur'an [The Holy Qur'an] (Al-Qāhirah: al-Ṭab'ah al-thānīyah, 1952).

Ameen, Abu'l-Mundhir Khaleel ibn Ibraaheem, *The Jinn and Human Sickness: Remedies in the Light of the Qur'aan and Sunnah*, trans. by Nasiruddin Al-Khattab, ed. by Dr Abdul Ahad (Riyadh, KSA: Darussalam, 2005).

Atkinson, James A. (ed.), *The Loves of Lailí and Majnún: A Poem from the original Persian of Nizami* (London: David Nutt, 1894).

Bürgel, Johann C., 'Love, Lust, and Longing: Eroticism in Early Islam as Reflected in Literary Sources' in Al-Sayyid-Marsot and Afaf Lutfi (eds), *Society and the Sexes in Medieval Islam* (Malibu, CA: Undena Publications, 1979), 81–118.

Clinton, Jerome W., 'A Comparison of Nizami's *Layli and Majnun* and Shakespeare's *Romeo and Juliet*' in Kamran Talatoff and Jerome W. Clinton (eds), *The Poetry of Nizami Ganjavi: Knowledge, Love and Rhetoric* (New York: Palgrave, 2000), 15–27. https://doi.org/10.1007/978-1-137-09836-8_2

des Epesse, Bertrand Thierry de Crussol, *La psychiatrie médiévale persane: La maladie mentale dans la tradition médicale persane* (Paris: Springer-Verlag France, 2010). https://doi.org/10.1007/978-2-287-99478-4

Dols, Michael, *Majnun: The Madman in Medieval Islamic Society* (Oxford: Oxford University Press, 1991).

El-Zein, Amira, *Islam, Arabs, and the Intelligent World of the Jinn* (Syracuse: Syracuse University Press, 2009).

Foucault, Michel, *Language, Madness, and Desire: On Literature*, ed. by Philippe Artières, Jean-François Bert, Mathieu Potte-Bonneville, Judith Revel, and Robert Bononno (Minneapolis: University of Minnesota Press, 2015).

Giffen, Lois A., *Theory of Profane Love Among the Arabs: The Development of the Theory* (New York: New York University Press, 1971). https://doi.org/10.1017/S002074380005176X

Hickey, Jason E.; Steven Pryjmachuk, and Heather Waterman, 'Mental Illness Research in the Gulf Cooperation Council: A Scoping Review', *Health Research Policy and Systems* 14 (2016): 14–59.

Kalpaklı, Mehmet, and Walter G. Andrews, 'Layla grows up: Nizami's Layal and Majnun "in the Turkish manner"' in Kamran Talatoff and Jerome W. Clinton (eds), *The Poetry of Nizami Ganjavi: Knowledge, Love and Rhetoric* (New York: Palgrave, 2000), 29–49. https://doi.org/10.1007/978-1-137-09836-8

Khairallah, As'ad E., *Love, Madness, and Poetry: An Interpretation of the Magnūn Legend*, Beiruter Texte und Studien, 25 (Wiesbaden: Franz Steiner Verlag, 1980).

Krachkovskiĭ, Ignatij Julianovič, 'Die frühgeschichte der erzählung von Macnun und Lailā in der Arabischen literature', trans. by Hellmut Ritter, *Oriens* 8 (1955): 1–50.

Kronfol, Ziad, Suhaila Ghuloum, and Alan S. Weber, 'Mental Health Practice. Country in Focus: Qatar', *Asian Journal of Psychiatry* 6 (2013): 275–77. 10.1016/j.ajp.2013.02.004

Lord Byron, George Gordon, *The Works of Lord Byron Complete in One Volume* (Francfort: H.L. Broenner, 1829).

Nizami [Ganjavi], *The Story of Layla and Majnun*, trans. by Rudolf Gelpke, E. Mattin, and G. Hill (London: Bruno Cassirer and Faber & Faber, 1966).

Plato, *The Works of Plato*, ed. by Irvan Edman (New York: Modern Library, 1927).

Poirier, Paul-Hubert, *L'hymne de la perle des actes de Thomas: Introduction, texte-traduction, commentaire* (Louvain-la-Neuve, 1981). https://doi.org/10.7202/400038ar

Seyed-Gohrab, Ali-Asghar, *Layli and Majnun: Love, Madness and Mystic Longing in Nizami's Epic Romance* (Leiden: Brill, 2003).

Seyed-Gohrab, Ali-Asghar, 'Leyli O Majnun', *Encyclopædia Iranica*, 2009, http://www.iranicaonline.org/articles/leyli-o-majnun-narrative-poem, accessed 24 December 2018.

Wahass, Saheed, and Gerry Kent, 'Coping with Auditory Hallucinations: A Cross-Cultural Comparison between Western (British) and Non-Western (Saudi Arabian) Patients', *The Journal of Nervous and Mental Disease* 185.11 (1997): 664–68. 10.1097/00005053-199711000-00002

Weber, Alan S., 'Folk Medicine in Oman', *International Journal of Arts and Sciences*, 4.23 (2011): 237–74.

Weber, Alan S., 'Expressive Arts Therapy in the Arabian Gulf: History and Future', *Journal of Arts in Society* 6.5 (2012): 55–66.

Weber, Alan S., 'Avicennian Psychology as Bridge Concept for Islamic Psychotherapeutic Intervention in the Arabian Gulf', unpublished paper presented at the 15th Biannual Conference of the International Society for Theoretical Psychology (ISTP), Santiago, Chile, 6 May 2013.

Weber, Alan S., 'Ibn Sīnā Cures a Prince Who Thinks He Is a Cow', *Hektoen Journal* 8.1 (Winter 2016), http://www.hektoeninternational.org, accessed 5 May 2019.

Wehr, Hans, *A Dictionary of Modern Written Arabic*, 3rd edn, ed. by J. Milton Cowan (Ithaca, NY: Spoken Language Services, 1976).

Zarshenas, Mohammad M., Zohreh Abolhassanzadeh, Pouya Faridi, and Abdolali Mohagheghzadeh, 'Sphygmology of Ibn Sina, a Message for Future', *Heart Views* 13.3 (2013): 155–58.

2 The Anti-Psychiatry Ethos in Samuel Beckett's *Murphy*

Shoshana Benjamin

The perception of Samuel Beckett as an iconoclastic author who explored the inner worlds of the outcast, the socially unfit, and the mentally deranged may incline one to place him among the supporters of what is known as the anti-psychiatry movement. And in certain respects, his early novel *Murphy* (1938), several chapters of which are set in a British mental institution of the 1930s, does reflect the radical outlook on mental health subsequently evolved by R.D. Laing, David Cooper, Thomas Szasz, Erving Goffman, Franco Basaglia, and Michel Foucault. This small and loosely affiliated group of psychiatrists, philosophers, and sociologists were the main movers for change in Britain, America, Italy, and France. Though diverse in their thinking on specific issues, they shared three core ideas which form what I refer to as *the anti-psychiatry ethos*: that conventional psychiatric attitudes and practices were harmful and degrading to those they were meant to help; that cordoning off the mentally ill in institutions was therapeutically and morally wrong; and that the commonly accepted distinction between sanity and insanity was invalid. In a famously provocative statement, Laing turned the distinction on its head, deeming those labelled insane to be sane, and the sane, including generals, heads of state, and the psychiatric establishment, insane. Insanity, according to Laing, was 'a perfectly rational adjustment to an insane world' (Seymour, Crain, and Crockett 53). Depending on the ideology of the beholder, its cause was alternately held to be the family, capitalism, or the inability of conformist societies to tolerate otherness. That mental illness might be a medical condition was dismissed by Szasz as a myth, and indeed, there was no scientific evidence for it at the time.

Though anti-psychiatry ideas had already emerged in the eighteenth century (Crossley 877), they ripened into a full-fledged ideology with a concrete mission for the practice of psychiatry only in the 1960s and 1970s, a period that sought to overthrow the status quo in virtually every area of public and private life. In the field of mental health, new paradigms for understanding and treating the mentally ill challenged traditional approaches to madness, with considerable success. Viewed against the background of these developments, Beckett's novel demonstrates with exceptional clarity what the anti-psychiatry movement was in revolt against and where it was headed. In this study I show that Beckett not only anticipated the movement but also provided a stinging critique of some of its central beliefs and practices. Thus, while not intended to frame a debate over the validity of an approach to mental illness that had yet to claim public attention, his novel about a young Irishman who views the world of the madman as infinitely superior to the ordinary world of normal human beings brings its strengths and weaknesses to light.

To give my discussion a concentrated focus, rather than looking at the spectrum of anti-psychiatry practitioners and spokesmen, I draw on R.D. Laing, commonly referred to as the father of the anti-psychiatry movement, for a characterization of its ethos. Although Laing is best known for his first book *The Divided Self*, written at the age of twenty-eight, my main reference source is his later retrospect *Wisdom, Madness and Folly*, published in 1985. *Wisdom* is the wiser work, a distillation of many years of reflection. It covers the first thirty years of Laing's life, from 1927 to 1957, the year he completed *The Divided Self*. The story of his struggle to liberate himself from the psychiatric dogma of the day sums up the anti-psychiatry ethos more succinctly than the earlier work, which is composed of case studies that complement and support his existentialist theories about the nature of schizophrenia and its etiology. I relate to that work as well, though more briefly. In *Wisdom* Laing speaks from the heart about his own personal experiences. The story of his metamorphosis from a tradition-bound psychiatrist to a passionate rebel has much in common with Beckett's tale of a nonconformist hero confronting a rigid, closed-minded establishment. Indeed, the similarity between Murphy, a small cog in a large organization who proves capable of making a difference, and the real-life professional who turned against the ideas he was trained in, raises the question of influence, which I deal with in my discussion. The key question is whether Laing read *Murphy* before writing *The Divided Self.*

My study is a two-pronged affair. It aims a) to determine where Beckett stands on the issues taken up by the anti-psychiatry movement, and b) to correlate those views with Laing's. The first task turns out to be somewhat complicated because *Murphy* does not speak with one voice: within the novel there is an implicit inner debate between the protagonist, through whose eyes we perceive the world of the insane, and the omnipresent and omniscient authorial narrator, who looks at Murphy and his ideas about madness with a critical eye. This higher consciousness enthusiastically embraces some of his character's ideas, but unequivocally rejects others—among them, fundamental and foundational anti-psychiatry beliefs. The *split consciousness* that pervades the work, that of the lower consciousness immersed in the action, and that of the higher consciousness observing and commenting on his thoughts, speech, and deeds, obliges us to sort out their points of convergence and divergence. Only thus may we determine where Beckett, or the novel as a whole, stands vis-à-vis the anti-psychiatry ethos.

What complicates the task is Beckett's use of free indirect discourse, a form of speech representation that enables the narrator to convey the thoughts, feelings, or states of mind of the character in the latter's native idiom, without using quotation marks or other signs of attribution. In instances of free indirect discourse, it is not always clear whether the narrator is speaking for the character alone, or for himself as well, and if for the character alone, how he regards what he reports. I have left the considerations that lead me to assign 'ownership' of the ideas I deal with outside of my discussion, since the text leaves no doubt as to where the narrator stands in those critical cases where the two diverge. For example, after pointing out a discrepancy in Murphy's belief system, he mockingly adds: 'So much the worse for him, no doubt' (76). The care he takes to distinguish himself from his protagonist—and I say *his* protagonist because we are dealing with a narrator who claims to be the author of the fictional story he relates—is evident from the start, as shown by the qualifying phrase 'as though' in these famous first lines of the novel: 'The sun shone, having no alternative, on the nothing new. Murphy sat out of it, as though he were free, in a mew in West Brompton' (1). The higher and comprehensive perspective of the narrator, implicitly equated with that of the author of *Ecclesiastes*, counters

Murphy's belief that his retreats into his mind (metaphorically conceived of as *sitting out of the sun*) free him from the bonds of the outer world.

My second concern is to correlate the diverging and converging views of the narrator and the protagonist with those of Laing. To anticipate, those of the radically minded Murphy dovetail with Laing's, while only some of the narrator's views tally with them.

Let me end this introduction with two comments. First, it was long thought that Beckett acquired his knowledge of mental institutions by having worked in one for a time. That proves to have been untrue. The background information for his portrait of asylum life is based on observations made during visits to his friend Geoffrey Thompson, then in resident psychiatric training at the Bethlem Hospital. The visits took place between February and October 1935; *Murphy* was begun in August 1935 and completed in June 1936. Beckett was also exceptionally well versed in philosophical and psychological theories of the mind and widely read on the subject of abnormal psychology. His friendship with James Joyce, whose daughter Lucia was treated, unsuccessfully, for schizophrenia in 1934 by Carl Jung, gave him a more personal firsthand perspective on mental illness. Jung believed that both she and her father were schizophrenics (Jones). Many years later, Beckett recalled his walks with Lucia in the gardens of the mental institution at Ivry-sur-Seine: 'Everything would be calm and peaceful and all of a sudden she would become extraordinarily violent and aggressive' (Knowlson and Knowlson 51).

Second, given the focus of my study, I should point out that the main theme of the novel is not madness but an acutely felt mind/body conflict experienced by the protagonist. The two themes intertwine, however, as Murphy comes to view madness as an escape route from the world of the body, which he regards as a prison, to the world of the mind, where he feels free. Going mad is the goal he pursues and momentarily achieves, only to discover that it is not the haven he hoped for. The larger mind/body issue is treated in my article 'Seen and Unseen Narratives in Beckett's Cryptic Novel *Murphy*' (Benjamin 2020).

Murphy's Introduction to Asylum Life

Three of the novel's thirteen chapters are set in the Magdalen Mental Mercyseat, a reputedly humane institution described as a 'hospital for the better-class mentally deranged' (87) and 'a sanatorium, not a madhouse nor a home for defectives' (160). Some 15% of its patients belong to the category of *certified*; these include psychotics cut off from reality. The main narrative circumstance that brings Murphy to the asylum is economic: in need of a job, he eagerly accepts an offer made by an acquaintance, a third-rate Dublin poet named Austin Ticklepenny, to replace him as a male nurse. Endowed with good critical intelligence and the capacity for independent out-of-the-box thinking, Murphy makes for an acute but, it needs to be stressed, imperfect observer. His ability to see things as they are is compromised by his major defect, which is willful blindness. Though serious in itself and for Murphy's fate, his tragic flaw affects only some of the many observations he makes as a fresh mind registering impressions of a new and strange environment. Moreover, the fact that he has blind spots is even beneficial for sorting out the sometimes converging, sometimes diverging views of narrator and character, as his falsifications of reality are caught by the supervising narratorial eye and explicitly characterized as misperceptions.

The fact that Murphy is new to the job and has no professional training or previous experience with the mentally ill is narratively significant, for it not only enables Beckett to make use of his inquisitive mind as an instrument of perception, but also provides him with a realistic motive for treating the reader to a virtual tour of the institution. Murphy and the reader are thus simultaneously introduced to the particulars of the asylum's physical layout, its institutional policies and practices, the kinds of people on the staff, the types of patients and their maladies, as well as the general routine governing day-to-day life in a well-appointed place with a nonetheless institutional odor of 'paraldehyde and truant sphincters' (167). Ticklepenny, Bim the head nurse, and his twin brother Bom, who is Murphy's immediate supervisor, each show him around the facility. Bom's character is summed up in one line: 'Bom was what is vulgarly called a sadist and encouraged what is vulgarly called sadism in his assistants' (238). Though sadistic behavior is alluded to in the account of asylum life, it is not highlighted or actually depicted. The corrupting influence of power and authority in institutions is, however, emphasized: Bim is at once Ticklepenny's boss and his homosexual master.

Among the interesting things we learn from these introductory tours, the no-mingling policy designed to keep staff and patients strictly separate stands out. A primary target of the anti-establishment revolt, it is indirectly referred to in this excerpt from Bim's initiation speech, in response to Murphy's innocent question, 'Are they all certified?' Bim barks back: 'That is not your business. [...] You are not paid to take an interest in the patients, but to fetch for them, carry for them, and clean up after them. All you know about them is the work they give you to do. Make no mistake about it' (160). Murphy does not so much rebel against the regulation as ignore it. Acting according to his own lights, he takes no heed of protocol, approaches the patients as worthy human beings and does his best to help them. Where the rule-governed efforts of his colleagues fail or require coercion, his benevolent initiatives meet with great success: 'One patient [...] refused to exercise unless accompanied by Murphy. Another, a melancholic with highly developed delusions of guilt, would not get out of his bed except on Murphy's invitation. Another melancholic [...] would only eat when Murphy held the spoon. Otherwise he had to be force-fed' (182). Murphy may not have violated the letter of the law, but he clearly breached a norm, hence the narrator points out: 'All this was highly irregular, little short of scandalous' (182).

That untrained, underpaid, and overworked menials with no experience of the mentally ill were barred from interacting with a population of deranged people is not difficult to understand. Real risks were involved, as Bim's instructions to the newly hired Murphy indicate: 'He would never lose sight of the fact that he was dealing with patients not responsible for what they did or said. He would never on any account allow himself to be affected by the abuse, no matter how foul and unmerited, that would be poured out upon him' (158). Some patients were prone to violent outbursts of rage. But the policy that Murphy breaches is not merely precautionary. Staff and inmates were kept apart because the latter were in effect regarded as belonging to a separate subhuman species. The medical supervisor at the asylum, Dr Angus Killiecrankie, appears to have been no different in attitude from the lower-ranking staff, though he has little contact with the patients. Lower-ranking staff members take care of their everyday needs. That remained the norm both during and after the anti-psychiatry revolt (see Abrahamson on Laing's limited interaction with patients).

The Question of Influence

Moving now from the fictional to the real world, an extreme form of the no-mingling policy was in effect at the psychiatric ward where Ronald Laing served as a conscripted psychiatrist in the British Army during the Korean War. Not only was social intercourse outlawed, but so too all talk and conversation between staff and patients and among the patients themselves. This was held to be for the good of the patients. Laing writes: 'The staff in the psychiatric wing had strict orders not to talk to the patients or to encourage the patients to talk to them, or to each other, or to themselves, or at all. No patient was expected to speak to a member of staff unless spoken to. Talking between patients was observed, reported and broken up. Pairing off was prevented' (Laing 1998, 100). Laing explains that the therapeutic philosophy behind the silent treatment was that talk 'aggravates the psychotic process. It is like promoting a haemorrhage in a haemophiliac' (Laing 1998, 100). It took some time before Laing, having only recently completed his training as a psychiatrist, dared to listen to his dissenting inner voice and to act on it within the restrictive army framework. And even then, after contravening the prohibition, he lacked the certainty that he was right and the experts wrong. His uncertainty extended to other methods of treatment as well: debilitating insulin treatments, electric shocks, and lobotomies. But he was seized by doubt: 'Maybe I was mistaken. How could the whole of psychiatry be doing the opposite of what I assumed psychiatry was about—treating, curing if possible, arresting the course of mental illness? Was Artaud right?' (Laing 1998, 106).

These statements from *Wisdom, Madness and Folly* are part of Laing's account of how he evolved a point of view so at odds with the established psychiatric doctrines he absorbed during years of study and training. Whether *Murphy* played a role in that evolution is an open question. The main reason to suppose it likely is the strong correspondence between Laing's views and those of Beckett's hero. Conversely, one reason for supposing the opposite is that the then one and only 1938 edition of the novel would have been hard to find in bookstores and libraries. Reviewed in the press by, among others, a myopic twenty-four-year-old Dylan Thomas, who panned it, *Murphy* was a commercial failure. Only after Beckett made a name for himself with the London performances of the English-language version of *Waiting for Godot* in 1955 did it attract attention. Significantly, Laing mentions Beckett in *The Divided Self*, but only in connection with the play, which he looks at through a psychiatric lens, briefly diagnosing the two tramps as if they were patients. He describes their existential predicament as arising from 'despair, terror and boredom of existence' (Laing 1964, 41). There is definitely room here for a second opinion, I might add. The 1957 Grove Press edition of *Murphy* came out too late for Laing to have read it before writing *The Divided Self*. But the early edition, while unknown to the general public, would probably have found its way to the offices of psychiatrists, psychoanalysts, and other kinds of mental health professionals. Geoffrey Thompson is a case in point. Though Beckett did not tell him he was writing a novel set in a mental hospital when he visited him at Bethlem (Knowlson 1996, 197), Thompson would surely have read the work of his good friend once it was published, and it would have been natural for him to recommend it to colleagues. The limited readership of the 1938 edition of *Murphy* would probably have included the staff at the Tavistock Clinic where Beckett spent nearly two years (1934–35) in thrice-weekly sessions of psychotherapy with Wilfred Bion. Years later, starting in 1956, Laing practiced psychotherapy at Tavistock and remained there until 1964. Could he have been unaware of the fact that Tavistock's most illustrious patient had written an unconventional psychiatrically themed novel that portrayed life in a mental hospital? Or that it paid special attention to schizophrenia, the type of madness that most interested Laing? Or that its protagonist was above all *a divided self*, 'split' between his inner and outer worlds (110)? And yet, as far as I have been able to determine, he nowhere mentions *Murphy*. I find the omission especially puzzling in view of the fact that he generously acknowledges the contributions made to his intellectual development by Sartre, Heidegger, Kierkegaard, and Hegel. It is however known that Beckett, Laing's senior by twenty-one years, did not read *The Divided Self* (Knowlson 2003, 16).

Murphy and Laing Compared

Let me now draw attention to the disparity between Murphy's immediate and unhesitating rejection of conventional psychiatric norms and Laing's comparatively slow progress to the same place. A likely explanation is that Murphy did not have to throw off years of training and indoctrination. Nor did he have to cope with the problem of deferring to expert opinion, as he looks upon the resident authorities, Bim and Bom, as knaves and fools. This does not mean, however, that Murphy comes to the asylum with an open mind. He is as doctrinaire as can be, but his doctrine is based on very different principles than those that animated Laing. Where Laing was above all a humanist who was appalled by the insensitivity, inflexibility, and indifference to suffering on the part of healthcare professionals, Murphy is philosophically committed to a dichotomous view of reality. For him, there are two worlds, *the little world of the mind* and *the big world of the body*. The opposition is that between the private inner world that he experiences while immersed in self-induced trance states, and the outer world, experienced during ordinary waking consciousness. Unlike daydreaming, which we just slip into, due preparation is a condition for Murphy's entry into his little world. That involves two hypnosis-inducing procedures, eye fixation and rhythmic rocking in a rocking chair. The reality that unfolds there is hallucinatory.

Perceiving a parallel between his inner-world experience and the mental state of his wards, he sees them as a select band of men who made the bold choice of opting for a life lived in the mind. He regards their choice as a rational one, justified by the advantages available to the madman. In a classically anti-psychiatry reversal of values, the narrator tells us that Murphy's experience as a 'rational being obliged him to call sanctuary what the psychiatrists called exile and to think of the patients not as banished from a system of benefits but as escaped from a colossal fiasco' (178). Murphy admires and respects the patients: 'Except for the maniac [...] the impression he received was of that self-immersed indifference to the contingencies of the contingent world which he had chosen for himself as the only felicity and achieved so seldom' (168).

By contrast, Laing never seriously advocated insanity even when defending it as a rational choice. In practical terms, however, their disparate attitudes led to the same end: a more humane treatment of a helpless population incarcerated in institutions run by people who are strict about rules but lacking in empathy. Regarding institutions per se, here we find another important difference. Laing considered the institution of the mental asylum an evil in itself, to be abolished and replaced by community-based care and hostels. Mental institutions served the purpose of enabling society to rid itself of unwanted people. Laing makes a compelling case against the unchecked power of the psychiatrist, far exceeding that of judges in criminal cases, to condemn a person, sometimes on the strength of one short interview, to months, years, or a lifetime of incarceration. The family oddball is henceforth a certified mental case with no legal or human rights and no say regarding the treatment he is subjected to. But for all the criticism leveled against the institutional care of the insane at the Magdalen Mental Mercyseat, there is no sign that Beckett believed in abolishing institutions or that he even considered the possibility. The issue is simply not raised in the novel.

Murphy and Laing are, however, in basic agreement about the function of the psychiatric institution. Laing lists three purposes: '1) Voluntary and involuntary incarceration, 2) Stopping undesirable states of mind and conduct, and 3) changing undesirable states of mind and forms of conduct into less undesirable and even desirable states of mind and conduct' (Laing 1998, 16). He follows this up with the pointed question: *undesirable to whom?* Beckett had already answered in Murphy's name: 'The function of treatment was to bridge the gulf, translate the sufferer from his own pernicious little private dungheap to the glorious world of discrete particles, where it would be his inestimable prerogative once again to wonder, love, hate, desire, rejoice and howl in a reasonable balanced manner, and comfort himself with the society of others in the same predicament' (177). 'All this was duly revolting to Murphy', the narrator adds, making it clear that he is representing Murphy's view, and it would seem, his own. Laing similarly took issue with the psychiatrist's mission of turning *them* into *us*, which he did not find objectionable when that was the patient's goal as well. Murphy's goal, however, is entirely different: he wants to become one of *them*.

How a sane man becomes or tries to become a madman is discussed in my other essay on *Murphy* (Benjamin 2020). The cardinal point is *mutual recognition*. Murphy concocts a scheme based on the Hegelian notion that the way to confirm one's identity—to validate that you are what you take yourself to be—is through the agency of an outside party, one qualified to judge whether you are what you believe yourself to be. Aiming to substantiate his belief that he is a man of the microcosm and of the microcosm alone, Murphy attempts to form a reciprocal relationship with his favorite patient, the self-immersed non-communicating schizophrenic Mr Endon. After trying and predictably failing to get him to acknowledge him as a kindred spirit, Murphy recognizes the futility of his enterprise, decides to leave the asylum, but meets instead with a freak accident. He dies while rocking his way into his beloved little world.

Where Murphy and Laing Go Wrong

Murphy regards the inner world inhabited by Mr Endon as a true counterpart of his treasured mental world. And in fact, the brief glimpses into

Endon's self-enclosed world line up well with the ideal state that Murphy wishes to achieve on a permanent basis. Here is an illustrative excerpt:

> Mr Endon was a schizophrenic of the most amiable variety, at least for the purposes of such a humble and envious outsider as Murphy. [...] His inner voice did not harangue him, it was unobtrusive and melodious, a gentle continuo in the whole consort of his hallucinations. The bizarrerie of his attitudes never exceeded a stress laid on their grace. In short, a psychosis so limpid and imperturbable that Murphy felt drawn to it as Narcissus to his fountain. (186)

Mr Endon, however, is an exceptional figure, far different from the other inmates. These Murphy misperceives under the influence of a deeply entrenched *confirmation bias*, a term coined in the 1960s for what was formerly known as *willful blindness*. The narrator highlights it in connection with Murphy's rosy early impressions: 'Nothing remained but to see what he wanted to see', he says. 'Nothing remained but to substantiate these [impressions], distorting all that threatened to belie them' (176). The fundamental error in Murphy's thinking, as discerned by the narrator, is that he equates his blissful trance states not only with the ideal world of Mr Endon but with the unenviable experience of the ordinary patient. The error bears consequences, since it causes him to ignore or minimize their pain and suffering. The narrator takes him to task on this: 'The frequent expressions apparently of pain, rage, despair and in fact all the usual, to which some patients gave vent [...] Murphy either disregarded or muted to mean what he wanted' (179). To the extent that he does take notice, he adopts the tactic of blaming their suffering on the intervention of their healers:

> But [...] even if the patients did sometimes feel as lousy as they sometimes looked, still no aspersion was necessarily cast on the little world where Murphy presupposed them, one and all, to be having a glorious time. One had merely to ascribe their agitations, not to any flaw in their self-seclusion, but to its investment by the healers. [...] Left in peace they would have been as happy as Larry. (179–80)

Murphy's tactic of blaming the suffering of the mentally ill on the healers may be seen as heralding the new age of anti-psychiatry, which accused conventional psychiatry of harming the insane, not through barbaric means such as chaining lunatics to walls, but by incarcerating them in institutions and subjecting them to forms of treatment that amounted to mistreatment. Unlike Murphy, Laing and his contemporaries did recognize the suffering of their patients and tried to alleviate it by means other than commonly employed psychiatric methods. To a considerable extent, the difference consisted in nothing more than treating patients as human beings deserving of respect, which entailed listening to them and talking to them. Laing points out the primacy of this approach to the mentally ill, identical in kind to that which scandalized Murphy's superiors at the Magdalen Mental Mercyseat: 'Whatever treatment they get, first and last, "we" should not forget to treat "them," however strange "they" are to "us," as "simply human" like ourselves' (Laing 1998, 7). The new philosophy further entailed abandoning the kinds of medical treatment that the psychiatrists would not have wanted administered to themselves.

But more controversial innovations were also tried out, of which Laing's daring but not unprecedented experiment at Kingsley Hall is probably the best known. In this residence established in 1965 for the psychotic and the schizophrenic, Laing attempted to implement an ideology that aimed at breaking down the distinction that separated *them* from *us* in the institutions he worked in. At Kingsley Hall, inmates and doctors shared a communal lifestyle, lived on the same premises, and ate at the same table. Cannabis and LSD were not in short supply. According to Sean O'Hagan, who interviewed Kingsley Hall 'survivors', the place was meant to be 'a refuge, a safe haven […] where there were no locks on the doors and no anti-psychotic drugs were administered. People were free to come and go as they pleased' (O'Hagan). All-night therapy sessions were held and role-reversal—patients taking the role of doctors and vice versa—was encouraged. The atmosphere was described by one former resident as *chaotic*. Unfortunately, the experiment did not fulfill its promise. No psychiatrist or therapist stayed on as a resident for long; Laing himself left after one year, though he continued to work there. In his sympathetic but not uncritical account of Laing and the anti-psychiatric movement, Zbigniew Kotowicz notes that Kingsley Hall closed down after the five-year lease on the building was up (Kotowicz 87). That is well known, but O'Hagan links the end with the rarely mentioned fact that two people jumped off the roof. The community soon disbanded. Laing made plans to go to Ceylon (now Sri Lanka) and India for a year. Kotowicz writes that his departure 'brought his career as a theoretician and militant of radical psychiatry to an end' (Kotowicz 87). But his later memoir shows him to have remained faithful to the anti-psychiatry ethos long afterwards as well.

On Divided Selves

Though the title of Laing's best-known work brings Beckett's existentially split protagonist to mind, the profile of Laing's schizophrenic type does not fit Murphy all that well. The critical differentiating factor is *sanity*: Laing's schizophrenics are insane schizoids; Murphy, to his regret, is a sane schizoid. The term *schizoid*, as defined by Laing, refers to 'an individual the totality of whose experience is split in two main ways: in the first place, there is a rent in his relation with his world and, in the second, there is a disruption of his relation with himself' (Laing 1964, 17). Murphy is unquestionably schizoid. He owns up to being divided between two selves dubbed *the mental Murphy* and *the physical Murphy* but, unlike the Laingian schizoid, he is at one and in harmony with his mental self. He is also not the helpless victim of the division within himself: he can enter his mental world at will and similarly exit it. Nor is he a wretch who experiences the 'despairing aloneness and isolation' ascribed to Laing's schizoid (Laing 1964, 17). He has friends and is romantically involved with a beautiful woman whom he needs and loves. Their relationship derails over her insistence that he get a job, not because he is incapable of sustaining a relationship with another human being.

Murphy's relationship to the outside world is nonetheless largely antagonist. He does not value the outer world, and he is not valued by it. His mere appearance elicits mockery, as for example when he applies for a job at a chandlery: '"'E don't look rightly human to me", says one chandler, "not rightly"' (77). Overall, the much-emphasized fact that Murphy is a divided self whose relationship with the outside world is out of joint, combined with the fact that he ardently wishes to go mad, makes him a good subject for testing Laing's theory about the process of going mad. The main plank in that theory is that adverse circumstances, such as growing up in a soul-crushing home, cause sane schizoids to transition into psychotic schizophrenics. And here, I suggest, it may enhance our appreciation of what fiction can do for the understanding of mental illness by looking at Beckett's novel about a divided self as a kind of laboratory where scientific hypotheses are tested, without danger of harm to living human subjects.

In this imaginary laboratory, the criterion for judging the validity of a hypothesis is the outcome of a narrative event or course of action. Outcomes are the equivalent of research results in that they are capable of confirming or invalidating hypotheses or established practices. For instance, Murphy's violation of the no-mingling doctrine may be construed as a test for the idea of mandating strict segregation of staff and inmates. His disregard for the rules, commendable on purely humane grounds, proves to be theoretically sound as well. His wards cooperate with him and feel better.

Regarding the etiology of schizophrenia, which *The Divided Self* sets out to explain, Laing's thesis that schizophrenics are formerly sane people who become insane in response to external factors finds no support in Beckett's laboratory of fiction. At best, Murphy experiences a brief psychotic episode while in a trance state during which unwilled sounds and images flood his consciousness. However, on the verge of descending into nightmarish depths, he manages to pull himself back to the outside world. That brush with madness convinces him that insanity is not an option for him.

Other examples of ideas tested and evaluated may be less consequential for the plot of *Murphy* but nevertheless demonstrate the usefulness of the laboratory concept. One is the idea propagated in textbooks of the period that psychotics are incapable of distinguishing among different items belonging to the same class:

> According to the text-book psychotic, with his tendency to equate those objects, ideas, persons, etc., evincing the least element in common, the patients should have identified Murphy with Bom & Co, simply because he resembled them in the superficial matters of function and clothing. The great majority failed to do so. (182)

Their failure to lump Murphy together with the other caretakers quashes this textbook notion.

A more important issue raised and settled in Beckett's laboratory is the question of whether insane people can form interpersonal relationships. According to Laing, a definitive feature of the conventional diagnosis of schizophrenia is the inability of insane people to form such relationships: 'The attribution to the other of an incapacity to form a bond was and is *the* basis for the diagnosis of schizophrenia', he writes (Laing 1998, 8; italics in the original). Arguing against Karl Jaspers and Manfred Bleuler, Laing took the opposite view: the 'unbridgeable gulf between some people and the rest of us' could, he maintained, be spanned (Laing 1998, 6). The same term, *gulf*, appears in two *Murphy* contexts: bridging the gulf between *them* and *us* as the function of treatment (177) and Murphy's experience of an abyss separating him from the patients (240). The latter, which occurs prior to his disappointing final encounter with Mr Endon, offers support for the conventional as opposed to the Laingian view about interpersonal relations.

Consider the evidence: after his successful first week, Murphy commences his second week, this time on night duty. Alone with the patients with no staff members around to define himself contrastively against, he occupies the role of a sane individual, categorically different and separate from his insane wards. The gulf is absolute: 'In short there was nothing but he, the unintelligible gulf and they. That was all. All. All' (240). The emphatically repeated 'All', together with Murphy's subsequent failure to reach and be reached by Mr Endon, means that from the standpoint of the novel, the gulf is truly unbridgeable.

This conclusion is of great consequence for Laing's conception of therapy. For what he sought was camaraderie with his patients, whether as a condition for or as an end goal of successful treatment: 'A therapeutic relationship', he writes, 'cannot exist without a primary human camaraderie being present and manifest. If it is not there to start with, therapy will have been successful if it is there before it ends' (Laing 1998, 30). In proto-Laingian fashion, Murphy gives camaraderie a heroic try, but fails to establish a reciprocal relationship with the self-immured, non-communicating Mr Endon. This is emphasized:

> Mr Endon would have been less than Mr Endon if he had known what it was to have a friend; and Murphy more than Murphy if he had not hoped against his better judgment that his feeling for Mr Endon was in some small degree reciprocated. (241)

Camaraderie proves unachievable in Beckett's laboratory of fiction.

I would now like to conclude this study by summing up my main findings. Having sorted out the views of Murphy and the narrator and compared them with Laing's, I ascribe the need for humane and respectful behaviour toward the mentally ill to both men, but not the Laingian idea of mental illness as an escape mechanism adopted by formerly sane persons to gain release from oppressive realities or irresolvable conflicts. Nor is support found for the anti-psychiatry notion that the healers are to blame for the suffering of the mentally ill. Left in peace, they would not be 'as happy as Larry'. It is noteworthy that Beckett offers no alternative explanation of the cause of schizophrenia. That is probably just as well, as its absence is in line with contemporary thinking.

According to the Mayo Clinic website entry on *schizophrenia*, 'It's not known what causes schizophrenia, but researchers believe that a combination of genetics, brain chemistry and environment contributes to the development of the disorder' (Mayo Clinic). By contrast, the once-popular explanations proposed with great assurance by Laing and his contemporaries have little support today. Anticipating Laing, Beckett developed the idea that there is such a thing as a sane schizoid and saw a clear line separating sane and insane types. The distinguishing factor is volition. Mr Endon's involuntary and permanent state of insanity and Murphy's voluntarily induced transient trances are categorically distinct, as demonstrated by the fact that Murphy fails to go mad, though not for want of trying. In addition, Beckett does not idealize or romanticize madness, though he does value inwardness per se, and probably not only for its own sake. There is a well-known connection between madness, the inner world, the unconscious and artistic creativity, but as it is not treated in the novel, I do not raise it here. As for the anti-psychiatry ethos in general, I believe it is clear that Beckett was far ahead of his time and saw beyond what the later generation of radical thinkers, whom he may have influenced, was able to perceive.

References

Abrahamson, David, 'R. D. Laing and Long-Stay Patients: Discrepant Accounts of the Refractory Ward and "Rumpus Room" at Gartnavel Royal Hospital', *History of Psychiatry* 18.2 (2007): 203–15. https://doi.org/10.1177/0957154X06073635

Basaglia, Franco, 'Breaking the Circuit of Control' in D. Ingleby (ed.), *Critical Psychiatry: The Politics of Mental Health* (Harmondsworth: Penguin Books, 1981), 184–92.

Beckett, Samuel, *Murphy* (New York: Grove Press, 1957).

Benjamin, Shoshana, 'Seen and Unseen Narratives in Beckett's Cryptic Novel *Murphy*', *Narrative* 28.1 (2020): 103–24. https://doi.org/10.1353/nar.2020.0000

Cooper, David, *Psychiatry and Anti-Psychiatry* (London: Tavistock, 1967).

Crossley, Nick, 'R.D. Laing and the British Anti-Psychiatry Movement: A Socio-Historical Analysis', *Social Science and Medicine* 47.7 (1998): 877–89. https://doi.org/10.1016/S0277-9536(98)00147-6

Foucault, Michel, *Madness and Civilization* (London: Tavistock, 1971).

Goffman, Erving, *Asylums: Essays on the Social Situation of Mental Patients and Other Inmates* (Harmondsworth: Penguin Books, 1970).

Jones, Josh, 'How James Joyce's Daughter, Lucia, Was Treated for Schizophrenia by Carl Jung', *Open Culture* (2017), http://www.openculture.com/2017/02/how-james-joyces-daughter-lucia-was-treated-for-schizophrenia-by-carl-jung.html, accessed 3 May 2022.

Knowlson, James, *Damned to Fame: The Life of Samuel Beckett* (New York: Simon and Schuster, 1996).

Knowlson, James, *Images* (Cambridge: Cambridge University Press, 2003).

Knowlson, James, and Elizabeth Knowlson (eds), *Beckett Remembering/Remembering Beckett* (London: Bloomsbury Publishing, 2007).

Kotowicz, Zbigniew, *R.D. Laing and the Paths of Anti-Psychiatry* (London: Routledge, 1997).

Laing, R.D., *The Divided Self: An Existential Study in Sanity and Madness* (Harmondsworth: Penguin, 1964).

Laing, R.D., *Wisdom, Madness and Folly* (Edinburgh: Canongate Books, 1998).

Mayo Clinic, *Schizophrenia—Symptoms and Causes*, www.mayoclinic.org/diseases-conditions/schizophrenia/symptoms-causes/syc-20354443, accessed 22 December 2020.

O'Hagan, Sean, 'Kingsley Hall: RD Laing's Experiment in Anti-Psychiatry', *The Guardian*, 2012, www.theguardian.com/books/2012/sep/02/rd-laing-mental-health-sanity, accessed 3 May 2022.

Seymour, Jack L., Margaret Ann Crain, and Joseph V. Crockett, *Educating Christians: The Intersection of Meaning, Learning, and Vocation* (Nashville: Abingdon Press, 1993).

Szasz, Thomas, *The Myth of Mental Illness* (St Albans: Granada, 1972).

3

Apartheid's Garden: Dismantling Madness in J.M. Coetzee's *Life & Times of Michael K*

Sebastian C. Galbo

J.M. Coetzee's novel *Life & Times of Michael K*, published in 1983, is unlikely to number among the major postcolonial works that explore madness within the contexts of political oppression. Perhaps more significant than any other of Coetzee's novels in summoning specters of madness is *In the Heart of the Country* (1977), in which the female protagonist, living on a remote Karoo homestead, is plunged into a nightmarish dreamscape of patricide, rape, and power relations that slowly blurs the reality–fantasy binary (see Collins). This chapter offers a reading of *Life & Times* as an extension of the author's preoccupation with madness in his earlier work. Specifically, I situate the novel within the context of the state-controlled labor, resettlement, and psychiatric camp complex established in South Africa's Apartheid era to imprison the mentally ill, the vagrants, political enemies, and other populations deemed criminal by the government. Within this context, madness operates as an unstable social and political construct perpetuated by Apartheid hegemony, mostly to codify otherness, justify extrajudicial incarceration, and control populations. By extension, I draw on the philosophy of Édouard Glissant who, in *Le discours antillais* (1981), defines madness as a reaction to the 'mental deprivation' perpetuated by racist ideologies (Glissant 212). Delirium, notes Glissant, embodies 'the psychotic violence of the radical choice of madness' (Glissant 292). Coetzee's novel similarly and vividly represents Apartheid's ideological construction of madness to politically designate alterity and control

Sebastian C. Galbo, 'Chapter 3: Apartheid's Garden: Dismantling Madness in J.M. Coetzee's *Life & Times of Michael K*' in: *Madness and Literature: What Fiction Can Do for the Understanding of Mental Illness*. University of Exeter Press (2022). © Sebastian C. Galbo. DOI: 10.47788/TJNQ3925 the colored South African populations. In *Life & Times*, however, because of its tenuous and protean construction, madness is also redefined as a mode of resistance by the very people it labels. Glissant's readings of madness provide a critical lens for (re)reading *Life & Times* in a way that paradoxically articulates madness as both a malleable political construct and an unlikely mode of counter-discourse.

'A Demented World': Madness and Apartheid

Clarification of the term 'madness' should be considered as it is applied to describe Coetzee's characters. Madness, as it is used in this discussion, is not a clinical or diagnostic term intended to define mental illness; rather, it describes broadly a set of performative behaviors, attitudes, and mindsets that challenge the oppressive political conditions that define their realities. The power of diagnostic categorization, to identify, or construct, individuals as mentally unstable, enables an oppressor to relegate those perceived to be political enemies or social undesirables to a controlled space of incarceration.

With this definition in mind, any close readings of Michael that define him as distinctly mad in the sense of mental derangement are, at best, reductive, as they risk oversimplifying the complex social and political factors that shape Michael's psychological character. Although it may be said that he suffers mentally, or suffers from mental ill-health, madness is too strong a diagnosis. Rather, Coetzee frames madness, or mental ill-health, on two interconnected levels. First, Michael can be read as a mentally suffering subject of Apartheid. Second, from a contrasting angle, Michael's 'feeble-mindedness' is also a social and political construct perpetuated by Apartheid discourse. Framing Michael as a character with mental suffering wrought by the political maladies of Apartheid goes hand in hand with Coetzee's incisive essay, 'Apartheid Thinking', in which he describes Apartheid ideology as a kind of 'free-floating, parasitic idea-system running the minds of its hosts' (Coetzee 1996, 35). Coetzee considers how 'madness spreads itself or is made to spread through a social body', viewing the cycles of germ and infection 'as an explanatory model for the communication of passions among masses of people' (Coetzee 1996, 180, 182). As a kind of germ-ridden miasma, Apartheid's sickly ideologies infected South Africa: 'ideas ("ideological" ideas) are not self-aware constructions used as means to ends, but instead float in the air, ready to infect whole societies' (Coetzee 1996, 183). In more colorful terms, André Brink characterizes Apartheid society in terms of widespread, seemingly incurable mental derangement: South Africa is a 'demented world'; a 'swamp of violence and hysteria'; 'an insane structure'; and a 'sickness of the mind' resembling 'psychosis' (Brink 152, 201, 205). Although Michael is not a perpetrator of Apartheid, he is nonetheless affected by the mental deprivation and dehumanization that render him a subhuman citizen of Apartheid rule.

Underlying Brink's epidemiological metaphors is a concern for how ideologies, like harmful contagions, take hold of, sicken, and deprive a society of sane and humane order, which begs the question: who, in fact, is *truly* mad—the oppressed or the oppressor? Tensions between binaries, such as sanity and madness, delusion and lucidity, are emphasized in Glissant's *Le discours antillais*: 'The analysis of what I call mental deprivation shows that its most obvious manifestations are not to be found in the pathological or the delirious, but in the *very texture of daily existence*, through the lack of any references to oneself' (Glissant 212; emphasis mine). Although Glissant refers specifically to postcolonial Martinique, he suggests that psychopathology slips from easy definition in places where the texture of everyday life is dictated by a politically enforced master–slave binary, that madness or mental ill-health is not intrinsic to the individual but to the sickly undulations of Brink's infected world.

To appreciate the applicability of Glissant's thinking, it must first be situated within its originally geographical and historical context, the Caribbean. A key theoretical pillar of Glissant's thinking is the notion of *detour*, a 'tactical and ambiguous' mode of resistance (Britton 25). As this chapter argues, detour is a condition of postcoloniality that transcends the Caribbean context and relates to South Africa. Detour circumvents 'obstacles rather than confronting them head on, and it arises as a response to a situation of disguised rather than overt oppression and struggle' (Britton 25). Detour, however, does not manifest as an act of flagrant subversion or an obstreperous capsizing of the status quo. As Britton notes, Glissant's detour is similar to Michel de Certeau's concept of *la tactique*, which, like the detour, 'is in fact a form of struggle appropriate to a specific situation in which there is not an overt struggle between two factions each of which aims to take power, but rather a (suppressed) opposition on the part of those who are suffering from the established order' (Britton 28). Although hegemony cannot be toppled outright, a detour can destabilize the master–slave relation, rendering it 'an unbalanced situation, never static, always in the process of being redefined' (Britton 28). As an oppositional tactic, the detour arises when 'the enemy cannot be attacked directly, the confusion is such that opposition is not coherent and organized; it is not even entirely conscious. Thus, the detour is itself marked with the alienation it is trying to combat. It is both an evasion of the situation and an obstinate effort to find a way around it' (Britton 26), a paradox that I argue defines Coetzee's approach as well.

It is worthwhile to consider what may be gained from using Glissant's theoretical framework to (re)read madness within the context of Coetzee's novels. After all, what bearing does a conceptional tool from Caribbean philosophy have on South African literary contexts, especially for reading work that responds critically to an entirely different set of political and social hegemonies? To draw on Glissant's work takes a cue from Derek Attridge's assertion that Coetzee's novels offer opportunities for expansive (re)interpretation. His literary work, writes Attridge, invites renewed 'engagement with the text that recognizes, and capitalizes on, its potential for reinterpretation, for grafting into *new contexts*, for *fission and fusion*' (Attridge 10; emphasis mine). To this point, as William Collins notes, 'Coetzee's work does manifest a thoroughgoing critique of not only South African apartheid, but also of the larger genus of political hegemony to which apartheid belongs' (Collins 47). Performing close readings under these unlikely lenses continues the polyphonic interpretations around his novels.

Constructing Madness: Apartheid Ideology and the Camp Complex in *Life & Times*

Driving the plot of *Life & Times* is a lulling kinetic energy, as it reads as a kind of melancholy paean to human mobility, to Michael's movement into and beyond the omniscient glare of state surveillance. Detour, as it works in the novel, is expressed as both a physical and political/linguistic maneuver. First, Michael enacts a peripatetic form of resistance as a fugitive of state control, as his propensities for circumvention (literal detours) carry him beyond the fringes of panoptic surveillance. Second, the political/linguistic dimension of Michael's detour is silence, regarded by his counterparts as a symptom of his apparent slow-wittedness; however, Michael's taciturnity works as a form of resistance, enacting a refusal to cooperate with the state while a workcamp prisoner and, later, as a patient at a medical clinic. For Michael, detour manifests as both spatial delinquency and linguistic resistance through silence.

Michael's physical deformity and inability to speak clearly and intelligently place him in a penumbra of alterity. Michael's status as Other is reinforced by several factors. His harelip, 'curled like a snail's foot', is described as 'disfigured'; his mind is not 'quick' (4), and he is 'committed to' the state-managed Huis Norenius, where he learns basic skills for employment alongside 'other variously afflicted and unfortunate children' (4). Nadine Gordimer writes, '[Michael] appears to be, and perhaps is, retarded—one of those unclassifiable beings that fascinated Dostoevsky, a "simple"' (Gordimer 2). Noting the deeper symbolism of the harelip, Ato Quayson writes: 'Michael K has a harelip but is inarticulate also because he is an underclass colored person in Apartheid South Africa' (Quayson 149).

Michael's silence, however, is also rooted in his father's absence. Although Michael's father is never identified, the specter of paternal control embodies the edicts that govern his childhood. As a student at Huis Norenius, he reveals that his father was 'Huis Norenius' and 'the list of rules on the door of the dormitory, the twenty-one rules of which the first was "There will be *silence* in dormitories at all times"' (104–05; emphasis mine). Of the twenty-one laws, Michael recalls the mandate commanding silence, internalizing this edict as an omnipotent surrogate paternal figure. Such institutions like Huis Norenius, Foucault writes, 'know where and how to locate individuals, to set up useful communication, to interrupt others, to be able at each moment to supervise the conduct of each individual, to assess it, to judge it, to calculate its qualities or merits' (Foucault 1995, 143). From an early age, silence was ingrained inextricably into Michael's perception of self and the world.

Michael's alterity is also shaped by a powerlessness to give an account of himself: 'there remained a gap, a hole, a darkness before which his understanding baulked, into which it was useless to pour words' (110). Further troubling Michael's world is South Africa's unstable political climate. Details of the civil war are vague—people are displaced, a corrupt military patrols, and prison camps are erected—but it is said that the fighting will establish whether 'minorities will have a say in their destinies' (157). Michael's mother, who is sick, resolves to return to her birthplace, Prince Albert, a far-flung cluster of homesteads in the Karoo, where she hopes to convalesce peacefully. She and Michael decide to make the journey together; however, their travel permits never arrive, likely lost in the abyss of state bureaucracy. Gathering his mother and their few possessions in a makeshift wheelbarrow, Michael attempts the arduous journey anyway but they are thwarted by armed government checkpoints. As his mother's condition deteriorates, she is hospitalized and dies, her body cremated before Michael gives hospital officials consent to do so.

Following his mother's death, Michael is vagrant, advancing along the lines of the novel's elliptical cycle of detour that carries him along the currents of departure and circumvention, capture and escape. He ignores the state-imposed curfew, is robbed by police, and loiters insouciantly in public places. Coetzee sketches Michael as a bewildered casualty of what Heidegger terms *Geworfenheit* (or 'thrownness'): the experience of being thrust into a world governed by inexplicably inscrutable and seemingly arbitrary laws (Coetzee 2007, 171; see Collins 49). David Attwell views the human experience of *Geworfenheit* as integral to a figure that is a constant throughout Coetzee's fiction—the 'displaced subject', an individual who is 'not one of the primary agents of colonization but who lives in the conditions created by such agents, and who endures the subjectivity this position entails' (Attwell 56). Undergirding *Geworfenheit* is a kind of frenetic madness itself, in which Michael experiences the exasperating disorder as a subject of Apartheid, with its attendant indignities, social codes, and bureaucracies that appear to be rarefied and immutable. Arriving to Prince Albert, Michael settles on the property of the ramshackle homestead and begins scavenging, hunting birds, nibbling roots, and, in a fit of wild hunger, slaughters a wild goat. He finds a package of pumpkin and melon seeds that he sows, marking 'the beginning of his life as a cultivator' (Coetzee 1985, 59). Immersed in the blanched world of the Karoo, Michael devotedly coaxes his crops to life. But the war encroaches on his hiding place and he absconds to a mountain cave where he hides and nearly starves. Wandering in a stupor of starvation, Michael is arrested by a patrol that incarcerates him in a government medical clinic. Here, Michael resists the institutional forces that attempt to classify, discipline, and incarcerate his body. His emaciated body and refusal to eat hospital food lead the hospital staff to conclude facilely that he has alcohol poisoning. The medical staff regard him suspiciously as an unruly vagrant: 'He had no papers on him, not even a green card. […] and charged with leaving his magisterial district without authorization, not being in possession of an identification, infringing the curfew, and being drunk and disorderly' (70). The state's medical gaze looks with suspicion on Michael as a half-starved vagrant from the veld.

At no other point in the novel does Coetzee depict the inscrutable machinery of *Geworfenheit* in such vivid terms, as Michael, a displaced subject, is funneled along the convoluted zigzags of state bureaucracy. He is eventually placed into a state resettlement/labor camp, Jakkalsdrif, which conjures sinister recollections of his childhood institutionalization at Huis Norenius. He asks the inmates and guards why he has been incarcerated, and is assured that the camp is not a prison but an example of the state's benevolence in reducing poverty, unemployment, and vagrancy. Michael asks questions that cast doubt on mass incarceration and provoke irritated puzzlement among the inmates, one of whom asks, 'But why should people with nowhere to go run away from the nice life we've got here?' (78). For Michael, individual freedom is greater than the safety offered through servitude to the state.

Historically, Jakkalsdrif resembles the labor, resettlement, and psychiatric camp complex that the South African government operated during Apartheid. Perhaps not unaware of the period's barbarous legislation, Coetzee illustrates the randomness of *Geworfenheit* by depicting the grim reverberations of the Involuntary Commitment Act of 1973, a law that allowed the South African government to detain citizens indefinitely in secluded labor camps and medical institutions.[1] As historian Alban Burke notes, this legislation was the 'ideal vehicle with which to remove persons and put them in an unknown place [like Jakkalsdrif] for a legally unspecified period of time without either their families or they themselves knowing where they were' (Burke 91; bracketed note mine). The establishment of labor and psychiatric camps was a government solution designed to separate political dissidents, the unemployed, and vagrants (specifically, those identified as '"idle or undesirable" Black South Africans') from White society (Burke 91). To be clear, 'Many of these people did not commit "crimes" but created a nuisance for the government. Alternative ways had to be found to "remove" these agitators and civil disobedients [*sic*] from society' (Burke 91). Through the Involuntary Commitment Act, government power coalesced around and criminalized alleged mental ill-health, vagrancy, and idleness. Discourses of madness, codified through this vein of legislation, moved to the foreground of everyday life and, collectively, played a salient role in defining and codifying the politically constructed sick and criminal colored South African body. The great sweep of this law, in all of its superbly arbitrary logic, functioned to target and incarcerate the colored body in a camp complex similar to that which Coetzee depicts.

Detained individuals were 'admitted to mental institutions[2] for various reasons—because they "broke curfew," if they were physically ill (going to general hospitals to seek medical treatment and subsequently being committed to psychiatric hospitals), or if they were considered dissidents' (Burke 91). Apartheid brands of psychiatry and rehabilitative disciplines were not diagnostic or therapeutic, but political, tools. Such legislation, viewed through the prism of the fictional Jakkalsdrif, reflects the kind of governmental practices that Foucault describes in his writings, specifically the creation of laws that advance a state's capacity to control human populations (Foucault 1995, 148). Historian Tiffany Fawn Jones summarizes, 'States can classify and confine patients indefinitely with the semblance of concern about social and individual well-being, even if its goal may be to control its labor force, manage the actions of certain of its citizens, or even its ideal of a modern, sanitary living space free from vagrants' (Jones 5). Under this new law, madness could be diagnosed arbitrarily, depending on whether the detained individual was deemed to be a vagrant or political enemy. Jones writes: 'Apartheid was a makeshift, complex entity that although it was about segregation, was more concerned about shielding white (Afrikaner) men from foreign (be it local or international) encroachment—we particularly see this when it came to policies regarding madness' (Jones 11). The Involuntary Commitment Act achieved two key results: first, it enabled the state to isolate unwanted populations, in extrajudicial spaces, from White society; and two, it empowered government authorities to politically construct and codify madness as a diagnosis that authorized indefinite institutionalization.

Jones clarifies, however, that these institutions and penal camps, as might be reasonably assumed, were not highly organized satellites of state control. Due to the immense bureaucracy of Apartheid government, and its attendant staff shortages and operational inefficiencies, 'state processes were obscure and inept' (Jones 178). She notes, 'Although the government did attempt, in vain, to deal with its disordered black population through repatriation strategies, the use of the judicial and prison system, and eventually by detaining them in contracted facilities, even in these areas, policies were confusing and obscure' (Jones 178). Such institutional variability gives the *Geworfenheit* that undergirds the Apartheid world an intense eraticism.

At Jakkalsdrif, inmates are transported from the camp to a farm where they perform backbreaking labor in an alfalfa pasture. The clinical ideology driving camp labor was the concept of so-called industrial therapy, a rehabilitative process believed by Apartheid authorities to help imprisoned individuals to better manage mental illness and/or proclivities for vagrancy through the numbing routines of simple, everyday toil (not unlike the curricula of Huis Norenius). According to Burke, colored South Africans were 'hired out to companies to perform labor without pay', fabricating cheap commodities, such as coat hangers, wire brushes, rubber leg guards for miners, mats, sheets, cloths, and aprons (Burke 92). One of Michael's fellow inmates describes, with historical accuracy, how the Apartheid camp system is enmeshed in the South Africa economy: 'from a gang in Jakkalsdrif a farmer gets a day's work blood cheap, and at the end of the day the truck fetches them and they are gone and he doesn't have to worry about them or their families, they can starve, they can be cold, he knows nothing, it's none of his business' (Coetzee 1985, 82). Of course, industrial therapy was a hollow euphemism for exploitive labor provided by those imprisoned in the Apartheid camp complex.

This government program had vast public health implications: 'The forced removals and "dumping" of millions of Black South Africans into small, disconnected, barren, poor reserve areas, bereft of adequate medical, psychiatric and public health services caused, amongst various other [sic], high mental-illness rates' (Dommisse, quoted in Burke 5). So-called patients, like Michael, 'were involuntarily detained in the facilities. Discharges from the hospitals were few, each one authorized only by the State psychiatrist' (Burke 92). Systemic erasure was key to ensuring that the horrific realities of the camps were kept strictly clandestine: 'No public record existed on how monies were spent on the camps and the secrecy surrounding the institutions was almost impenetrable' (Burke 92). In 1970, the Citizens Commission on Human Rights investigated and exposed[3] the cruelties of these so-called psychiatric camps, compiling and submitting a report on the findings to the World Health Organization and the Red Cross; however, the South African government swiftly amended the Mental Health Act so that it was a criminal offense to document, report, photograph, or sketch psychiatric hospitals, camps, or inmates (Burke 92). Institutional censorship swept government activities into secrecy.

For the others, however, Jakkalsdrif is comfortably insulated from the outside world of hunger and discord, and Michael's questions are perceived as subversive threats, especially by camp guards: 'You climb the fence and I'll shoot you' (Coetzee 1985, 85). Michael's seemingly naïve questions provoke disquiet among the other inmates, one of whom asks: 'First time, Jakkalsdrif. Second time, Brandvlei. You want to go to Brandvlei, penal servitude, hard labor, brickfields, guards with whips?' (78). Another guard tells Michael that it is for his own good that he is in the camp: 'If I let you out now, in three days you'll be back pleading to be let in' (85). Michael is viewed as mad insofar as he poses questions of escape and freedom that challenge the inmates' passivity: 'Why have I been sent here? How long do I have to stay? [...] Why do people stay here?' (75 and 78). But these are not the mutterings of a restive vagrant eager to overthrow South Africa's penal order—Michael views the workcamp as another incomprehensible obstacle of *Geworfenheit*, an extension of Huis Norenius disguised as a benevolent institution, veiled as a disciplinary tool used to control a maligned population.

Michael recalls a Jakkalsdrif police captain who called the camp inmates parasites: 'the camp at Jakkalsdrif, a nest of parasite hanging from the neat sunlit town, eating its substance, giving no nourishment back' (116). He reflects, 'it was no longer obvious which was host and which parasite, camp or town. If the worm devoured the sheep, why did the sheep swallow the worm' (116). For a gardener who is thought to be incapable of lucid expression, Michael provides an appreciably eloquent metaphor—a mutually destructive symbiosis between government and citizenry, wherein the sated state fails to nourish an emaciated body politic. Michael becomes a stark corporeal allegory for the South African body politic—gaunt and sickly, 'nothing but bone and muscle', his body swept from society into the camp complex (101). These are the distinct echoes of Coetzee's aforementioned essay, 'Apartheid Thinking', and Brink's epidemiological metaphors. Although Michael may not be able to clearly articulate the question, his line of reasoning poses the question: what is truly mad—to resign oneself unthinkingly to a society crumbling to civil war and dehumanizing ideologies; or to flee a 'demented world' governed by racist ideology?

Michael's questions carry out *la tactique*, puncturing the collective silence of the inmates who have acquiesced to state control; but his aberrant questions are understood by the other inmates to be at drastic odds with the political realities of South Africa. An inmate remarks sententiously, 'You're a baby [...]. You've been asleep your whole life. It's time to wake up. Why do you think they give you charity, you and the children? Because they think you are harmless, your eyes aren't opened, you don't see the truth around you?' (89). Michael, if not perceived by the other inmates as mad, is infantilized as a disempowered manchild oblivious to political exigencies (which oddly anticipates Gordimer's own objections to Michael's alleged passivity, described below). Enacting another literal detour, Michael flees the camp, walking in 'great loops' and 'trembling sometimes with the thrill of being free' (97). Michael, in the act of escape, views himself in increasingly diminutive forms, something too insignificant to be noticed and conquered by the Other, 'as a speck upon the surface of an earth too deeply asleep to notice the scratch of ant-feet, the rasp of butterfly teeth, the tumbling of dust' (97). Back at the homestead, detour is expressed poignantly in Michael's earthen burrow. Foraging for food at night and sleeping during the day, Michael becomes subterranean and nocturnal, increasingly intoxicated by the sweet odors of groundwater, the leaves of veld bushes, the flinty gusts of summer petrichor: 'He was learning to love idleness [...] as a yielding up of himself to time' (115). Cultivating his vines, Michael keeps alight the wan flame of cultivation—in a moment of tearful exaltation, sinking his teeth into grilled pumpkin, Michael intones an imperative: 'All that remains is to be a tender of the soil' (113). Gordimer challenges this simple dictum, criticizing Michael's turn from South Africa's political exigencies to focus, passively, on gardening: 'It's better to live on your knees, planting something?' (Gordimer 6). In contrast, rejoins Sally-Ann Murray, 'is Gordimer not wrong to imagine that Coetzee was naively constraining the field of social action by depicting K as a gardener?' (Murray 46). Especially within the context of the Apartheid camp system, the action of gardening, of cultivation, *is* a revolutionary gesture because its aim is to locate human subsistence, and ultimately survival, outside of the sphere of power, wherein incarcerated subjects rely solely on the state for nourishment and where they must tend crops that are not their own, but belong to those who profit from state-enforced labor.

Michael, as one of Coetzee's displaced subjects, distances himself from the political conditions that constitute the very human experience of *Geworfenheit*. Summarizing Glissant, Britton writes that '*deviance is also a detour*—an alienated way to find a way around alienation' (Britton 91; emphasis mine). What Michael seeks is to live in quiet reciprocity with the earth, exercising simple cultivation—a skill conspicuously anachronistic during war. At this juncture of the novel, it is perhaps helpful to understand detour not only as a literally physical peripatetic maneuver to evade state authority, but as, in the words of Martin Munro, a kind of 'sensibility' (Munro 118). According to Munro, detour 'marks a *temporary reawakening* of a sensibility that has apparently been assimilated into the discourse of domination' (Munro 118; emphasis mine). The sensibility, which has not been assimilated, is Michael's vigilance to the abiding fragility of human survival, the ability to respond sufficiently to the human needs that existentially precede the elaborate but unsteady scaffolding (what Foucault terms 'a grid of practices'; Foucault 2008, 3) of *Geworfenheit*. It is an awareness that once society reconfigures this scaffolding, attention is due to what will sustain the course of its new direction—turning to essential vocations, like agriculture, that bind humans together in interdependent communities. Aware of this sensibility, Michael admits that 'there must be men to stay behind [from war] and keep gardening alive, or at least the idea of gardening; because once that chord was broken, the earth would grow hard and forget her children' (Coetzee 1985, 109). For Michael, if all were swept into the vacuum of war, if no one lingered behind the front lines to tend the soil, who, in the end, could lead others to start anew? to rebuild? to return closest to our very origins, earth?

'A different kind of food': Detour, Hunger, and Starvation

Severely malnourished on his pumpkin diet, Michael is arrested again by a military patrol and committed to an infirmary at a 'rehabilitation camp'. In the second part of the novel, Coetzee shifts the narration to a first-person account from the perspective of a camp medical officer responsible for Michael's convalescence. The medical officer, with the skeptical irreverence of a conscientious objector, views the camp's routines with a mordant cynicism: 'Do any of us believe in what we're doing here? I doubt it. […] We ply them [prisoners] with items from the brass band repertoire and show them films of young men in neat uniforms demonstrating to grizzled village elders how to eradicate mosquitoes and plough along the contour' (134). This first-person narrator's account reads as a kind of wartime journal, wherein the jaded medical officer airs his political sarcasms and clinical reflections. Though sympathetic to his patient, the officer assumes a clinical condescension afforded by the authority of the medial gaze, noting that '[Michael] is a person of feeble mind […]. He ought to be in a protected environment weaving baskets or stringing beads, not in a rehabilitation camp' and that he resembles 'someone out of Dachau' (131, 146). Unlike his colleagues, he doubts the rehabilitative aims of industrial therapy, quipping that Michael's recovery is important 'so he can rejoin camp life and have a chance to […] shout slogans and salute the flag' (133). The officer has a vague premonition that Michael will elude rehabilitation, that something ineffable accounts for his emaciated body.

The centrality of food and nourishment to individual social/political intelligibility, as well as claims to sanity, is especially pronounced in this section of the novel. Michael jests about his malnourished, skeletal body: 'I could become a jockey too, at my weight' (130). Enacted by a 'feebleminded' vagrant incarcerated in another camp, Michael's self-starvation is not a grandstand objection to Apartheid indignities. Instead, denying the camp's food is an intuitive refusal of the state—bodily nourishment will not be derived from consuming morsels doled out by the camp complex. After Michael collapses during mandatory camp exercises, he refuses a feed bottle: 'It's not my kind of food' (145). Warned that he will die of starvation, Michael gives a 'repulsive, sharklike' smile (147). Is it the harelip that twists grotesquely to form a smile or Michael's mocking grin in the face of willed atrophy that repulses the officer? The longer Michael refuses food, the more the officer views him as a kind of prehistoric specimen, a patient who defies definitive medical diagnosis. The officer catalogues a series of objectifying comparisons that represent Michael as eluding recognizable clinical taxonomies: 'a human soul above and beneath classification' (151); 'creature left over from an earlier age' (151); 'coelacanth' (151); 'last man to speak Yaqui' (151); 'stick insect' (149); 'obscurest of the obscure' (142); 'original soul' (151); 'figure of fun' (149); 'clown' (149); 'wooden man' (149); and 'wraith' (154). Readers are inclined to sympathize with the medical officer's disdain for the camp but, through the medical gaze, he remains complicit in perpetuating Apartheid ideology by constructing Michael as an unknowable, 'feebleminded' Other in need of institutionalization.

Aside from rejecting hospital food, Michael resists cooperating with interrogators who suspect him of abetting rebel forces by leveraging silence and his perceived idiocy (140). Suspecting Michael of growing vegetables for insurgents, the interrogators demand an account of his action, to which he says, 'I am not in the war' (138). Michael has no regard for political exigencies: 'He will not speak and commit himself over to an authoritative narrative, just as he will not engage in political struggle and give himself over to abstract principles' (Chesney 312). Asked about who the vegetables were for, he responds with gnomic utterances: 'What grows is for all of us. We are all the children of the earth' (Coetzee 1985, 139). The medical officer notes that in Michael's elusive exchanges with the interrogators, he smiles 'craftily' (141). It is especially interesting that the medical officer notes the scarce occasions when Michael smiles, and they are noted when Michael refuses hospital food and tells interrogators that he cannot provide an account of himself ('I am not clever with words'; 139)—these few occasions he does grin are when he is decidedly uncooperative with the state, when the lacunae of his own story become a source of frustration for authorities.

Camp officials dismiss Michael's responses as the ravings of a half-starved 'simpleton': 'He should have been shut away in an institution with high walls, stuffing cushions or watering the flower-beds' (141). That Michael defies medical comprehension and refuses to cooperate with interrogators gives rise to the officer's increasing frustrations to understand his patient. His frustration gives way to angry shouting, 'What the hell *is* your kind of food?' (145). The officer's obsession drives him (unsuccessfully) to arrange a fraudulent discharge; he promises Michael that he will not force a feeding tube; and he procures a butternut squash from a market outside of the camp (which Michael also refuses). Coetzee does not demonize the medical officer, but depicts him as a conflicted bureaucrat who doubts the efficacy of the camp system (not unlike the Magistrate of Coetzee's novel *Waiting for the Barbarians*, 1980). As Jones notes, 'Certainly, South African mental institutions were spaces where human rights abuse occurred and where the state detained some of its opponents. [...] But mental health practitioners as a group did not give blanket support to the racialized ideas of apartheid' (Jones 21). Indeed, 'It is suspect to suggest that all practitioners were instruments of the state' (Jones 178). This frustration culminates in a letter, wherein the officer wrestles introspectively with his clinical relationship with Michael—what the officer grasps for, like the interrogators, is a perfectly scrutable account of Michael's life ('I want to know your story'; 149). For the medical officer, the lacuna of Michael's story is his vexed relationship with food: 'Another thing I would like to know is what the food was that you ate in the wilderness that has made all other food tasteless to you. [...] Was it manna?' (151). Michael's pumpkins are not eucharistic morsels promising salvation; they are the forms of sustenance that he has labored to harvest of his own toil, not the food prepared and offered up by the Other.

How might Michael's self-starvation be appreciated, then, if not understood as a political protest? Abstaining from camp food gives Michael agency over his incarcerated and politically constructed body. As a mode of resistance, writes Sarah Ilott, starvation can enact a powerful 'refusal of the Other or the outsider' (Ilott 5). This notion of barring the Other in a refusal to eat parallels a key observation made by Maud Ellmann as she articulates starvation not as a symptom of madness but as 'the only means of saving subjectivity from the invasion of the other in the form of food'; however, she notes, the grim fallout of starvation is that, through deprivation, the self is ultimately destroyed 'in the very process of confirming its identity' (Ellmann 30). Food, offered by the state, is viewed as a kind of contagion-ridden material from which Michael refuses to derive nourishment. Only by planting, harvesting, and ingesting his own food is he free from being inhabited by the Other—in starvation, the Other is always on the outside, circling, probing, unable to enter the self's body. Refusing to incorporate the Other's food, Michael is not, in turn, consumed by the Other or the camp complex; his body remains obdurate and fibrous, not receptive to the Other's nutrition. To be nourished by the state is to be enslaved to the state, to pass through its bowels ('the intestines of war'; 135). With clinical certainty, the officer writes: 'I asked myself: why will this man not eat when he is plainly starving? […] I slowly began to understand the truth: that you were crying secretly […] for a different kind of food, food that no camp could supply' (163–64). Michael seeks nourishment not from the state and its camps, but from the veld, that windswept *tabula rasa* that remains uncontaminated by the contagions of a sick, maddened state. Detour, as expressed through the deviance of self-starvation, enables Michael to maintain agency and control of his subjectivity.

Conclusion

Viewed through the lens of Glissant's theory, specifically the notion of detour, Coetzee's novel frames madness not as a clinical condition, but as a social construction, as well as a symptom of mental deprivation perpetuated by racist and politically oppressive ideologies. Glissant's theoretical tools invite readers to scrutinize the nonsensical and the aberrant, suggesting that madness does not mark an impasse to interpretation, but calls readers to be attuned to its instabilities, possibilities, and dissonances. Coetzee's *Life & Times* represents the lived experiences of one colored South African man against the historical backdrop of the Apartheid camp complex system. Situated within this historical context, Coetzee's novel examines the far-reaching implications of how discourses of madness were constructed to diagnose, incarcerate, and institutionalize subjects of Apartheid government, particularly targeting those deemed as vagrants and dissidents.

Notes

1. Some of these 'psychiatric camps' and 'mental hospitals' were established at abandoned mining sites (Burke 92).
2. Remarkably, historical statistics reveal that by 1976, 'admissions to these "private" psychiatric hospitals had increased by 400 percent over a 10-year period' (Burke 91).
3. The Church of Scientology's publication, the *Peace and Freedom* magazine, claimed that the camps were labor institutions concerned with only economic productivity (Jones 1). Another criticism appeared in a 1975 column printed in a Johannesburg periodical, the *Sunday Times*. Entitled 'Millions Out of Madness', the article stated that the camps were redolent of 'Dickensian workhouses' (quoted in Jones 1).

References

Attridge, Derek, *J.M. Coetzee and the Ethics of Reading: Literature in the Event* (Chicago: University of Chicago Press, 2004). https://doi.org/10.7208/chicago/9780226818771.001.0001

Attwell, David, *J.M. Coetzee: South Africa and the Politics of Writing* (Berkeley: University of California Press, 1993).

Brink, André, *Map Makers: Writing in a State of Siege* (London: Faber & Faber, 1983).

Britton, Celia M., *Edouard Glissant and Postcolonial Theory: Strategies of Language and Resistance*, New Word Studies Series (Charlottesville: University of Virginia Press, 1999).

Burke, Alban, 'Mental Health Care During Apartheid in South Africa: An Illustration of How "Science" Can Be Abused' in J.T. Parry (ed.), *Evil, Law and the State: Perspectives on State Power and Violence*, At the Interface / Probing the Boundaries [Book 24] (New York: Editions Rodopi BV, 2006).

Burke, Alban, 'Mental Health Care During Apartheid in South Africa: An Illustration of How "Science" Can Be Abused', http://citeseerx.ist.psu.edu/viewdoc/download?doi=10.1.1.522.5771&rep=rep1&type=pdf, accessed May 2019.

Chesney, Duncan McColl, 'Toward an Ethics of Silence: Michael K', *Criticism* 49.3 (2007): 307–25. https://doi.org/10.1353/crt.0.0036

Coetzee, J.M., *In the Heart of the Country* (New York: Penguin Books, 1977).
Coetzee, J.M., *Waiting for the Barbarians* (London: Vintage, 2004 [1980]).
Coetzee, J.M., *Life & Times of Michael K* (New York: Penguin Books, 1985).
Coetzee, J.M., *Doubling the Point*, ed. by D. Attwell (Cambridge: Harvard University Press, 1992).
Coetzee, J.M., *Giving Offense: Essays on Censorship* (Chicago: University of Chicago Press, 1996).
Collins, William, 'Restoring Madness to History in J.M. Coetzee's *In the Heart of the Country*', *MediaTropes* 4.2 (2014): 46–67.
Ellmann, Maud, *The Hunger Artists: Starving, Writing and Imprisonment* (Boston: Harvard University Press, 1993).
Foucault, Michel, *Discipline and Punish: The Birth of the Prison*, trans. by A. Sheridan (New York: Vintage Books, 1995 [1977]).
Glissant, Édouard, *Le discours antillais*, trans. by J.M. Dash as *Caribbean Discourse: Selected Essays* (Charlottesville: University of Virginia Press, 1989; original: Paris: Éditions du Seuil, 1981).
Gordimer, Nadine, 'The Idea of Gardening: *The Life and Times of Michael K*', *New York Review of Books* 3.6 (2 February 1984): 1–6.
Ilott, Sarah, *New Postcolonial British Genres: Shifting the Boundaries* (New York: Palgrave Macmillan, 2015). https://doi.org/10.1057/9781137505224
Jones, Tiffany Fawn, *Psychiatry, Mental Institutions, and the Mad in Apartheid South Africa* (New York: Routledge, 2012). https://doi.org/10.4324/9780203129555
Munro, Martin, *Exile and Post-1946 Haitian Literature: Alexis, Depestre, Ollivier* (Liverpool: Liverpool University Press, 2007). https://doi.org/10.2307/j.ctt5vjng1
Murray, Sally-Ann, 'The Idea of Gardening: Plants, Bewilderment, and Indigenous Identity in South Africa', *English in Africa* 33.2 (2006): 45–65.
Quayson, Ato, *Aesthetic Nervousness: Disability and the Crisis of Representation* (New York: Columbia University Press, 2007).

4 Sniffs and Dribblers: *Poppy Shakespeare* and the Identities of Madness

Clare Allan

'Since Prisons and Madhouses exist, why somebody is bound to sit in them'—so wrote Anton Chekhov in his short story, 'Ward No. 6' (Chekhov 421), and it is this quotation which forms the epigraph of my own novel, *Poppy Shakespeare*, written after ten years spent sitting in a variety of North London madhouses, and also in some sense my passport to a new identity outside them.

The role of identity in our experience of mental distress and in our perception and treatment of those with mental health problems forms a central concern of *Poppy Shakespeare*, and in this chapter I will discuss the ways in which narratives of identity inform and shape the world of the novel and the experiences of its characters. I will consider what purpose such narratives serve, and to what extent fictional approaches to understanding mental distress might contribute to current conversations about the validity of psychiatric diagnosis and the categorizing of mental health problems as distinct psychiatric conditions. Further, I will argue that in enabling the reader temporarily to inhabit the 'mad' identity, literature, and in particular the novel, can serve as an important instrument in helping to dismantle the artificial barrier between madness and sanity, and to rehabilitate what Goffman calls the 'spoiled identity'.

The Function of Madness

The identity of Madness, and of the Mad person, as alien, other, by turns hilarious, embarrassing, and terrifying, is established very early. Certainly, I remember quips about Madness and the threat of becoming Mad, or of being revealed as a Mad person, often formed the basis of taunts and teasing in the primary school playground. 'The second sign of madness is hairs on the palm of your hand!' 'What's the first sign?' 'Looking for them!' Shrieks of laughter as the hapless target hastily lowered their hand. 'The little white van is going to take you away…'

This was in the Seventies, before all the anti-stigma campaigns—Time to Change,[1] Heads Together,[2] and Mental Health Awareness Weeks,[3] and heaven knows what else. But I'd be surprised if children don't continue to joke in this way.

For the concept of 'Madness' serves an important function. A function so important that, to misquote Voltaire, if Madness did not exist, we would have to invent it. Because if Madness did not exist, then Sanity could not exist either. And it is this, I would contend, that makes people so uneasy.

We sometimes refer to the intangible nature of mental illness—the fact that Madness cannot be diagnosed, for example, by means of a blood test. An MRI cannot be used to confirm a diagnosis of schizoaffective disorder. But this, it seems to me, is not the issue. The much greater concern is that there is no blood test to prove that you are *not* Mad. Every so often, the discovery of a potential genetic link to a particular diagnosed disorder causes great excitement: 'Scientists open the "black box" of schizophrenia with dramatic genetic discovery' trumpeted the *Washington Post* in January 2016 (Nutt). By contrast, the well-established correlation between levels of social and financial inequality and levels of mental ill health[4] receives scarcely any coverage at all. This latter, which, unlike our genetic make-up, we could as a society actually do something about, offers none of the reassurance of a hypothetical definitive test: order your self-testing kit online, send off your mouth swab and six weeks later, we'll text you your results. Pee on a stick—one line and you're normal, two lines and we're sending the little white van … Such tests, of course, do not exist and never can exist. Because mental illness, or mental distress, or mental health problems—or whatever imprecise term we grope for to try and pin down this amorphous collection of human thoughts, feelings, behaviours, and experiences—is inevitably the consequence of a multitude of intersecting, interconnecting factors: social, biological, experiential, and so on.

Moreover, Madness is a cultural construct quite as much as a medical one. What are categorized as abnormal or undesirable beliefs, feelings, or behaviours are determined by cultural and political assumptions and expectations. In *The Female Malady: Women, Madness and English Culture 1830–1980*, Elaine Showalter persuasively argues not only that much of what was diagnosed as mental illness in women was a consequence of women's struggle to reconcile a desire for freedom and autonomy with their culturally conditioned beliefs as to appropriate female behaviour, but also that when women deviated from the gendered norms they were labelled aberrant by a male psychiatric system which served to uphold, and indeed enforce, those same culturally conditioned beliefs. Even today, certain diagnoses carry a marked gender bias. Borderline Personality Disorder, for example, is diagnosed three times as often in females as it is in males. The history of the relationship between psychiatry and politics is chequered to say the least. The use of psychiatric detention for political ends in the Nazi era, the USSR, and China is well known. Instances in the USA are less so. In *The Protest Psychosis: How Schizophrenia Became a Black Disease*, psychiatrist Jonathan Metzl describes how African Americans were diagnosed with schizophrenia at the Ionia State Hospital in Michigan in response to their civil rights ideas.

Perhaps then it is hardly surprising that no one has yet designed a scanner (or indeed a human being) capable of computing the many subjective variables to come up with a reliable, definitive, objective calculation as to whether an individual is Mad or not. Hardly surprising, but unfortunate certainly. For if there is one thing almost everyone appears to agree on (I will return to that 'almost') it is that to be considered Mad is undesirable. Because to be judged Mad is to be judged 'other', to be judged, in some fundamental sense, not quite a human being; to be in possession, in short, of a 'spoiled identity', to borrow Erving Goffman's phrase. And so we find ourselves in a precarious position, deeply concerned lest anybody might suspect us of Madness, yet without any conclusive means of asserting our Sanity. And in the absence of determining features to distinguish the Mad from the Sane, it is imperative that we assign some, and quickly, before anyone suspects what we all deep down know in some sense to be true: that in that hidden, interior, private world, we are all of us more or less barking.

Such ideas about stigma and the nature and purpose of stigma are hardly new. My thoughts have been shaped and influenced by any number of writers, but perhaps above all by James Baldwin, who went to Paris to in some sense escape the black identity America imposed on him, or at least to gain enough distance to be able to examine it, and in doing so discovered that this identity was not as distinct as he had up to that point imagined. In his late essay, 'Freaks and the American Ideal of Manhood', Baldwin says:

> Freaks are called freaks and are treated as they are treated—in the main, abominably—because they are human beings who cause to echo, deep within us, our most profound terrors and desires [...] But we are all androgynous, not only because we are all born of a woman impregnated by the seed of a man but because each of us, helplessly and forever, contains the other—male in female, female in male, white in black and black in white. We are a part of each other. Many of my countrymen appear to find this fact exceedingly inconvenient and even unfair, and so, very often, do I. But none of us can do anything about it. (Baldwin 828–29)

There are similarities in the experience of any stigmatized group, but there are clearly differences too. Blackness is visible. Madness is not. And moreover, blackness is an identity that somebody is born with, born in, quite literally the colour of one's skin. To become mad, or perhaps to recognise one's madness, involves a change of identity, a crossing of the border from the world of the Sane into the world of the Mad.

Normalizing Madness: Writing into 'the Other'

In *Poppy Shakespeare*, it is the eponymous heroine who crosses the Madness border, where she is greeted by the narrator, N, a day patient who, like a vernacular Virgil, guides her ever deeper into the spiralling world of the Abaddon psychiatric hospital, an infinitely tall tower, in which each floor houses patients madder than the one below it—a tower so tall, it is rumoured that from the upper floors, you can see right round the world and back in through the windows behind you. Poppy is outraged at the new identity: 'It's not that I've got a problem with mental illness, it's just there's nothing the matter with me. Do you know what I'm saying!' (Allan 60), convinced that she must have been assigned it by mistake, and determined to rid herself of it as quickly as possible. Meanwhile N, who has been in the system since 'before [she] was even born' (Allan 3), is in turn unable to comprehend that anyone would wish to discard the single badge of identity she herself uses to validate her existence and place in the world.

Which brings me back to that 'almost'. Almost everyone appears to agree that to be considered Mad is undesirable. Everyone, that is, apart from those who have nothing else. Everyone, apart from those for whom Madness provides a sense of being part of a community, of having a place in the world: in short, of belonging. And a community of 'outcasts' is particularly strong. Yes, you might infuriate each other, but there is an implicit understanding, an understanding that cannot be shared by anyone outside the community. You are in it together. The world has 'othered' you, and you, in turn, now 'other' the world. That's a very strong bond.

In the novel, the first floor of the Abaddon houses the Dorothy Fish psychiatric day hospital, whose patients live in the community, which is to say in council flats on the nearby Darkwoods Estate. I remember showing a draft of an early chapter to a friend, who commented that he thought it would make better sense if the patients stayed at the hospital all the time. He thought the situation would be clearer for the reader if the doors were locked and the patients were therefore physically prevented from leaving. This was useful feedback as it crystallized for me the challenge that I faced. How to convince the reader not only that the day patients willingly attend each day, but that they are desperate to do so? That despite the apparent emptiness of day after day, and month after month, and year after year spent sitting in the Abaddon common room on two rows of vinyl-covered chairs with the stuffing poking through the rips in the seats, and a dead plant in the corner, there is literally nothing they would rather do than climb the hill to the Abaddon each morning? This is hard for an outsider to understand. Indeed, Poppy herself, initially at least, shares my friend's confusion:

> 'It's just generally speaking,' Rosetta said, 'day patients aren't compulsory, we're here on a voluntary basis.'
> 'You mean you *choose* to come!' said Poppy—thought *I* was slow on the uptake.
> 'We come 'cause we need to,' Rosetta said.
> 'They say I've got to stay a month,' said Poppy. 'So they can work out what's wrong. I told them there *wasn't* anything wrong! I can't stay a month, do you know what I'm saying!'
> 'Why can't she stay a month?' asked Sue, but Verna just shook her head.
> (Allan 79)

It is not locked doors or walls or fences that keep the patients of the Dorothy Fish from leaving, it is something much more powerful. What keeps them there is a sense of belonging to a community, coupled with a conviction that they cannot exist outside it. For the patients of the Dorothy Fish, the prospect of discharge is the worst thing they can imagine. The Dorothy Fish is their identity and to be discharged is to be cast out, to lose that identity as surely as an angel cast down into hell. To be discharged is in a very real sense to cease to exist.

As a writer, what I was attempting to do was to take the reader into that community, not as a spectator but as a participant, to have them experience it for themselves. I remember reading Martin Amis's reverse-told novel, *Time's Arrow*, on a train, and the jolt when I stepped down onto the platform and discovered that the world was in fact moving forwards. I wanted the reader to inhabit the Mad identity so completely that the world outside the hospital seemed other. I wanted them to know what that was like, not because they'd read a psychology textbook, or indeed a paper in a journal, but because they had been there themselves. (Some readers already had, of course, and for them I wanted the novel to be both a celebration of our world and a critique of it.)

But how to accomplish this? How to sneak the reader across the border, a border closely guarded on both sides by assumptions, preconceptions, stereotypes, and above all by barbed-wire certainty that those on the other side must be 'other'? For me, the answer was found through voice, and specifically through the voice of the narrator, N. It was through N's voice that I attempted to show both her individuality (she is not just a Mad person, she is N) and her very ordinary humanness, her self-deception, bluster, bravado, courage, and vulnerability. It was also through N's voice that I tried to convey the absolute normality of the Mad world from her perspective. Because voice is not just about who is speaking; it is also, crucially, about who is being spoken *to*—whether this be literally or in the speaker's imagination. The assumptions a narrator makes about the knowledge, experience, and interests of the person to whom they are telling a story are one of the most powerful ways in which they reveal themselves to the reader. N has been in the system, as she tells us more than once, since 'before [she] was even born'. She comes from a long line of 'dribblers', spent her childhood in and out of care, as her mother was repeatedly hospitalized, finally ending her life when N was twelve. Shortly after this, she found herself in 'this unit for fucked-up kids':

> After that it was like I never looked back. By thirteen I been diagnosed with everything in the book. They had to start making up new disorders, just to

have me covered, then three days before I turned seventeen, they shipped me
up to the Abaddon to start my first six-month section. (Allan 4)

A narrator such as N who, until she meets Poppy, has never known anyone from outside the system ('sniffs' in the Abaddon vernacular) will naturally assume that she is telling her story to somebody from her world. She will no more feel the need to explain this world, to translate it for 'outsiders', than I would feel the need to explain that in the sentence, 'I drove through a red light', the red light was telling me to stop, just in case a reader from Mars should happen to stumble across it. For me, the writer behind the curtain, this situation naturally presented challenges. I needed the reader to understand the mechanics of this fictional world, but to understand them from the inside, as a long-term patient would, rather than as a visitor clutching a guidebook. One solution was, of course, the introduction of Poppy, and tasking N with showing her around, which both allowed Poppy to ask questions on behalf of the reader, as it were, and N to express her surprise that Poppy didn't already know. Too much of this could easily feel clunky though, and as much as possible I left the reader to put the pieces together. In my experience, readers tend to understand far more implicitly than many writers think they do. One of the most frequent comments I make in the margins of my students' work is LRWO: 'Let the reader work it out'. Explaining is distancing.

Another factor influencing N's narration is that the story is not told in present tense, but rather from a more experienced perspective. N is looking back at events from a point where she has begun to encounter the world beyond the hospital, and I tried to capture a sense of her attempting to acknowledge the possible Sniffs among her readership, while still secure in her conviction as to their 'otherness':

> At the time all this happened I was going to the Dorothy Fish, which in case you don't know is a day hospital, and in case you don't know what one of *them* is, it's this place where you go there every day and when it shuts at half-four you go back down the hill to your flat on the Darkwoods Estate. (Allan 5)

Finally, I think it is important to acknowledge that not everything needs to be clear. The reader does not need to understand every aspect of the fictional world, any more than I understand every aspect of the 'real' one. Too often 'truth' is sacrificed for 'clarity', it seems to me (diagnosis being a case in point), but the truth is invariably muddy and to filter it into a crystal clear, readily drinkable version performs a disservice. For me, the fundamental truth was the reality of the narrator. The reader must not be looking at N, but rather through N, at the world. Every decision I made as a writer had to come second to that.

Of course, there are many different identities on each side of the Mad/Sane border. Though to those on the one side, the Madness or Sanity of those on the other might seem to be their defining characteristic, within each world individuals must find other means of distinguishing themselves from each other and asserting their difference. The Abaddon is a finely graded hierarchical community, not just in terms of the staff—who range from the all-powerful, invisible Dr Diabolus, who is rumoured to sit on a golden throne, to Minimum Wage, the cleaner—but also in terms of the patients. As the patients move down through the floors of the Abaddon, they are permitted greater freedoms, an allusion to types of behaviour therapy, or as N puts it: 'It was all meant to get you to lay off the mad stuff and start acting normal, like showing a dog a treat to make it sit' (Allan 6). Though the patients boast about how high up the tower they've gone, the universal goal is to reach the Dorothy Fish, which, in the words of N, 'was the best of both worlds: you was getting the help but you done what the fuck you wanted' (Allan 7). This creates tension between the 'flops', or inpatients, and the 'day dribblers', who, in their determination never to be discharged, are blocking their places. As happens with any identity border, those on the one side begin to assign attributes of identity to those on the other. This is most obvious as the novel progresses and flops start to take the places of newly discharged day patients:

> So there we all are one afternoon, what's left of us, and the flops down the sides—disgusting they was to be perfectly honest, even Jacko the Penguin said they made him feel sick, and he'd *been* a flop till the week before. 'Like vultures,' said Tadpole [a former flop], 'that's what they are!' 'No self-respect!' said Curry Bob. 'Waiting to pick our bones,' said Tadpole. (Allan 303)

But the day patients must also find ways of measuring themselves against each other. Under threat of discharge, they clutch their identity badges ever tighter. Medication, suicide attempts, benefit rates, traumatic histories even—all become currency, ways of assuring themselves, and each other, that they are entitled to their identity, and at least as entitled as the person sitting next to them.

And the hospital is, of course, measuring patients too. For how else can they demonstrate the efficacy of their madness-reducing treatments? Which brings us back to the thorny problem of how to measure something as intangible, as subjective, as mental distress. The answer to this provides the main drive for the plot of *Poppy Shakespeare*, for unbeknown to her, Poppy has been placed in the Abaddon not because she is mad, but because she is the very definition of 'normal'. She is to serve as a living yardstick against which the insanity of the patients can be measured. Poppy, desperate to be discharged, discovers that her only hope is to employ a specialist lawyer to prove that she is normal. But the lawyer can only take Poppy's case if she is in receipt of Mad Money, which she cannot obtain unless she proves she is mad. Caught in the world of the hospital, and under the tutelage of N, inevitably Poppy's mental health begins to deteriorate, prompting the mass discharge of patients who are consequently deemed to have got better, and winning the hospital an award for excellence of care.

Diagnosis and Empathy

So far, so satirical, though I have to say that in the UK at least, what seemed the wildest satire a decade ago is being rapidly overtaken by reality. My point is that measuring things distorts them. It may be necessary in some situations, but we should never kid ourselves that measurement equates to understanding. Measurement is driven by a need for clarity, a clarity which often belies the complexity of the actual situation. The problem occurs when we mistake the measurement for the truth. Take psychiatric diagnosis, for example. We think of diagnoses as though they exist as actual entities, rather than concepts with which we attempt to clump together particular patterns of behaviour and thought, aka 'symptoms'. Diagnoses are a way of looking at 'a thing'; they are not 'a thing' in themselves. Or to put it another way, the diagnosis exists in the mind of the perceiver, not in the person perceived. But that is not how they are commonly thought of. Not by the public, not by the media, not by most mental health professionals, and it is certainly not how they are experienced by the diagnosed patient themselves. Despite the fact that even experienced clinicians, who have received extensive training in applying the diagnostic criteria, only agree on a broad diagnostic category around 50% of the time (Cooke 22), a diagnosis quickly becomes a symbol of identity, and, in some cases—personality disorders, for example—a decidedly toxic one.

In writing *Poppy Shakespeare*, I avoided referring to the patients' diagnoses. So powerful are these labels, I was concerned that if I used them, it would make it harder for the reader to relate to the characters as individual people. (There is an occasional exception, for example Schizo Safid, where the diagnosis has been requisitioned to form part of a patient's name.) In my experience, diagnoses facilitate neither genuine understanding nor empathy, and this feeling is shared by many other service users: 'I was told I had a disease ... I was beginning to undergo that radically dehumanising and devaluing transformation ... from being Pat Deegan to being "a schizophrenic"' (Campbell 22).

Empathy relies on some sense of commonality. One human being projects themselves into the consciousness of another. The process of dehumanization makes genuine empathy impossible, a fact that has been exploited throughout history with horrific consequences:

> Thinking sets the agenda for action, and thinking of humans as less than human paves the way for atrocity. The Nazis were explicit about the status of their victims. They were Untermenschen—subhumans—and as such were excluded from the system of moral rights and obligations that bind humankind together. (Smith 12)

Empathy also necessitates recognizing another person as an individual, rather than as a type. You cannot project yourself into the consciousness of a group, for the simple reason that a group doesn't have a consciousness. Diagnoses inevitably group patients together. That, after all, is their purpose.

In recent years NHS England has also introduced so-called clustering, as a means of grouping patients together according to their rated needs. The following description is taken from its Mental Health Clustering Booklet.

What is a Cluster?

NHS England describes a cluster in the following way:

> In this context a cluster is a global description of a group of people with similar characteristics as identified from a holistic assessment and then rated using the Mental Health Clustering Tool (MHCT). The clusters allow for a degree of variation in the combination and severity of rated needs. However, as the clusters are statistically underpinned, definite patterns in the MHCT ratings exist for each of them. These ranges are indicated by the colour coded

grids (Appendix 3) and are supplemented by the contextual information on the left hand side of each page, which is particularly useful when reviewing the appropriateness of previous cluster allocations. (NHS England 3)

Statistically underpinned or not, my personal experience of clustering was that I was expected, after years of building a relationship with a trusted psychiatrist, to start afresh with somebody else, when the shiny new Mental Health Clustering Tool assigned me to a different cluster.

Some patients find a diagnosis helpful, at least at first. For some it can come as a relief, a sort of stamp of validity, a confirmation that something is 'really wrong' and it's not just a question of needing to pull oneself together. A badge of identity can also be useful, not least in terms of accessing welfare support and disability benefits. And of course, we need to be able to group things together in order to talk about them at all. But such groupings have no objective meaning in and of themselves. Rather, they take on meanings according to the particular 'language game' we are playing, to borrow Wittgenstein's phrase. The problem comes when we fail to acknowledge the context of the game, or forget that we're playing one altogether and start viewing diagnoses as unassailable facts.

Poppy Shakespeare is of course a novel, in itself another sort of language game. It is a shaped, constructed, artificial world. It represents a point of view, if you like, as opposed to any sort of 'objective' reality. In *Poppy*, the patients are as one in their belief that they cannot exist outside the hospital. Reality is of course much more diverse and much less tidy, but the fact remains that once a person crosses the Madness border, it is very easy for the world outside to start to slip away. Behaviours that might seem perfectly within the normal range outside may start to be seen as symptoms of a disorder, by mental health professionals, by friends and family, and most destructively of all by the person themselves. You need think only of David Rosenhan's famous 'Thud' experiment, one of the inspirations for the novel, to witness this in practice.

None of which is to suggest that mental distress isn't real, or that people experiencing mental distress are not in need of support; quite the opposite. But mental distress, or mental illness, or mental health problems (you can pick your own signpost) are experiences; they are not identities. And as experiences, they are not exclusive to any particular group, do not belong in a separate 'not quite human' category. Indeed, it is the conflation of mental distress with the identity of the Mad person that stops people from recognizing the fact that they need help, as well as enabling the systematic underfunding of mental health services. In England mental ill health accounts for almost a third of the so-called disease burden, but receives just 13% of the NHS budget.

Beyond Fiction: Living the Spoiled Identity

In my own life, I found that once I became a patient, and despite the fact that I was already published, my writing ambitions were seen as delusional. My parents were called in to be told that the family needed to adjust their expectations of me, adjust presumably to my spending a lifetime in hospital, or perhaps at best in the community, shuffling between day centres and depot injections. At no point during the years I spent in a day hospital and on the wards did anyone ever refer to the future, beyond the next few days perhaps, or the end of my current prescription. I was twenty-six years old when I crossed the border from sniff to dribbler and yet not once, not ever, can I remember anyone asking me what I wanted to do with my life. It was taken as read, at least as I understood it, that a mental health patient was who I was, and all I was, and all I ever would be.

It took me a long time to get into the system, partly because I did not recognise what I was experiencing as being connected to mental health. The world had stopped turning. This was a fact. It had nothing to do with my state of mind. But it was also because I did not fit the image I had, the image I had absorbed from my culture, of what a mentally ill person was. I did not fit what I perceived as the Mad identity. Even as I walked through the doors of my real-life Abaddon, I remember my fear that they would be able to tell, to spot that I wasn't really mad, and turn me away.

And if there's one thing harder than getting into the system, it's getting out of it. In the novel, it is Poppy who enables this for N by providing her with a model of a different way of being, and also by failing to recognize her Mad identity, something which offends N immensely at first, but later perhaps enables her to visualize herself in a different way. The novel ends with N discharged, and if not quite in the world of the sniffs, certainly on the cusp of it.

When you finish writing a novel, you have to let go of your characters. Which is not to say their lives do not continue, but they do so in private—unrecorded, freed from the printed page. From time to time though I do still catch myself worrying about N. How is she faring ten years on? How does she navigate the multiple perils of her spoiled identity? What does she say when people ask about her past? Is she working? What did she put on her CV? My own passage out of the system was guided, indeed enabled, by a wonderful social worker to whom the novel is in fact dedicated. I hope N has someone to help her, someone to discuss such issues with. Though with the decimation of social care in the UK under so-called austerity measures, I'm afraid I rather doubt it.

For me, as I mentioned at the beginning, Poppy served as a sort of passport to the world outside the system. It gave me a new identity, but, in a case of sort of dual nationality, I did not, or at least not fully, relinquish the old one. It seemed important to me in talking about Poppy, and also in the column about mental health I started publishing in *The Guardian*,[5] to be open about my own experience and the way it had shaped my outlook.

But this was not a straightforward thing to do. For while my coming out enabled me to form many positive connections, most particularly with other dual nationals, inevitably at times I was viewed, am viewed, through the distorting lens of my Mad identity. There is a need for people to locate my difference in order to distinguish themselves as sane, as normal, not the sort of person who could ever wind up on a psychiatric ward. For example, at the time of *Poppy Shakespeare*'s publication, and in my first ever interview with a national newspaper, I managed when expressing myself rather forcefully to lean back in my chair so far that I toppled over backwards onto the floor. Writing in *The Times*, the journalist Emma Cook described the incident thus:

> In Allan's writing, her descriptions of acute mental illness can be disconcertingly at odds with her rational demeanour when you meet her *which is what makes it disturbing to listen to* [my italics]. One can't help wondering to what extent she still feels she has to present a 'face' to the world. At one point during the interview, she tilts back on her chair and slips, quite unexpectedly, flat on her back. For a second, her expression is pained, helpless. We both laugh as she picks herself up, but we are embarrassed, *more so than normal* [my italics], and I wonder why. Is it her awareness that she lost control? Then the calm surface returns and we feel secure again. (Cook 17)

In the UK, the Equality Act of 2010[6] prohibits employers from asking about an applicant's mental health before making a job offer in most circumstances. Whilst this change was certainly long overdue and extremely welcome, the fact that such legislation is needed is indicative of the impact a 'spoiled identity' can have on the way a person is perceived. The best one can hope for across the border is to successfully pass incognito. But not only does this create considerable anxiety in the person obliged to live undercover, inventing extended periods of travel to account for the gaps on their CV, it also blinds employers to the full breadth and range of an applicant's experience when assessing them for a job.

Writing as an Instrument of Change

The irony is that for all my official qualifications, my stamps of suitability, it is my experience of inhabiting the Mad identity that I draw on at least as much as anything else in my teaching and writing practice. For writing (and reading) fiction is all about crossing identity borders: borders of gender, colour, class, profession, and nationality, to name but a few. The novelist is a sort of identity trafficker, their ultimate mission to smuggle the reader across the border of the individual self. 'Ask yourself', I say to my students, 'what is your character's "normal"? What is so ordinary to them that they fail to notice it? And how are you going to take the reader inside that normality?'

Dismantling borders takes time, of course—time and persistence and a variety of tools and approaches. Perhaps the most a novelist can hope to achieve is a barely perceptible chip in the border wall. Certainly, the Mad identity is not going to crumble easily. A question I have been repeatedly asked at book festivals, where I am sometimes invited to speak at events with such titles as 'Life on the Outside', is whether Poppy was 'really mad'. But I remain convinced that such chips have value and that small though the novelist's chisel may be, its job is a crucially important one. For it is above all the novel which, in conveying individual, subjective experience, is able to challenge the very notion of collective identity. It is the novel which enables the reader to cross the border, to become 'the other', and in doing so, perhaps to realize that the fear of madness is above all a fear of recognition—and perhaps, just perhaps, to dare at last to acknowledge that when they looked at the Mad person, they were looking at themselves all along.

Notes

1. https://www.time-to-change.org.uk
2. https://www.headstogether.org.uk
3. https://www.mentalhealth.org.uk/campaigns/mental-health-awareness-week

4. For a rigorous analysis of the impact of income inequality on levels of mental ill health, see Wilkinson and Pickett 63–73.
5. Clare Allan, 'It's my life', *The Guardian*, 2006–2018, https://www.theguardian.com/society/series/itsmylife
6. Equality Act 2010, c.15, http://www.legislation.gov.uk/ukpga/2010/15/section/60.

References

Allan, Clare, *Poppy Shakespeare* (London: Bloomsbury, 2006).

Amis, Martin, *Time's Arrow* (London: Jonathan Cape, 1991).

Baldwin, James, 'Freaks and the American Ideal of Manhood' in *Collected Essays* (New York: Library of America, 1998; first published in *Playboy*, January 1985), 814–29.

Campbell, Peter, 'Surviving the System' in T. Bassett and T. Stickley (eds), *Voices of Experience: Narratives of Mental Health Survivors* (Chichester: Wiley Blackwell, 2010). https://doi.org/10.1002/9780470970362.ch3

Chekhov, Anton, 'Ward No. 6', trans. by B. Guilbert Guerney, in C. Neider (ed.), *Short Novels of the Masters* (New York: Cooper Square Press, 2001), 386–438.

Cook, Emma, 'One Day She Lost the Plot', *The Times*, 25 March 2006, Body and Soul: 17.

Cooke, Anne (ed.), *Understanding Psychosis and Schizophrenia* (London: British Psychological Society, 2014).

Goffman, Erving, *Stigma: Notes on the Management of Spoiled Identity* (New Jersey: Prentice-Hall, 1963).

Kirk, Stuart A., and Herb Kutchins, 'The Myth of the Reliability of the DSM', *Journal of Mind and Behaviour* 15 (1994): 71–86.

Metzl, Jonathan M., *The Protest Psychosis: How Schizophrenia Became a Black Disease* (Boston: Beacon Press, 2011).

NHS England, *Mental Health Clustering Booklet (V.5.0)* (NHS England Publications Gateway Reference: 04421, NHS England Publications, 2016). https://doi.org/10.1136/bmj.i4023

Nutt, Amy Ellis, 'Scientists Open the "Black Box" of Schizophrenia with Dramatic Genetic Discovery', *Washington Post*, 27 January 2016 [online], accessed 2 May, 2022, https://www.washingtonpost.com/news/speaking-of-science/wp/2016/01/27/scientists-open-the-black-box-of-schizophrenia-with-dramatic-genetic-finding/.

Rosenhan, David L., 'On Being Sane in Insane Places', *Science*, New Series, 179.4070 (19 January 1973): 250–58. https://doi.org/10.1126/science.179.4070.250

Showalter, Elaine, *The Female Malady: Women, Madness and English Culture 1830–1980* (London: Virago, 1987).

Smith, David L., *Less Than Human: Why We Demean, Enslave and Exterminate Others* (New York: St Martin's Press, 2011).

Wilkinson, Richard, and Kate Pickett, *The Spirit Level: Why Greater Equality Makes Societies Stronger* (New York: Bloomsbury, 2010).

Wittgenstein, Ludwig, *Philosophical Investigations*, trans. by G.E.M. Anscombe (New York: Macmillan, 1958).

Part II
Literary Theory and Experiencing Mental Illness

5. Reading Shattering Minds and Extended Selves in Virginia Woolf's *Mrs Dalloway*

Anna Ovaska

> In this book I have almost too many ideas. I want to give life & death, sanity & insanity; I want to criticise the social system, & to show it at work, at its most intense. (Woolf 1978, 248)

In a recent article, 'What Does It Mean to Be Mad?', literary narratologist Porter Abbott (Abbott 18) reminds us that 'madness' is often used as a label for something that appears as 'unpredictable' or 'obscure' from the outside. It is employed to categorize something that puzzles and disturbs us, something that breaks the illusion that we can 'read' other minds, leaving us in a state of distress. In other words, to interpret another person as mad is to deem them unintelligible and 'other'—and it is also a way to protect ourselves from madness, from the uncertainty and chaos it represents. In *Mrs Dalloway* (1925), one of the seminal portrayals of 'madness' in modernist literature, Virginia Woolf fights against this very basic human tendency to label and push away what appears as threatening. As she writes in her diary from the time when she was working on the manuscript: 'I adumbrate here a study of insanity & suicide: the world as seen by the sane & the insane side by side' (Woolf 1978, 207). She states that she wants to 'give life & death, sanity & insanity' and 'to criticise the social system, & to show it at work' (Woolf 1978, 248). She aims to depict madness from the inside—as understandable and meaningful in the context of a person's life and experiential world—and to show how our experiences are shaped by the environments and the societies we inhabit.

In this chapter, I discuss the fictional minds Woolf created in *Mrs Dalloway* from the perspective of current cognitive theories which emphasize the embodied, enactive, embedded, and extended nature of the mind, experience, and subjectivity (cf. Varela, Thompson, and Rosch; Colombetti and Krueger). I suggest that long before the '4E' views were formulated, Woolf managed to bring to focus the way we are entangled with one another and our cultural and material circumstances. From today's perspective, the theories can in turn help to illuminate Woolf's narrative techniques and their effects on readers.[1] I argue that Woolf shows the way we are tied to one other, supported by our environments and other people, and also shattered—for example, due to traumatic events. She portrays all minds as precarious, and thus she contests the borders of 'normal' and 'abnormal'. I also focus on readers' engagement with the fictional minds created in her novel: the way we are invited to encounter the experiences of others while at the same time maintaining a respectful distance to another and remaining aware of our own bodies and our own situatedness in the world we inhabit. Furthermore, I suggest that Woolf's writing warns us of appropriating the experiences of others and pushes us to reflect on the ways mental illnesses are understood in the society and culture, as well as our own experiences of distress and shattering.

Many critics of *Mrs Dalloway* have noted that Woolf gives Septimus Warren Smith, the young First World War veteran and the other main character of the novel, experiences that are similar to the ones she herself was going through at times of mental distress: Septimus hallucinates birds singing in Greek and his mind is controlled by thoughts of madness, suicide, and death. Septimus is often read through different psychological frames and diagnoses: he is understood to be suffering from trauma caused by the Great War, from repressed homosexuality, or, alternatively, he is interpreted as a schizophrenic or as a manic-depressive character.[2] However, I do not want to suggest here any specific diagnosis for Septimus and I would argue that it often makes little sense to try to 'diagnose' fictional characters. That said, one of Woolf's many accomplishments in *Mrs Dalloway* was that, long before post-traumatic experiences were properly understood, she was able to imagine and convey to her readers what the soldiers returning from the war might have been going through. Woolf, in other words, created experiential, phenomenological knowledge of feelings of shattering and loss of self inflicted by trauma. Most importantly, she portrayed mental distress and illness as tied to worldly circumstances and to social structures, and sought to describe the ways traumatic events can alter lives and experiential worlds. As is often noted, Woolf also explored in *Mrs Dalloway* her own distrust of doctors, based on her experiences of medical treatment (e.g. Scott xxxv). One of the threads of Woolf's social critique is thus directed against the mistreatment and stigmatization of those of us who suffer from mental illness: against the efforts to silence 'others' in order to protect 'ourselves'.

As Woolf suggested in her diary, she studies in the novel the world from the perspectives of 'the sane & the insane side by side'. She places Septimus alongside other characters like Clarissa Dalloway, Peter Walsh and others who are arguably 'sane'—or who at least maintain an image of sanity in the society. At the same time, she shows that the borders between 'sanity' and 'insanity' are never clear-cut. She portrays all her characters, not just Septimus, as entangled with the world and with others: intermingling and losing boundaries between the self and the world in different ways, some of them painful and traumatic, some not—and all part of life. She refuses to label or silence experiences of mental illness and distress and instead seeks to convey experiences of shattering, delusions, and hallucinations to her readers. She invites us to attune to the experiences of her characters: to listen to the pain and the pleasures, the distress and joy they go through, and to recognize the ways the characters are tied to one another and shaped by their worlds.

To implement her plan of exploring the world from different perspectives, Woolf developed a new method for constructing fictional characters and narrating their experiences: a 'tunnelling process', as she called it in her diary (Woolf 1978, 272). In another entry, she elaborates: 'I dig out beautiful caves behind my characters [...] The idea is that the caves shall connect, & each comes to daylight at the present moment' (Woolf 1978, 213). Like Joyce in *Ulysses* three years earlier, Woolf focuses on one day (a day in June 1923) that is shared by all her characters, and creates a narrative structure in which the readers are invited from one character's experiential world to the next as the moments and hours of the day pass. Bonnie Kime Scott has described how the changes of perspective are constructed in the 'tunnelling process': 'Transitions between characters often occur via an experience of the present moment that they share—hearing the tone of one of the many chiming clocks, or the alarming backfire on Bond Street, or watching an airplane doing skywriting far above. These are all forms of connecting in the present moment, as called for in the "tunnelling process'" (Scott xlix). In other words, Woolf connects the characters through the 'tunnels' or 'caves' she creates. Below the 'surface', the characters' pasts are opened up in memories and flashbacks. Sometimes the tunnels intersect, and we are invited to moments and places that the characters have shared in the past. At the time of narration, the tunnels 'come to daylight' to a shared space and time, and we are shown how the characters perceive the world from their different perspectives: the skywriting, the car backfiring, the church bells, Big Ben, and finally Clarissa's party. Furthermore, the 'surface', the time of narration, is also where readers are taken from one tunnel to the next: moved from one character's experiential world to another.

In the following, I focus on how Woolf depicts her characters' minds as embodied and interacting with the environment and other people, and how she solicits the readers' experiences of being in the world, in space and time, in order to invite us inside the experiential worlds of her characters. To clarify the effects of Woolf's 'tunnelling' method and the way she portrayed the human mind intermingling with the world, I draw on the 4E theories which likewise emphasize the embodied, enactive, embedded, and extended nature of the mind.

The Embodied, Enactive, Embedded, and Extended Mind

According to the 4E perspectives, the mind is not produced solely by the brain, but it is rather a result of our sensorimotor interaction with the world. Mental processes are enacted by the whole living organism that is embedded in its environment (Varela, Thompson, and Rosch; Colombetti). A minded creature is thus understood as an embodied being that is situated in the world, partly constituted by its environment, and extending into the world. Or as phenomenologist Thomas Fuchs puts it, emphasizing the role of interpersonal relations: 'The individual mind is not confined within the head, but extends throughout the living body and includes the world beyond the membrane of the organism, especially the interpersonal world of self and other; this is also the world in which mind and brain are essentially formed' (Fuchs 2009, 221). The mind is supported by its social environment, by other people, as Fuchs suggests, but also by the material world, by tools, instruments, and objects of nature that can become a part of one's 'affective scaffolding' (Colombetti and Krueger), regulating one's emotions and cognitive capacities, affording possibilities for action or restricting one's movements.

The understanding of the mind as embodied, enactive, embedded, and extending into the world has consequences for the way we understand mental disorders. The mind is not confined to the skull, and neither are mental disorders 'inside the head'. Rather, they are changes in the way we are in the world: in the way we navigate or make sense of our environments and in the possibilities the world affords us. As philosopher of mind Giovanna Colombetti suggests, borrowing the term *Umwelt* from biologist Jakob von Uexküll: 'psychiatric disorders are to be understood as shifts in sense-making, resulting in an extraordinary and therefore often disconcerting *Umwelt*' (Colombetti 1097). Mental disorders are, in other words, alterations in our embodied being in the world and our ways of interacting with other people and the environment. For example, the traces of traumatic experiences can manifest themselves in the way one is able to act in the world and engage with other people. Trauma involves a loss of trust in the world and others, in the support they provide, which results in changes in one's sense of time and space, for example in distressing flashbacks or even in delusions or hallucinations (cf. Fuchs 2012; Ratcliffe).

The way one interacts with and is supported by one's environment could be exemplified with Woolf's description of how Clarissa Dalloway experiences herself as extending into the world and other people. In the following passage, Clarissa's mind is given to us through Peter (her former lover), who is focalizing the scene:

> But she [Clarissa] said, sitting on the bus going up Shaftesbury Avenue, she felt herself everywhere; not 'here, here, here'; and she tapped the back of the seat; but everywhere. She waved her hand, going up Shaftesbury Avenue. She was all that. So that to know her, or any one, one must seek out the people who completed them; even the places. Odd affinities she had with people she had never spoken to, some woman in the street, some man behind a counter—even trees, or barns. (Woolf 2004, 135)

The way Clarissa's experience is scaffolded by the bus seat and by the things around her is thematized in Peter's memory of her. The structure of consciousness representation in the passage is quite complex: Clarissa is shown to us through Peter as he remembers how Clarissa, when they were young, used to have these strong, 'odd' experiences of affinity with people, objects and places—some 'woman' or a 'man', even 'trees' and 'barns'. The scene is a very explicit example of Woolf's understanding of the mind and subjectivity as embedded in and extending into the world. When reading *Mrs Dalloway* from the perspective of the 4E theories, we can notice how Woolf repeatedly shows her characters as intermingled with the world and with one another in various ways: in the way they experience themselves in the world, in the way their thoughts and memories are constructed, and even in the way the characters are portrayed through one another. One feature of Woolf's technique is the way she invites her readers to adopt the perspectives of the different characters in turn: as discussed, they all share the same world and the same time, one day in London after the First World War, and they are linked to one another through the 'tunnels', either in their thoughts or through the connections offered by the narrative design. We are invited to imagine how they are scaffolded in different ways in the same world and time. Let us now look more closely at how Woolf portrays the characters' experiential worlds becoming altered.

Altered Experiential Worlds

As suggested, Woolf depicts Septimus's world from his perspective, and the readers are invited to follow the way he experiences his body and his surroundings. In a famous scene—the 'mad scene', according to Woolf (Woolf 1978, 272)—in Regent's Park, Septimus feels his body merging with the world around him. Septimus and his wife Rezia are at the park and Woolf's figural third-person narration renders Septimus's point of view:

> But he [Septimus] would not go mad. He would shut his eyes; he would see no more. But they beckoned; leaves were alive; trees were alive. And the leaves being connected by millions of fibres with his own body, there on the seat, fanned it up and down; when the branch stretched he, too, made that statement. The sparrows fluttering, rising, and falling in jagged fountains were part of the pattern; the white and blue, barred with black branches. Sounds made harmonies with premeditation; the spaces between them were as significant as the sounds. A child cried. Rightly away a horn sounded. All taken together meant the birth of a new religion—
>
> 'Septimus!' Said Rezia. He started violently. People must notice. (Woolf 2004, 18)

Septimus feels the leaves and the branches as part of his body and his experience. From a psychological perspective, Septimus's experience of being connected to the world comes close to what phenomenological psychiatry has described as the 'delusional mood'—an atmosphere of curious meaning which precedes psychotic hallucinations or delusions (see Jaspers 98). Louis Sass describes this altered state of experiencing the world: 'Every detail and event takes on an excruciating distinctness, specialness, and peculiarity—some definite meaning that always lies just out of reach, however, where it eludes all attempts to grasp or specify it' (Sass 52). In Septimus's experience, the borders between the self and the world are breaking down, and the world takes on a curious meaning. The experience is framed as 'madness' in Septimus's thoughts, but through negation ('he would not go mad'). At first, the feeling has a positive, even comforting tone: a 'birth of a new religion'. The atmosphere of horror emerges only moments later when we encounter him hearing voices—sparrows singing in Greek—and finally experiencing a hallucinatory flashback of his fallen friend resurrecting from the dead: 'There was his hand; there the dead. White things were assembling behind the railings opposite. But he dared not look. Evans was behind the railings!' (Woolf 2004, 20). Woolf shows Septimus interacting with the world: extending into the world, but also shattering inside it. The distressing hallucination is tightly connected to material objects. In the scene, 'madness' is not ultimately something unintelligible or obscure, but rather it is full of meaning: it is an altered way of being in the world in which the traumatic past is enacted in the present as delusions and hallucinations.

From a narratological perspective, Dorrit Cohn (Cohn 133–34) has described passages like the one quoted above as a 'hazy region' where inner and outer fictional realities are intertwined. When reading passages like this, it becomes difficult to separate the description of environment from the representation of characters' perceptions and consciousness: the two are almost the same. Through such narrative technique in which the character's consciousness and the description of environment are intertwined, Woolf is able to create an impression of how the borders between an experiencing mind and its environment are breaking down. As Herman (Herman 2011, 244) suggests, Woolf invites her readers not only to thematize Septimus's experiences—to observe Septimus or 'diagnose' him—but to enact what it feels like to go through psychotic experiences.

Septimus's 'mad scene' is a very explicit example of the way a character's mind and the fictional world are intertwined on the level of narration, but there are similar instances throughout the novel. In the park at the same time, with Septimus and Rezia, is young Maisie Johnson who has just arrived in London. For a short moment, Woolf's narration leaves Septimus and takes the readers 'inside' Maisie's mind:

> And Maisie Johnson, as she joined that gently trudging, vaguely gazing, breeze-kissed company—squirrels perching and preening, sparrow fountains fluttering for crumbs, dogs busy with the railings [...]—Maisie Johnson positively felt she must cry Oh! (for that young man on the seat had given her quite a turn. Something was up, she knew).
>
> Horror! Horror! she wanted to cry. (She had left her people; they had warned her what would happen.) (Woolf 2004, 22)

Maisie briefly encounters Septimus and Rezia and sees the same sparrow fountains and railings as they do, and like Septimus, she too suddenly experiences an inexplicable feeling of horror that penetrates her thoughts. Her feeling of being far away from home and the insecurity caused by her loneliness seem to manifest in an altered experiential world. Her experience is more mundane and common than Septimus's, but just like for Septimus, the world around her is altered—and this is also emphasized by the fact that Maisie's experience is in part triggered by Septimus whose distress Maisie seems to recognize.

Later, Septimus's and Maisie's experiences are juxtaposed with Peter's who, too, has arrived at Regent's Park. He is sitting on a bench, falling asleep:

> A great brush swept smooth across his [Peter's] mind, sweeping across it moving branches, children's voices, the shuffle of feet, and people passing, and humming traffic, rising and falling traffic. Down, down he sank into the plumes and feathers of sleep, sank, and was muffled over. (Woolf 2004, 49)

As in Septimus's and Maisie's scenes, Woolf shows Peter's mind and his environment as intermingled: the description of the environment brings forth Peter's mind and the environment is constructed through Peter's mind. There is no way to separate the two. And as Peter's consciousness disappears when he falls asleep, the narration is also paused and the section ends. From the readers' perspective, the merging of the description of physical environment and the representation of consciousness creates an effect of a mind extending into its environment. In Septimus's and Maisie's scenes, this is framed as distressing, but Peter's passage evokes an atmosphere of tranquillity.

Through Septimus, but also through the other focalizing characters (Clarissa, Maisie, Peter), Woolf is able to explore experiences in which the borders between the self and the world become hazy and in which the world takes on new meanings. She creates moments in which the mind is shattering (Septimus) and scenes of momentary distress and horror (Maisie), but also aligns them with moments of, for example, falling asleep (Peter). Woolf's narration solicits the readers' experiences of being bodily, affective subjects embedded in the world. She invites us to reflect upon the ways we are entangled with our environments and with one other. She often constructs characters who are going through experiences of suffering and trauma in order to remind us of the precariousness of the human mind, but it is important to note that not all Woolf's examples of being merged with the world are framed as distressing nor pathological: as the 4E theories suggest, all cognition is supported or 'scaffolded' by the environment, the material and social worlds, and intersubjective engagements.

Another important characteristic of Woolf's way of constructing minds is that not all characters whose lives and experiential worlds she opens for the readers are portrayed in a positive light. A good example of this is Lady Bruton, one of the socialites of the novel, whose political plans are portrayed briefly. Let us look at a passage in which Woolf shows her falling asleep after a meeting with Richard Dalloway and Hugh Whitbread. Like Peter earlier, Lady Bruton is somewhere in between daydreaming and sleeping, and the narrator describes how she experiences Richard and Hugh as connected to her:

> And they went further and further from her, being attached to her by a thin thread (since they had lunched with her) which would stretch and stretch, get thinner and thinner as they walked across London; as if one's friends were attached to one's body, after lunching with them, by a thin thread, which (as she dozed there) became hazy with the sound of bells, striking the hour or ringing to service, as a single spider's thread is blotted with raindrops, and, burdened, sags down. So she slept. (Woolf 2004, 99)

During her luncheon with the two men, Lady Bruton is presented to the readers in quite a negative light. We have learned that Hugh and Richard are summoned to help Lady Bruton to write an opinion piece for the *Times*, which promotes a eugenicist plan to send young women and men of 'respectable' background to Canada. The passage evokes an ambiguous mood. It could be read either as a thematization of the way Lady Bruton's experiential world is scaffolded by the men helping her, or in a more sinister interpretation, the 'thread' could be read as a metaphor for Lady Bruton's power: she is a spider spinning its webs. Yet, even though we are invited to take distance from the lady's worldview and politics, her experiences are nonetheless brought to us from her perspective, inviting us to recognize the way she, too, is entangled with her environment on many levels: material, intersubjective, and socio-cultural.

Encountering Others

The characters of *Mrs Dalloway* are connected to one another through complex structures: they inhabit the same time and space, and they share perceptions and memories of the same moments and events. Both in her diary and in the novel Woolf thematizes the ways people are affectively scaffolded by one another and the world around them, with metaphors like the 'tunnel', the 'cave', and the 'thread'. She creates techniques of consciousness representation in which characters are portrayed through one another's perceptions and memories, and which capture the way we go 'in and out of each other's minds without any effort', as Peter recalls himself and Clarissa doing when they were young (Woolf 2004, 54–55). In other words, she explores some of the very basic forms of intersubjective engagement: the way we experience others and understand them effortlessly through our bodies, expressions, and the worlds we share, and also the way our experiences are formed and scaffolded by intersubjective relations. However, at the same time Woolf creates moments in which intersubjective connections fail and engaging with others causes suffering.

This is shown especially through Septimus. His tragedy is that the others in the storyworld can neither recognize nor acknowledge his experiences. Dr Holmes claims that 'there is nothing the matter with him' (Woolf 2004, 58, 79). Sir William Bradshaw recognizes the shell shock but has an ideological position that appears as more important than actually caring for Septimus: 'Sir William said he never spoke of "madness"; he called it not having a sense of proportion' (Woolf 2004, 85). His solution is to take Septimus out of sight, to a 'home' where he will be 'taught to rest' (Woolf 2004, 85–86). Paradoxically, Sir William's refusal to name Septimus's condition as 'madness' appears as a form of violence: as a repudiation of his experiences.[3] Neither doctor will listen to Septimus: both seek to negate his experience, by denying that he is ill and by sending him away, and Woolf shows how their actions ultimately lead to Septimus's death. Not even Rezia, the person who knows Septimus best, can understand what he is going through. She only knows that the doctors fail them and perceives her husband's suffering. The readers are ultimately left with a heavy responsibility: we alone are given an access to Septimus's experiential world.

At the end of the novel, Clarissa tries to imagine what Septimus had been going through. She never meets him but hears about his death from Sir William at her party. What follows is a scene in which Clarissa re-enacts Septimus's death:

> He had killed himself—but how? Always her body went through it first, when she was told, suddenly, of an accident; her dress flamed, her body burnt. He had thrown himself from a window. Up had flashed the ground; through him, blundering, bruising, went the rusty spikes. There he lay with a thud, thud, thud in his brain, and then a suffocation of blackness. So she saw it. But why had he done it? And the Bradshaws talked of it at her party!
>
> She had once thrown a shilling into the Serpentine, never anything more. But he had flung it away. They went on living (she would have to go back; the rooms were still crowded; people kept on coming). They (all day she had been thinking of Bourton, of Peter, of Sally), they would grow old. A thing there was that mattered; a thing, wreathed about with chatter, defaced, obscured in her own life, let drop every day in corruption, lies, chatter. This he had preserved. Death was defiance. Death was an attempt to communicate; people feeling the impossibility of reaching the centre which, mystically, evaded them; closeness drew apart; rapture faded, one was alone. There was an embrace in death.
>
> But this young man who had killed himself—had he plunged holding his treasure? 'If it were now to die, 'twere now to be most happy,' she had said to herself once, coming down in white. (Woolf 2004, 163)

In her figural narration, Woolf lays out everything that goes through Clarissa's mind in only a couple of seconds: Clarissa imagining Septimus dying, her memories of her youth, thoughts about death, and a memory of citing Shakespeare a long time ago. The passage begins with a description of a bodily simulation: 'Always her body went through it first'. The narrator never actually describes Septimus's suicide in such detail, but we get to 'see' it when Clarissa bodily re-enacts the death in her imagination. However, the powerful, painful image is then undermined by Clarissa's petty distress that someone would ruin her party by talking about a suicide (a kind of duality that is typical for Woolf, as we saw also in Lady Bruton's scene). Then the narrator describes big, gnomic thoughts that are flickering in Clarissa's mind: 'Death was an attempt to communicate'; 'There was an embrace in death'. Finally, a line from *Othello* appears: the words, 'If it were now to die, 'twere now to be most happy' transport Clarissa to her youth, to the one summer that she, Peter, and Sally spent together before she married Richard.

As the readers of *Mrs Dalloway* often notice, the connection, even affinity, between Septimus and Clarissa is crucial for the composition of the novel. The main characters never actually meet, but Woolf portrays their lives as entangled in many ways. They go through similar experiences of suffering—even though we are guided to understand that Septimus's pain is inflicted by the war, whereas Clarissa's experiences are connected to her role as a woman in post-Victorian society. However, from Peter we learn that Clarissa, too, has experienced a trauma: she has witnessed her sister die in an accident. Some critics have suggested that Septimus functions as a 'scapegoat': he dies so that Clarissa does not have to.[4] The passage above can thus be read (at least) in two ways: either Clarissa trivializes Septimus's death, or his death opens something important in her, a personal and social understanding. Perhaps Clarissa's mistake is that she appropriates Septimus's experiences, subsuming them into her own.[5] A different reading is, however, also possible: without ever meeting him, she recognizes Septimus's distress and understands what the war has done to a generation of young men, while simultaneously going through her own pain. Throughout the novel, Woolf makes Septimus and Clarissa repeat the same sentences and have similar thoughts and experiences. By creating the affinity between Clarissa and Septimus and emphasizing the way the human mind is shaped by its environment and other people, the description of mental distress gradually grows into the social critique Woolf had planned: 'I want to give life & death, sanity & insanity; I want to criticise the social system, & to show it at work, at its most intense' (Woolf 1978, 248). Her statement in the diary works in binaries, but the novel itself contests the juxtaposition between 'sanity' and 'insanity'. Instead of drawing a line between Septimus and the others, Woolf invites her readers to reflect on the ways our immersion in the world and our sense of self is precarious, and how both illness and health are bound to social and material circumstances.[6]

Reading in Space and Time

In an early essay, 'Reading' (*c*.1919), Woolf describes reading as an embodied and situated activity:

> [A]nd somehow or another, the windows being open, and the book held so that it rested upon a background of escallonia hedges and distant blue, instead of being a book it seemed as if what I read was laid upon the landscape not printed, bound, or sewn up, but somehow the product of trees and fields and the hot summer sky, like the air which swam, on fine mornings, round the outlines of things. (Woolf 1988, 142)

For Woolf, reading is a spatial and bodily experience. When we read, we are attuned to the experiences of others and to the storyworlds, while at the same time remaining in our own bodies and worlds (and in our individual ways of being extended into and scaffolded by our environments). As Kate Flint suggests, Woolf's views on reading reveal an ambivalence which also 'haunts' her thoughts on intersubjective relations: 'Reading texts, like knowing people, requires the simultaneous play of closeness and objectivity, the desire to merge with another and the desire to keep oneself separate' (Flint 188). This can also be read as an ethical statement: we need to recognize the difference between the self and the other, and the fact that we can never fully know what another person is experiencing. There is a strange overlapping or layering of space and time: for example, me reading *Mrs Dalloway* in Helsinki, in the summer heat or winter darkness, about Septimus sitting in Regent's Park in London after the war, or Clarissa opening the French windows in Bourton as a young woman two decades before the war. The book functions as an extension of my experiential world: it carries some of my affective states the way an instrument carries the affective states of its player (cf. Colombetti and Krueger). Such experiences would not be possible without the coupling between the reader and the book. When I read, I feel with Woolf's characters, Septimus, Peter, Clarissa, Maisie Johnson, and Lady Bruton, but at the same time I do not lose awareness of my own body and my own embeddedness in the world, nor do I lose the awareness of their fictionality or of the materiality of the book (cf. also Kuzmičová).

The basic elements of narrative—perspective, time, space, and metaphors—tap into our basic ways of being in the world. Narratives solicit the readers' experiences of being bodily, affective agents embedded in the world. This is one of the reasons why narrative fiction is so powerful in its ability to convey experiences—even when there are no words to describe them. David Herman illustrates the interaction between the reader and the text as follows:

> Interpreters of narrative do not merely reconstruct a sequence of events and a set of existents, but imaginatively (emotionally, viscerally) inhabit a world in which, besides happening and existing, things matter, agitate, exalt, repulse, provide grounds for laughter and grief, and so on—both for narrative agents and for interpreters working to make sense of their circumstances and (inter) actions. (Herman 2009, 119)

In addition to 'inhabiting' a narrative world, there is an 'intersubjective contact made possible by stories', as one of the founders of narrative medicine, Rita Charon (Charon 158), puts it. For Charon, this contact between readers and fictional characters (as well as readers and authors, and readers and other readers) is made possible through close reading: through close attention to the words, silences, sensory detail, metaphors, allusions, space, time, and perspective of the story. 'Every word counts', she writes, 'keeping track of temporal, spatial, metaphorical, allusive, affective, structural aspects' of a text (Charon 180). By showing (and, in effect, constructing) the world from her characters' perspectives one after another, Woolf invites her readers to attune to the ways experiences emerge in an interaction between the subjects and the worlds they inhabit. With the 'tunnelling' structure, she invites us to *read closely*: to keep track of the changing perspectives and the ways the characters move in space (London) and time (from one hour to the next; from the present to the past), and also the ways they are connected through space and time. Woolf merges the representation of consciousness and the description of environments, and uses her 'tunnelling' method to create the effect of the extended mind: a mind formed and shaped by its environment, entangled with others and the world. Moreover, she invites us to reflect upon our own experiences and to compare them with those of the characters we read about.

As philosopher Alva Noë (2015) suggests, drawing on the 4E perspective, art is a practice that investigates the ways we are shaped by the things we do and the worlds in which we are embedded. The purpose of art is not to 'trigger' experiences, but rather to direct our attention: to make us look closely at works of art, the world, others, and ourselves. Literary narratives are special in the way they can focus our attention to subjective experiences and entanglements of bodies, times, and spaces (the 'tunnels' and 'caves' that connect us in time and space). Woolf, especially, is a writer who creates experiential worlds, studying intersubjective relations and the subjects' embodied being in the world. Her writing teaches us that our minds extend into the world: we are tied to one another in complex ways and the past lives in the present, in one's bodily memories and in the spaces one inhabits. This also means that mental illness is not 'inside the head'. Like all experience, experiences of distress and suffering are ways of making sense of the self, the world, and others. By switching character perspectives, Woolf challenges the boundaries between 'sanity' and 'insanity' and 'normal' and 'abnormal', directing the readers' attention to the precariousness of the human mind and to the ways minds can become shattered when their scaffoldings in the world are altered—for example due to traumatic events.

Notes

1. In this, I follow David Herman (Herman 2011, 249) who has discussed the modernist portrayals of the human mind and experience as embodied by and interacting with the world—rather than turning 'inward' as is often suggested. As Herman puts it: 'Modernist writers can be viewed as [...] explorers of the lived, phenomenal worlds that emerge from, or are enacted through, the interplay between intelligent agents and their cultural as well as material circumstances' (Herman 2011, 265–66; see also Ovaska). Patricia Waugh has also discussed the way *Mrs Dalloway* undermines 'the Cartesian distinction between the objective and subjective, or inside and outside': 'In *Mrs Dalloway*, everything, including the composite self that emerges out of the connection between Clarissa and Septimus, is distributed and non-localizable; it becomes impossible to say whether thoughts, sounds, feelings, exist within or outside the mind (for even the chimes of Big Ben are carried on the atmosphere as vibrations into the very core of the body)' (Waugh 203). The understanding of Woolf as an explorer of the ways that subjects are entangled with their worlds also underscores the social and political aspects of her writing. In *Mrs Dalloway*, one of her explicit aims was, as we saw, to show the social system 'at work', and as early as in 'Modern Fiction' (1919/21) she implied the political aims of her modernism, criticizing Joyce's *Ulysses* for being 'centred in a self which, in spite of its tremor of susceptibility, never embraces or creates what is outside of itself' (Woolf 1984, 162; cf. also Scott li–lii).

2. For example, Suzette Henke (1981b) and Jesse Wolfe (2005) have written about the questions of repressed sexuality in *Mrs Dalloway*. Karen DeMeester (1998), in turn, has emphasized the trauma caused by the war. DeMeester also underlines the difference between the interpretations of Septimus as a schizophrenic and as a trauma survival: 'Critics who have diagnosed Septimus as schizophrenic […] have failed to recognize that Septimus suffers not from psychological pathology but from psychological injury' (DeMeester 653).
3. For example, Karen DeMeester (1998) has discussed trauma in *Mrs Dalloway* in relation to the ways those suffering from shell shock were stigmatized after the First World War. As Molly Hite (2010) points out, both doctors are portrayed in an extremely satirical light, inviting readers to distance themselves from them.
4. In fact, Woolf originally planned that the novel would end in Clarissa's death. See e.g. Henke 1981a; Wolfe. On Woolf's writing process, see Bonnie Kime Scott's introduction to *Mrs Dalloway* (Scott, xlvii–l).
5. For example, in Elizabeth Abel's (1989) reading Clarissa's grief is not really for Septimus but rather for herself. See also Hite 254.
6. This is also an important theme in Woolf's well-known essay 'On Being Ill' (1926), in which she writes about illness as a fundamental part of life.

References

Abbott, H. Porter, 'What Does It Mean to Be Mad? Diagnosis, Narrative, Science, and the DSM' in Robyn Warhol and Zara Dinnen (eds), *The Edinburgh Companion to Contemporary Narrative Theories* (Edinburgh: Edinburgh University Press, 2018), 17–29. https://doi.org/10.1515/9781474424752-005

Abel, Elizabeth, *Virginia Woolf and the Fictions of Psychoanalysis* (Chicago/London: University of Chicago Press, 1989).

Charon, Rita, 'Close Reading. The Signature Method of Narrative Medicine' in Rita Charon et al. (eds), *The Principles and Practice of Narrative Medicine* (New York: Oxford University Press, 2017), 157–79. https://doi.org/10.1093/med/9780199360192.003.0008

Charon, Rita, 'A Framework for Teaching Close Reading' in Rita Charon et al. (eds), *The Principles and Practice of Narrative Medicine* (New York: Oxford University Press, 2017), 180–207. https://doi.org/10.1093/med/9780199360192.003.0009

Cohn, Dorrit, *Transparent Minds: Narrative Modes for Presenting Consciousness in Fiction* (Princeton: Princeton University Press, 1978). https://doi.org/10.1515/9780691213125

Colombetti, Giovanna, 'Psychopathology and the Enactive Mind' in K. W. M. Fulford, Martin Davies, Richard G.T. Gipps, George Graham, John Z. Sadler, Giovanni Stanghellini, and Tim Thornton (eds), *The Oxford Handbook of Philosophy and Psychiatry* (Oxford: Oxford University Press, 2013), 1083–102. https://doi.org/10.1093/oxfordhb/9780199579563.013.0063

Colombetti, Giovanna, and Joel Krueger, 'Scaffoldings of the Affective Mind', *Philosophical Psychology* 28.8 (2015): 1157–76. https://doi.org/10.1080/09515089.2014.976334

DeMeester, Karen, 'Trauma and Recovery in Virginia Woolf's *Mrs Dalloway*', *MFS Modern Fiction Studies* 44.3 (1998): 649–73. https://doi.org/10.1353/mfs.1998.0062

Flint, Kate, 'Reading Uncommonly: Virginia Woolf and the Practice of Reading', *The Yearbook of English Studies* 26 (1996): 187–98. https://doi.org/10.2307/3508657

Fuchs, Thomas, 'Embodied Cognitive Neuroscience and Its Consequences for Psychiatry', *Poiesis Prax* 6 (2009): 219–33. https://doi.org/10.1007/s10202-008-0068-9

Fuchs, Thomas, 'Body Memory and the Unconscious' in Dieter Lohmar and Jagna Brudzinska (eds), *Founding Psychoanalysis Phenomenologically: Phenomenological Theory of Subjectivity and the Psychoanalytic Experience* (Dordrecht: Springer, 2012), 69–82. https://doi.org/10.1007/978-94-007-1848-7_4

Henke, Suzette A., 'Mrs Dalloway: The Communion of Saints' in Jane Marcus (ed.), *New Feminist Essays on Virginia Woolf* (Lincoln: University of Nebraska Press, 1981a), 125–47.

Henke, Suzette A., 'Virginia Woolf's Septimus Smith: An Analysis of "Paraphrenic" and Schizophrenic Use of Language', *Literature and Psychology* 31.4 (1981b): 13–23. https://doi.org/10.1007/978-1-349-05486-2_6

Herman, David, *Basic Elements of Narrative* (Chichester, UK/Malden, MA: Wiley-Blackwell, 2009). https://doi.org/10.1002/9781444305920

Herman, David, 'Re-Minding Modernism' in David Herman (ed.), *The Emergence of Mind: Representations of Consciousness in Narrative Discourse in English* (Lincoln, NE: University of Nebraska Press, 2011), 243–72. https://doi.org/10.2307/j.ctt1df4fwq

Hite, Molly, 'Tonal Cues and Uncertain Values: Affect and Ethics in *Mrs Dalloway*', *Narrative* 18.3 (2010): 249–75. https://doi.org/10.1353/nar.2010.0003

Jaspers, Karl, *General Psychopathology Vol. I–II* (Baltimore/London: The Johns Hopkins University Press, 1963).

Kuzmičová, Anežka, 'Does it Matter Where You Read? Situating Narrative in Physical Environment', *Communication Theory* 26.3 (2016): 213–347. https://doi.org/10.1111/comt.12084

Noë, Alva, *Strange Tools: Art and Human Nature* (New York: Hill & Wang, 2015).

Ovaska, Anna, *Shattering Minds: Reading Experiences of Mental Distress in Modernist Finnish Literature* (Helsinki: Finnish Literature Society, forthcoming).

Ratcliffe, Matthew, *Real Hallucinations: Psychiatric Illness, Intentionality, and the Interpersonal World* (Cambridge, MA: MIT Press, 2017). https://doi.org/10.7551/mitpress/10594.001.0001

Sass, Louis A., *Madness and Modernism: Insanity in the Light of Modern Art, Literature and Thought* (Cambridge, MA: Harvard University Press, 1994).

Scott, Bonnie Kime, 'Introduction' in Virginia Woolf, *Mrs Dalloway*, ed. by Mark Hussey (Orlando: Harcourt, 2005), xxxv–lxviii.

Varela, Francisco J., Evan Thompson, and Eleanor Rosch, *The Embodied Mind: Cognitive Science and Human Experience* (Cambridge, MA: MIT Press, 1991). https://doi.org/10.7551/mitpress/6730.001.0001

Waugh, Patricia, 'Precarious Voices: Moderns, Moods, and Moving Epochs' in David Bradshaw, Laura Marcus, and Rebecca Roach (eds), *Moving Modernisms: Motion, Technology, and Modernity* (Oxford: Oxford University Press, 2016), 191–216. https://doi.org/10.1093/acprof:oso/9780198714170.003.0014

Wolfe, Jesse, 'The Sane Woman in the Attic', *MFS Modern Fiction Studies* 51.1 (2005): 34–59. https://doi.org/10.1353/mfs.2005.0018

Woolf, Virginia, *The Diary of Virginia Woolf, Vol. 2: 1920–1924*, ed. by Andrew McNellie and Anne Olivier Bell (London: Hogarth Press, 1978).

Woolf, Virginia, 'Modern Fiction' (1919/1921) in *The Essays of Virginia Woolf, Vol. 4: 1925 to 1928*, ed. by Andrew McNeillie (London: Hogarth Press, 1984), 157–64.

Woolf, Virginia, 'Reading' in *The Essays of Virginia Woolf, Vol. 3: 1919–1924*, ed. by Andrew McNeillie (London: Hogarth Press, 1988), 141–61.

Woolf, Virginia, *Mrs Dalloway* (London: Random House, 2004 [1925]).

Woolf, Virginia, *On Being Ill* (Ashfield, MA: Paris Press, 2012 [1926]).

6 Spill the Words: Speechlessness and Creativity in the Writing of Janet Frame

Mary Elene Wood

In New Zealand writer Janet Frame's 1961 novel *Scented Gardens for the Blind*, characters struggle with speech and language. In particular, they wrestle with the difficulty of bringing traumatic experience into language, of breaking out of the isolation and suffering that accompany the silences of trauma, and of creating new languages and ways of being that can help re-establish social connections. By reading *Scented Gardens* through the lens of the writing of American psychoanalyst and memoirist Annie G. Rogers, we can begin to see that the language of schizophrenia—so often seen as meaningless by psychiatrists, an opaque symptom of brain dysfunction—can at times hold the seeds of recovery.

Both Frame and Rogers were diagnosed with schizophrenia in their youth. Janet Frame lived in New Zealand state mental institutions for eight years during the mid-twentieth century, underwent numerous electroshock treatments, and was slated for pre-frontal lobotomy before a hospital director discovered her talents as a writer (Frame 1989, 222–23).[1] The psychiatrist subsequently canceled the surgery, released her from the institution, and helped arrange a place for her to have the time and space to write. She went on to become one of New Zealand's most celebrated and admired twentieth-century writers. Annie G. Rogers spent many years in and out of American mental hospitals in the 1980s before finding psychoanalysts who helped her work through the difficulties of her traumatic past, which she survived by creating new ways of perceiving

Mary Elene Wood, 'Chapter 6: Spill the Words: Speechlessness and Creativity in the Writing of Janet Frame' in: *Madness and Literature: What Fiction Can Do for the Understanding of Mental Illness*. University of Exeter Press (2022). © Mary Elene Wood. DOI: 10.47788/ZEIP9285 within an isolated, often distressed existence. Before emerging out of psychosis, she focused her energies on translating a 'celestial language' that only she could understand (Rogers 2016, 138). She eventually re-entered the social world and its shared realities, transforming delusion into art through painting and writing.

After her long struggle with acute experiences of psychosis, Rogers went on to become a respected specialist in child and adolescent psychology, with a keen ability to parse the metaphors and meanings of language labeled psychotic (Rogers 2007, 12–13). Such language has historically usually been dismissed by American psychiatrists as the white noise of neurobiological misfirings or chemical imbalances.[2] Rogers' first book, *A Shining Affliction: A Story of Harm and Healing in Psychotherapy*, published in 1995, tells the story of her first psychotic break and her early experiences working with children in severe emotional distress. This early memoir is her best known, but it is her two later books, *The Unsayable: The Hidden Language of Trauma* (2007) and *Incandescent Alphabets: Psychosis and the Enigma of Language* (2016) that grapple most profoundly with the kinds of speech and communication struggles that Janet Frame portrays in her fiction. Using Lacanian psychoanalytic theory that, according to Rogers, speaks directly to her own experience of psychosis, Rogers finds a way to break through the isolation and often indecipherable speech of her adolescent patients. The literal enactment of linguistic forms that characterized her experience of psychosis gives way to an understanding and mastery of the figurative possibilities of speech and language. She writes, 'My language now works through metaphor. I am not literally conversing with a ghost, and this ghost is not my father's ghost, but a character I have created' (Rogers 2007, 143).

I don't wish here to present Rogers' work as theory applied to Frame's fiction. Rather, I see their writings as engaged in conversation; both Rogers, using memoir, and Frame, using the form of the (often autobiographical) novel, explore the conundrums of speech and silence that can accompany traumatic experience and profound mental and emotional distress. Within both writers' stories, trauma and the accompanying mental and emotional suffering are often labeled by psychiatrists and other clinicians as 'schizophrenia' and then viewed through the limited lenses of neurobiology and genetics. Their work intersects at the nexus of trauma and the endangered subject, for whom language and speech—the pathways of communication and connection with others—must be navigated with care, sometimes with evasion, often with silence, lest the subject be destroyed.

In this chapter, I examine the ways that both writers use language itself to show how speech is both inadequate and necessary to communicate the experiences of those living with schizophrenia. Because Rogers bases so much of her approach in Lacanian psychoanalysis, I begin with a brief overview of tensions between brain science and psychoanalysis in twentieth- and twenty-first-century understandings of mental illness. I move from there to examine the ways that Rogers and Frame explore both the failures and possibilities of speech as a pathway to human connection that can lead out of schizophrenia's isolation. I then turn to Jane Bennett's concept of 'vibrant matter' as a useful lens through which to read Frame's and Rogers' rejection of mechanistic neurobiological understandings of human consciousness. The chapter ends with an exploration of forms of creativity beyond rational speech—painting, drawing, poetry—through which those living with schizophrenia can actively shape the material world and communicate what cannot be spoken in ordinary rational discourse.

Psychoanalytic Theory, Schizophrenia, and the Limitations of Brain Science

It might seem as if the turn to brain science and genetic programming as explanations for mental illness is a fairly recent phenomenon. However, at the time Janet Frame was writing in the 1950s and early 1960s, neurological explanations of and treatments for what were considered severe mental illnesses, such as schizophrenia and manic depression (as it was called at the time), were already well on their way to displacing more psychosocial understandings of mental suffering. The use of pre-frontal lobotomy as a treatment for schizophrenia, popularized by Portuguese neurologist António Egas Moniz in the mid 1930s and performed liberally in Europe and the USA throughout the 1940s and 1950s, is itself evidence that during this period mental illness was seen as located in a defective brain. Neurologists seized on and exaggerated Sigmund Freud's fraught claim that psychoanalysis could not successfully treat psychosis, using that to shore up their descriptions of psychosis as rooted in brain disease.[3]

Yet practitioners continued to use psychoanalytic theories and methods to treat psychosis throughout the twentieth century and into the twenty-first. Harry Stack Sullivan, Frieda Fromm-Reichmann, and Gregory Bateson, to name a few important clinicians and researchers from the mid-twentieth century, are often now vilified for developing approaches that blamed the mother for schizophrenia and other psychoses; yet their theories went well beyond such simplification, exploring the psychosocial dynamics that contributed to human psychological development.[4] In a 1950 collection titled *Mid-Century Psychiatry*, based on conference proceedings from the Institute for Psychosomatic and Psychiatric Research and Training at the University of Illinois and published simultaneously in the USA, England, and Canada, one paper puts forward the promise of neurophysiology to explain human behavior while another urges psychotherapists to push psychoanalysis, while maintaining its basic theoretical tenets, beyond the framework of the Oedipus complex.

As I will show in more depth below, Annie G. Rogers found in Lacanian psychoanalysis in particular a way out of her isolating and frightening experiences of thought distortion, paranoia, and hallucination. Where neuropsychiatry would see such symptoms as meaningless in their content, mere signs of brain disease, the psychoanalytic approach of Rogers' therapist would dive straight into them, seeing their disentanglement and the re-establishment of right relations between signifier and signified as key to her recovery. In her own reading of Jacques Lacan's seminars on psychosis, especially *Seminar III: The Psychoses*, Rogers finds a framework for constructing her memoirs of illness and recovery, which explore how traumatic experience severed her from everyday social communication and how the unpacking of her language itself led her, and eventually her own psychotherapy clients, back to both art and the social world.

I do not have space here to extrapolate on Lacan's complex theory of the Imaginary and the Symbolic and their relationship to language, or to discuss how these theories emerged from Freudian psychoanalysis. My main interest here is in how Rogers was drawn to and used these ideas and how we can then read Frame's work as well through Rogers' lens, particularly as it reveals the relationship between language, creative expression, and recovery from the isolation of schizophrenia. The most important aspect of Lacan's approach for Rogers is that in psychosis the individual fails to enter the social order, an entry that should happen with the acquisition of language, when signifier and signified become divided. For example, most people know that the word 'apple' is not itself an apple and that in order for the word to lead us to the fruit that we eat, we need to be successfully embedded in a complex web of social and linguistic interactions and understandings. For the person in psychosis, the word 'apple' loses its ability to signify the fruit itself. The word loses its metaphorical status and both fruit and word become defamiliarized, frightening, uncanny. For Rogers, faulty childhood development can cause this defamiliarization and so can trauma. To return to the social world and to language as a more-or-less secure, meaningful system, the signifier must be returned to its place; speakers must once again be able to recognize themselves as not the victims of language but its wielders, as creators of metaphor and image. At the same time, for both Rogers and Frame, the person with experience of psychosis retains the trace and memory of this collapsed linguistic system, a system in which the material world reveals its liveliness. As artists and poets, these individuals can communicate to others, if partially and obliquely, the nature of this experience and this world.

The Failures of Speech as Path to Recovery

Janet Frame's novel *Scented Gardens for the Blind* begins as the story of Vera, a middle-aged woman in New Zealand whose daughter Erlene has gone silent and whose husband Edward has fled to England, abandoning his own wife and daughter in order to study obsessively the genealogy of a family unrelated to him. Ignoring the catastrophe of his daughter's complete withdrawal from language, he seeks to establish an orderly history of English descent far from his own family and the New Zealand landscape which always signifies, in Frame's fiction, both at-homeness and alienation from the imperial center. In contrast to her husband, Vera struggles to understand her daughter's withdrawal, saying, 'She was not going to speak to anyone. She could not speak if she wanted to, because every time she opened her mouth to say something, her voice, in hiding, reminded her that there was nothing to say, and no words to say it' (Frame 1980, 31). Frame's description—via Vera—of Erlene's silence resonates with Rogers' observation, based on her reading of psychoanalytic theorist Jacques Lacan, that 'In relation to unconscious questions about his existence, his very place in the world, the psychotic falters—as if he has no name, no place, in the cultural, symbolic world. That position is foreclosed, and it creates a hole, a crater, in language' (Rogers 2016, 37–38). In Frame's novel, the source of this foreclosure is Erlene's dramatic disconnection from her parents, who have turned away from her; their disconnectedness in turn arises from the ruptures and violences of history—war, genocide, imperialism, the threatened nuclear disasters of the early 1960s—specters that hover in the background throughout the novel. As in most of her novels, Frame links personal trauma to historical and intergenerational violence, oppression, and poverty. Vera reflects:

> the pent-up weight of words had fallen; the world was at last muffled by the drifting centuries of its own speech. There was no longer need or power to speak. There was only sleep left, numbness too deep for dreaming; the cellulose culture; the nerve ends permed and lacquered like unmanageable hair; there was only Death, with the everlasting words falling and melting, people and words, paper and snow, falling in great drifts, concealing tracks and roads and railway lines, cutting off communication; words falling all day and night blocking the doors of speech, and what use was it for people to proclaim themselves people […]? (Frame 1980, 235–36)

The failure of speech is not just a personal one; it is as if the world has collapsed in upon itself and communication has become impossible.

In her efforts to reach her daughter, Vera turns away from familiar language to the languages of the body and land. In the interior monologue that characterizes the greater part of *Scented Gardens for the Blind*, Vera recounts:

> So I placed before me a diagram of the human head neck and chest, drawn to scale, with the tunnels of speech and breath so gay in their scarlet lining; and ignoring the arrows darting from right and left to stab at the listed names of the blue and red and pink territory, I moved my finger, walked it along the corridor, trying to find the door into speech, but the diagram did not show it, somewhere in the rain, the book said, an impulse in the rain letting the words go free, sympathetic movement of larynx lips tongue, the shaping of breath, and even then, the book said, it may not be speech which emerges, it may only be a cry such as a bird makes or a beast lurking in the trees at night, or, loneliest of all, not the cry of a bird or beast but the first uttering of a new language which is understood by no one and nothing, and which causes a smoke screen of fear to cloud the mind, as defense against the strangeness. (Frame 1980, 10)

A peculiar strangeness emanates from the unfamiliarity of this new, emerging language, a form of speech that is not representable in medical diagrams but that comes from the body—'larynx lips tongue'—from the continuity of the human body with other living forms—'a bird or beast'—and from the land itself—'the trees at night', 'the rain'. As her absent husband searches for a distant, unconnected history and genealogy, Vera seeks with longing for a new kind of language that is alive, yet fragmented, intensely alien, causing 'a smoke screen of fear to cloud the mind'. Despite this fear, the new form of speech is potentially generative of possibility, of new 'sympathetic movement'. Fear clouds the mind but clouds bring rain, 'letting the words go free'.

Like Frame, Rogers draws attention to the generative potential of the fragmented body and the fragmented, mute subject as the very construction of a path out of silence and social disconnection. For Rogers, Lacan's version of Freud's theory of the unconscious provides a framework for understanding how the body tries to speak what ordinary language cannot hold. Rogers writes that 'we all carry unconscious traces of the body in fragments, and the body as Imaginary. We forget these early experiences, but the person who is psychotic has direct access to the Imaginary body' (Rogers 2016, 39). In Rogers' understanding, as well as in her experience as she narrates it, repressed responses to trauma make themselves heard through signifiers that have become detached from their common meanings in everyday communication. As a practitioner, Rogers learns to listen to her child and adolescent patients in a new way, just as her analyst listened to her. She writes:

> Listening for the unsayable directly required another shift in my thinking. I was used to thinking of silences as long pauses or refusals to speak about something particular. However, to hear the unsayable I had to consider *words* as revealing both a conscious narrative about experience and an unconscious one.
>
> I began to hear in a new way. Every sentence we speak is continually surrounded by what is not said and may in fact be unsayable. Ironically you can only hear the unsayable through what is *said*. I then began to underline negations, evasions, erasures, and omissions in transcripts, making notes in the margins, listening for another melody within the spoken story. (Rogers 2007, 61; italics in the original)

According to Rogers, in psychosis, language loses its ability to form social connections and in so doing takes on an 'incandescent' materiality. Because regular meanings are inadmissible in the subject's social environment, language itself has become useless as communication and transforms into form without content. In other words, letters, words, phrases become objects in themselves rather than conveyers of messages. Rogers clarifies this shift by comparing language to music:

> In psychosis, it seems that language and music change places. In the place of silently scanning words and sentences to find the meanings others also may hear and converse about, one is lost in language and sometimes cannot follow what is said. It is not possible to keep track of plausible meanings unfolding in a sentence. What then? Rather than listening to language as mute, language becomes musical, a series of sounds addressed to the listener and filled with significance. One searches in vain for a lost code that will scan, deliver meaning to language as enigma. To find such a code, one must create language, or notations, of another order. (Rogers 2016, 80–81)

In Frame's *Secret Gardens of the Blind*, the silent Erlene, Vera's daughter, thinks about language in just this way:

> With words in a language, nouns, verbs, adverbs, sentences clipped like hedges and lawns into strange shapes that surprise you in the dark? Sentences with the growth cut back; or like wild bush where there's a struggle among the plants to get first to the sun? Words which climb other words and feed upon them or blossom on them, like clematis? Dim green sentences with yellow shadows? (Frame 1980, 181)

I make the comparison here between Rogers' memoir and Frame's novel not so much in order to apply Lacan's theory of the unconscious to Frame's work, but instead to emphasize the movement both writers make towards locating recovery from psychosis in the very struggle with language and communication that often marks experiences of profound mental and emotional distress. For both writers, the intent listening to another can help move the person in distress from mute isolation to the agency of art and creation. Rogers writes, 'For the psychotic structure, incandescent alphabets carry the *jouissance* of the subject, and when they are used to make a new social link, we see a construction that is *not delusion*' (Rogers 2016, 175; italics in the original). The word 'jouissance' here refers to the pleasure, even ecstasy that artists can discover in the act of creation, if they are able to experience that act as creativity rather than as a nightmarish reality inflicted upon them from without. In a sense, according to Rogers, if those labeled psychotic can learn to see themselves as artists, as creators, assuming some degree of agency over the imaginative products that seem to appear out of nowhere, they can begin to re-enter the social world, a world in which artists produce art and poets produce poetry.

For Frame, as for Rogers, those diagnosed with psychosis are (sometimes literally) dying to be heard, to be seen, to be understood. Frame's character Vera, who, like her daughter Erlene, is labeled as psychotic, literally hammers to make herself heard: 'Lately I have found myself suddenly hammering with my fist upon the table, here, where I write this, or upon the panels of the door, as if a gesture of violence may help me to break into the silence of everything around me, to ransack and spill the words which lie trapped there' (Frame 1980, 215). Both the table and the door are social objects, the one a place where people gather and the other an entryway into social spaces. The ransacking and spilling of words becomes art to the extent that the hailing of others can here find a response.

For Frame, the approaches of psychiatry, as represented in the novel, fail in their meager, inept attempts at this intentional listening. Frame writes, through Erlene's words:

> And what about Dr. Clapper, snipping pieces of everyone and trying to fit them upon himself, wearing disguises, running in and out of people as if they had no power to resist him, as if they were water instead of walls, and why didn't he understand when Erlene tried to tell him with secret signals that people were stones and castles and prisons and it would take a bomb to get them to open the front door one inch; and that one could not so easily remove the skin of people as if their minds were buckets of boiled milk only waiting to be skimmed and skillied, adulterated, diluted, changed? (Frame 1980, 233–34)

As Rogers claims, what is needed to help someone in acute mental and emotional distress is an attuned kind of listening to the signs and signals of the body, of dreams, of fragments of speech and gesture. Attunement to such signs and signals became of less and less interest to much of psychiatry from the time of the novel's writing in 1961 up to the present day. As American psychologist Gail A. Hornstein writes in her book *Agnes's Jacket*:

> Simplistic theories of chemical imbalances and the rote administration of toxic and often ineffective drugs make little sense as ways of understanding or responding to the intense fear or anguish that lead patients to seek help. But should psychiatrists' lack of imagination continue to constrain our own thinking? (Hornstein 274)

Consciousness as Vibrant Materiality

While there are many similarities between Rogers' view and Frame's in *Scented Gardens for the Blind*, I don't want to obscure some important differences. While Rogers' writing is firmly grounded in psychoanalytic theory, which is firmly focused on the human psyche, Frame's novel resists being subsumed within a human-centered model of conscious and unconscious mind. In Frame's world, the New Zealand landscape and the material objects and beings that inhabit it have a sentience and substance beyond the parameters of the human mind. Erlene and Vera create a new language not only from the stuff of the fragmented body and subject, but from that of the living, breathing matter that surrounds them. Vera cries out:

> Oh, I must urge the furniture to speak, and the walls, and the trees; my clothes, my food, all objects must speak; it is a panic; anything to drown the final silence of the human race! What use is the silence? Even now as I look out of the windows I can see the mounds of rotting words, the foul steam arising from them as, like compost, they generate their own fertile vapors and powers ... you see? There is no end, growth must emerge from them, perhaps I too shall walk all over the land scattering the dead words upon the soil and watching for the plants which grow from them, all the new trees which will shelter us from the sun and the fires in the sky. It is a new Eden: the growth of articulate speech from the silence that fell like a shroud upon the language. (Frame 1980, 216)

Such a vision reverberates with Jane Bennett's descriptions of a vital materialism in *Vibrant Matter: A Political Ecology of Things* (2010), where she proposes that '*All* forces and flows (materialities) are or can become lively, affective, and signaling. And so an affective, speaking human body is not *radically* different from the affective, signaling nonhumans with which it coexists, hosts, enjoys, serves, consumes, produces, and competes' (Bennett 117).

This vibrant materiality pervades Frame's novel, as in the passage above. Vera reflects, 'I have stroked the furniture, touching it gently as an archaeologist may caress a newly discovered piece of stone knowing that in the end if it is cared for, it will give up its secret, it will speak its language to him' (Frame 1980, 215) and, later, she listens for 'the true sound rising at last from ice and marshland, ancient rock and stone' (Frame 1980, 227).

To read Frame's words through the lens of Bennett's 'vibrant matter' is not just imposing a contemporary theoretical approach onto a mid-twentieth-century text. Psychological researchers from this period were also interested in what they saw as the psychobiological reverberations between the human organism and its environment. Anthropologist and psychologist Gregory Bateson in particular was interested in the embeddedness of humans in a myriad web of influences that ranged from creatures and things in the nonhuman world to internal bodily processes. Bateson wrote that 'the individual mind is immanent but not only in the body. It is immanent also in pathways and messages outside the body; and there is a larger Mind of which the individual mind is only a sub-system' (G. Bateson 468). Bateson's daughter Mary Catherine Bateson remarked that her father was interested in 'the pattern which connects all living things, recognizing in our own mental processes of thought and learning a pattern which connects us to the biosphere rather than an argument for separation' (M.C. Bateson 21).

Other critics have noted the importance of material objects in *Scented Gardens for the Blind*, yet they primarily see the material world as threatening, an intrusion of outside reality into Vera's protected inner realm. Andreia Sarabando claims that 'the relationship between human bodies and inanimate things is stressed and represented as hostile, the surroundings of the character both setting her mood and embodying her feelings' (Sarabando 608). For Vera, 'that which surrounds her is felt as threatening because it is free of the disciplinary authority of the eye and of the hand' (Sarabando 608). Sarabando offers good evidence for this claim, citing Vera's view of 'the terrible flowing and surrounding' that emanates from the things around her (cited in Sarabando 608).[5] Sarabando's reading is convincing, but at the same time I would say that this 'terrible flowing and surrounding' contains possibility as well as threat. These objects represent a terrifying breakdown of order and boundaries, yet they also embody hope for a new kind of language, a new communicative power.

Yet it would be hard to deny that Frame leaves us with questions about the sources of creative power that in *Scented Gardens for the Blind* can provide a way forward out of delusion, social isolation, and emotional distress. At the end of the novel, we suddenly discover that it is actually Vera, Erlene's mother, who has been silent for thirty years, locked inside a mental institution with no outward signs of recovery. She has no daughter, no husband, no family.

While vibrant matter pervades the novel, we find that it has been brought into being only through Vera's imagination, an imagination that has been locked in silence for decades, with almost no visible connection to the external world. And yet, paradoxically, the reader has been drawn into this world as if it were real, has met its characters, has felt its raw emotions.

Not knowing until the end that the whole story was in Vera's mind in a sense tricks the reader into seeing Vera as a sane and perceptive narrator, before the stigma of institutionalization and diagnosis have a chance to take hold. The reader sees Vera as a storyteller like any other, if only she can find someone to listen to her story. Frame thus underscores the possibility, put forth by Rogers as well, that the creative powers at work in extreme mental distress—what gets labeled in clinical settings as psychotic delusion—can be transformed into art embedded in a social world. Crucial to this transformation is the active participation of a listener, someone who hears the hammering on the table or at the door and believes that the silent or incomprehensible subject has a story to tell and a wholly original way to tell it.

At the same time, Frame pushes beyond Rogers' idea that psychotic delusion can transform into art or poetry, suggesting that maybe there is, after all, sentience in the table, the wall, the black beetle that crawls along the ledge. The risk here is twofold. On the one hand such a suggestion runs into the danger of conflating madness with creativity, a move that Frame has elsewhere deplored as simplistic and ignorant of the suffering and banality that usually go along with diagnosed mental illness.[6] On the other hand, such an assertion risks returning Vera to the madhouse in the reader's mind, reconstructing her as an example of psychosis whose language holds no meaning in the social world. Yet I would suggest that Frame successfully walks the tightrope between those two damning possibilities. Several decades earlier than Bennett, Janet Frame created characters who, yes, have been traumatized by both historical and personal experiences, but whose vision of and words about the sentience of matter nonetheless come across as more than a symptom of psychosis. These characters offer us, rather, philosophy, presented, developed, and argued (as Bennett presents, develops, and argues similar ideas) before the reader knows that Vera is in a mental hospital. Frame thus forces her reader to see Vera as philosopher rather than madwoman, and thus to consider her thoughts about the vibrancy of the material world as a rethinking of the nature of matter rather than as the ravings of madness or even as metaphors for an unbalanced, divided psyche.

Creativity and Mind as Matter

If we read Rogers' memoirs back through Frame's character of Vera, we can recognize anew Rogers' own penchant for assigning power to the material presence of words even after she has undergone transformation from psychotic to artist and poet. Rogers develops this understanding of the sentience and vibrancy of material things in the chapters of *Incandescent Alphabets* that focus on art by people in mental institutions throughout history. Here she presents most of the artworks as unknowable yet powerful and often beautiful. Of a painting by Dwight Mackintosh, she writes, 'Above these intricate figures the text floats, word-like and unreadable. In this image I read, again, the incandescent alphabets of an Imaginary body; a new language of seeing, drawing, and considering what it is to be human' (Rogers 2016, 68). She does not deconstruct this creative work with psychoanalytic interpretations, or if she does, it's only in the most minimal way. She respects its opacity as well as the power of its materials and techniques.

And this is perhaps a path to treatment as well, this respect for the at times unreadable presence of the art itself. At The Lavender Door, an art studio connected to Austen Riggs Center in Stockbridge, Massachusetts (a psychiatric treatment center based in psychotherapy), the space is designated as an 'interpretation free zone' where residents attend workshops, learn from working artists, and create their own artworks, without being pressured to have these works analyzed or 'read' for truths about their mental and emotional state (Beatty).

Recent explorations of the relationship between creativity and mental illness call attention to both the therapeutic value of artistic expression and the dangers of seeing artwork by 'the mentally ill' as a window into a troubled soul. Daniel Wojcik points out the following in *Outsider Art: Visionary Worlds and Trauma*:

> Art therapy was in some ways sparked by the work of Morgenthaler and Prinzhorn, both of whom emphasized the value of the patients' work *as* art and as genuine aesthetic ability and accomplishment. Advocates of art brut and outsider art were similarly influenced by Prinzhorn and Morgenthaler, with the focus on the artistry and authenticity of the mentally ill person's work, not on the therapeutic value of the creative process. (Wojcik 59)

Hans Prinzhorn (1886–1933) was a psychiatrist and art historian at the University of Heidelberg's psychiatric clinic who collected the art of patients diagnosed with psychoses. Walter Morgenthaler is the author of *A Psychiatric Patient as Artist* (1921), which focused on the art of his patient Adolf Wölfli. Both commentators troubled the assumption that art created by those in mental institutions or with a diagnosis of mental illness was somehow a different kind of art, an art that could give the viewer access to a different kind of mind, the mentally ill mind. It is precisely this assumption that Frame counters by hiding Vera's status as mental patient, and that Rogers counters by declining to interpret paintings in the light of the artists' diagnoses.

Artist Susan Aldworth came up against the conundrum of how to think about creativity and the diagnosis of mental illness when she created the Reassembling the Self exhibit at the Waterside Arts Centre in Manchester in 2015 (originally at the Hatton Gallery in Newcastle in 2012). As artist in residence at Newcastle University's Institute of Neuroscience, Aldworth worked with two artists living with schizophrenia—Camille Ormston and Kevin Mitchinson—to create this exhibit based on their work. While living with schizophrenia and its distorted perceptions is central to the exhibit itself, Aldworth walks a fine line (successfully, I would say) between presenting the two artists as interesting precisely because they are living with schizophrenia and insisting that they are artists first, who have a unique ability to portray the material disruptions and interconnections among mind–brain–body–self.

For Aldworth, as for Frame and Rogers, it is not the supposed fact of mental illness that makes these artists worthy of attention but their particular insight, as artists, into the material nature of body, brain, and consciousness and the connectedness of these elements to other forms of matter. Aldworth herself states in an interview with *Mancunion* that, after having a brain scan for a suspected hemorrhage, she realized, 'This brain landscape was worth exploring as an artist. And also, the imagery of the scans was uniquely beautiful. It left me wondering what is human consciousness? How is it summoned up from the 3 pounds or so of flesh of the brain?' (quoted in Rofman). Like Janet Frame, Aldworth and her co-exhibitors explore the materiality of consciousness; her use of the phrase 'brain landscape' betrays the sense that the brain is matter like other matter out beyond the body, that the brain has contours as does the land. To live with schizophrenia, as do her collaborators Ormston and Mitchinson, is to live with the enigma of the material brain, an enigma best explored and expressed through creative expression that always butts up against the unsayable.

Frame's novel and Rogers' memoirs, read in light of one another, offer the creative expression of those struggling with psychoses (whether artwork, writing, or just spoken language) as both a pathway to communication and a gesture of glowing opacity, a testament to the power of creativity to move both artist and viewer/reader/listener beyond the limitations of ordinary language without sacrificing human connection. Read this way, the creative expressions of those labeled mad or psychotic gesture towards the social world and may even offer hidden keys to more direct communication, to stories of trauma and other forms of suffering—yet they may also offer just themselves, their power, beauty, and luminosity.

Notes

1. In 1989, Braziller published *An Autobiography*, which compiled Frame's three autobiographical volumes *To the Is-Land* (1982), *An Angel at my Table* (1984), and *Envoy from Mirror City* (1985). For further discussion of the often elusive relationship between Frame's novels and autobiographical work, see Ash; Mercer; King; and Unsworth.
2. Studies of language use by patients diagnosed with schizophrenia tend to look to impaired brain structures and functions as the primary cause. See, for example, Kuperberg, who refers to the mostly widely accepted causes as 'abnormalities in the structure and function of semantic memory' and 'general executive function deficits'.
3. See my discussion of Freud and psychosis in Wood 2013.
4. See Sullivan; G. Bateson; and Fromm-Reichmann.
5. See also Wevers.
6. See Frame 1982, 112: 'There is an aspect of madness which is seldom mentioned in fiction because it would damage the romantic popular idea of the insane as a person whose speech appeals as immediately poetic; but it is seldom the easy Opheliana recited like the pages of a seed catalog or the outpourings of Crazy Janes who provide, in fiction, an outlet for poetic abandon.'

References

Ash, Susan, '"The Absolute, Distanced Image": Janet Frame's Autobiography', *Journal of New Zealand Literature* 11 (1993): 21–39.

Bateson, Gregory, *Steps to an Ecology of Mind: Collected Essays in Anthropology, Psychiatry, Evolution, and Epistemology* (Chicago: University of Chicago Press, 2000 [1972]). https://doi.org/10.7208/chicago/9780226924601.001.0001

Bateson, Mary Catherine, 'Angels Fear Revisited: Gregory Bateson's Cybernetic Theory of Mind Applied to Religion-Science Debates' in Jesper Hoffmeyer (ed.), *A Legacy for Living Systems: Gregory Bateson as Precursor to Biosemiotics* (Dordrecht: Springer, 2008). https://doi.org/10.1007/978-1-4020-6706-8_2

Beatty, Aaron, 'Art in our Midst', *Austen Riggs Center Webpage*, 14 January 2014, www.austenriggs.org/blog-post/art-our-midst, accessed 15 December 2020.

Bennett, Jane, *Vibrant Matter: A Political Ecology of Things* (Durham, NC: Duke University Press, 2010). https://doi.org/10.1215/9780822391623

Frame, Janet, *Faces in the Water* (New York: George Braziller Inc., 1982 [1961]).

Frame, Janet, *Scented Gardens for the Blind* (New York: George Braziller Inc., 1980 [1963]).

Frame, Janet, *An Autobiography* (New York: George Braziller Inc., 1989).

Fromm-Reichmann, F., *Principles of Intensive Psychotherapy* (Chicago: University of Chicago Press, 1960). https://doi.org/10.7208/chicago/9780226221274.001.0001

Hornstein, Gail A., *Agnes's Jacket: A Psychologist's Search for the Meanings of Madness* (New York: Rodale, 2009).

King, Michael, *Wrestling with the Angel: A Life of Janet Frame* (Auckland, NZ: Viking, 2000).

Kuperberg, Gina R., 'Language in Schizophrenia Part 1: An Introduction', *Lang Linguist Compass* 4.8 (2010): 576–89. https://doi.org/10.1111/j.1749-818X.2010.00216.x

Lacan, Jacques, *The Psychoses: The Seminar of Jacques Lacan, Book III (1955–1956)*, ed. by J.-A. Miller, trans. by R. Grigg (New York: Norton, 1997).

Mercer, Gina, '"A Simple Everyday Glass": The Autobiographies of Janet Frame', *Journal of New Zealand Literature* 11 (1993): 41–47.

Rofman, Roberta, 'Reassembling the self: The art of schizophrenia', *Mancunion*, 25 February (2015), https://mancunion.com/2015/02/25/reassembling-the-self-the-art-of-schizophrenia/, accessed 2 May 2022.

Rogers, Annie G., *A Shining Affliction: A Story of Harm and Healing in Psychotherapy* (New York: Penguin, 1995).

Rogers, Annie G., *The Unsayable: The Hidden Language of Trauma* (New York: Ballantine Books, 2007).

Rogers, Annie G., *Incandescent Alphabets: Psychosis and the Enigma of Language* (London: Karnac Books, 2016).

Sarabando, Andreia, '"The dreadful mass neighbourhood of objects" in the Fiction of Janet Frame', *Journal of Postcolonial Writing* 51.5 (2015): 603–14. https://doi.org/10.1080/17449855.2015.1072888

Sullivan, H.S., *Schizophrenia as a Human Process* (New York: Norton, 1962). https://doi.org/10.1080/17449855.2015.1072888

Unsworth, Jane, 'A Reflection on Theories of Autobiography with Reference to the Work of Janet Frame' in Julia Swindells (ed.), *The Uses of Autobiography* (London: Taylor & Francis, 1995), 13–24.

Wevers, Lydia, 'Self Possession: "Things" and Janet Frame's Autobiography' in Jan S. Cronin and Simone Drichel (eds), *Frameworks: Contemporary Criticism on Janet Frame* (New York: Rodopi Press, 2009), 51–65.

Wojcik, Daniel, *Outsider Art: Visionary Worlds and Trauma* (Mississippi: University Press of Mississippi, 2016).

Wood, Mary Elene, *Life Writing and Schizophrenia: Encounters at the Edge of Meaning* (New York: Rodopi Press, 2013). https://doi.org/10.1163/9789401209434

7 Pronominal Shifts and the Confusion of Self with Not-Self

Alice Hervé

Notable among the challenges of representing madness in literature are the two prerequisites of clarity and plausibility. For while literature has the ability to portray incoherent events and emotions, and to feature so-called mad characters, mad narrators, and illogical actions and assumptions, the creative writer must also construct personalities and domains that are credible and comprehensible. This study examines persistent and widespread methodologies that facilitate the portrayal of madness in fiction—principally in first-person fiction—and directs attention to their credibility, or authenticity, and the ways in which they may further our understanding of actual mental distress. In particular, comparisons will be made with applicable data from select psychopathological research in order to suggest how theories of anomalous self-experience provide a valuable analytical focus with which to examine the literature of madness.

Like literature itself, literary madness is wide-ranging, and may include neuroses, psychoses, and countless other categories of psychologically aberrant behaviour. Nevertheless, there are identifiable narrative devices and stylistic techniques that can overcome the problems of depicting mental distress in fiction, and these mechanisms and strategies have been disseminated and are replicated, albeit in different forms, in a wide variety of literary works. One widespread and persistent device for articulating a sense of alienation is the pronominal shift—the substitution of one pronoun for another in a way that is inappropriate, or bizarre. By replacing a first-person singular voice with first person plural, or with second or third, while retaining the original focalization, this mechanism functions to simply and coherently signpost a character's alienation. In relation to the theme of diminished selfhood (or to the term *ipseity disturbance* proposed by Louis Sass), compare the clinical record of a prodromal schizophrenic patient who stated: 'my I is disappearing' (Sass and Parnas 438).

As a notable literary example of the pronominal shift, Margaret Atwood's 1969 novel, *The Edible Woman*, features an unambiguous illustration. The disaffected narrator, Marian, slips out of first person and into third for more than half the novel. First-person narration is not re-established until the final pages, when she is said to be 'back to so-called reality' and announcing unequivocally that she has been restored to 'the first person singular' (Atwood 1983, 281, 278). The two stages of the pronominal shift here—one into third person and one out again—are bold and effective, and the sudden changeover of the narrative point of view is an unmistakable ploy to accentuate the protagonist's alienation. The focalizer throughout the novel is Marian—that is to say that the reader retains a privileged insight into her thought processes, only the point of view changes from first person to third.

The confusion of self with not-self is another notable technique that is capable of meeting the requirements of both clarity and authenticity, and conforms to the sort of self-anomalies that come under the umbrella of ipseity disturbances. A loss of subjectivity can diverge in many different fictional directions. Parts of the body, perceptions, actions, and attributes may be described as objectified, alien, or otherwise apart, so that in effect there are many variations on this theme, all capable of portraying a sense of a misplaced or misrecognized sense of being. These include the symbolic displacement of madness into doubles, mirror images, and even inanimate objects. However, these fractured identities need not necessitate a reflection or a secondary manifestation; they can also be represented by an assumption of the body as a thing deteriorating, splintering, or disintegrating. Darian Leader claims, in his extensive study of madness, that 'the disintegration of the body is common in psychosis', and several literary texts employ a symbolic level of fragmentation to represent this kind of psychic alienation (Leader 45).

One of the most emblematic devices employed to suggest a loss of ego boundaries is the specular image. A reflection is simultaneously alike and altered, and the idea of self/other is frequently played out in fiction in front of a reflective surface. The mirror is a space of 'you or me', as Leader himself emphasizes, and 'mirror situations can be of great danger both for the psychotic subject and to those around them' (Leader 313). Profound ontological insecurity, self-estrangement, and depersonalization can be expressed in this way. Perhaps this is why, for many literary psychotics, the mirror is envisaged as a trap. 'I reverse the mirror so it's toward the wall', says the narrator of Margaret Atwood's *Surfacing*, 'it no longer traps me' (Atwood 1972, 137).

First-Person Narratives

Pronominal shifts and the confusion of self with not-self most commonly feature in first-person fictions, most notably in texts where homodiegetic or autodiegetic narrators necessitate long passages of the vocalized or interiorized mad voice. I use Gérard Genette's classifications here. Homodiegetic narration is where the narrator is also a character in the story world, and autodiegetic narration is where the narrator is the chief protagonist (Genette 245). These first-person narratives typically involve two related perspectives—the experiencing agent and the narrating agent—and as Ansgar Nünning has noted, 'since the first-person narrator remembers what the narrated I knew, experienced, thought, and felt, the character perspective of the experiencing I is embedded in the cognitive domain of the narrating I' (Nünning 218). There may be spatiotemporal distancing, but essentially any distortions or limitations in this cognitive domain will be shared. If the exposition of madness in these texts is constructed in a way that is too comprehensible, it may not convey to the reader an impression of authentic character or narrative, and if it is made to seem authentic (inarticulate or frenzied), it may not be comprehensible. Hence the necessity to balance authenticity with lucidity is amplified in these first-person texts.

Exacerbating this difficulty is the impediment of language. For while writers cannot communicate without words, the mad, frequently, cannot communicate with them. Since psychosis severs the conceptual links needed for conventional social interaction, the mad voice does not necessarily say what it means or mean what it says, and common parameters of meaning are frequently altered or ignored. The authentic voice of the mad narrator is therefore inevitably unreliable; it is also potentially inarticulate. In narratives which contain long passages of monologic prose, devices for representing madness without compromising coherence are particularly valuable.

Throughout history, it has been the fate of the mad to be subjugated, censored, and sometimes deliberately misheard. Roy Porter described this as the 'oblivion or erasure of the voices of the mad' (Porter 235). The categories of first-person fictions that habitually ask the reader to engage with character as much as or more than story or discourse can open up avenues of understanding around a mad character that are not so easily traversed in actual encounters. They can take the bizarre and the incoherent and weave a pattern with it that, if not entirely rational, is at least comprehensible, and they can give madness back its voice. But before looking at literary examples, I would like to examine some of the authenticated indicators of madness that translate well into first-person narratives, and provide a useful analytical focus.

Clinical Evidence of Anomalous Self-Experience

The pronominal shift, as noted, involves the substitution of one pronoun for another in a way that is bizarre or incongruous. This is not to say that inappropriate use of pronouns is in itself a sign of psychosis. In the United Kingdom it is not unusual for people of a certain rank and standing to speak of their singular selves in the plural. However, changing pronouns without changing focalization as a signifier of madness is a phenomenon with a medical, as well as a literary, history. Allan Ingram writes of an eighteenth-century patient, Hannah Allen, who moved 'disconcertingly between a first and third person narrative' (Ingram 29); and R.D. Laing recorded a patient in the twentieth century who suffered 'a confusion of self with not-self', and spoke of herself 'in the first, second, or third person' (Laing 196). In a more recent example, Josef Parnas records the case of a schizophrenic patient who stated 'my first-personal life has been lost and is replaced by a third-person perspective' (Parnas 223).

Schizophrenic disorders, in particular, are known to involve profound alterations of mental states, and changes in the experience of subjectivity. Sass and Parnas have argued that schizophrenia can best be understood as a self-disorder, or ipseity disturbance. They describe ipseity as 'the experiential sense of being a vital and self-coinciding *subject* of experience or *first-person perspective on the world*' (Sass and Parnas 428; italics in the original). An ipseity disturbance is double-faceted, they suggest, with two fundamental and complementary components: hyperreflexivity and diminished self-affection. The first involves self-alienation, where the subject may experience itself as an external object; and the second is characterized by a diminishment of self-presence—that is to say in 'the implicit sense of existing as a vital and self-possessed subject of awareness', to the point of believing that actions, feelings, and thoughts are 'under the control of some alien force' (Sass and Parnas 428, 431).

Later research examined the extent to which depersonalization disorder (DPD), a condition quite distinct from schizophrenia because it is non-psychotic, could be characterized by analogous forms of diminished selfhood. The research concluded that there were important parallels, and that depersonalization encompassed some, but not all, of the 'self-anomalies' seen in schizophrenia (Sass et al. 432). The advantage of being a writer of fiction is that symptoms need only be suggestive of madness in a very general sense. There is no need to classify them as schizophrenia, DPD, or any other category of mental distress. It is not even necessary to engage in the debate about whether diagnoses can pick out discrete diseases at all. It is pointless to speak of literary characters as if they were real people, or to expect literary madness to follow the precise swerves and curves of medical reports. It is rare, in fact, for an author to proffer a diagnosis, and quite common to encounter a surprising amount of comorbidity.

Nevertheless, clinical descriptions of ipseity disturbances—where phenomena that are usually experienced subjectively are instead experienced either with no distinction between subject and object, or entirely objectively—can help to explain why devices such as the pronominal shift and the confusion of self with not-self can be effective signifiers of madness in literature, as well as offering ways of understanding some aspects of mental distress itself. It is of interest, therefore, that patients in the abovementioned 2013 study experienced indicators of depersonalization that included 'identity confusion', 'distorted first-person perspective', 'ontological anxiety', 'morphological change', 'mirror-related phenomena', 'psychophysical misfit or incongruence', 'feelings of extraordinary creative power or insight', and a sense of 'bodily disintegration' (Sass et al. 435). These characteristics are also manifest in the literatures of madness.

Literary Evidence of Diminished Selfhood

Margaret Atwood's 1972 novel *Surfacing* proposed that madness is 'only an amplification of what you already are' (Atwood 1972, 80). In *Alias Grace*, published twenty-four years later, she wrote, 'when you go mad you don't go any other place, you stay where you are. And somebody else comes in' (Atwood 1997, 37). These two disparate views—albeit from the same author—exemplify the sort of diversity that literary madness encompasses and even embraces. The fictional examples in this study are numerous in order to demonstrate the persistence and pervasiveness of indicators of madness, similar to those evident in the clinical research cited above (although all of them predate it).

As well as being confirmed by the empirical evidence, shifting pronouns as a narrative technique has a robust fictional history as an indicator of the disaffected psyche. Literary custom, rather than medical research, is often a determining factor with such categories of symptomatology. Pronoun displacement is, after all, a familiar practice for an author who, as Maurice Blanchot observed in *The Space of Literature*, inevitably moves 'from the first to the third person' whenever they write (Blanchot 133). An early example of a slippage of perspective can be found in the novel *Clarissa*. This eighteenth-century epistolary work by Samuel Richardson is narrated primarily through the letters of the eponymous heroine. When grief and despair overwhelm her, she is provoked amidst her otherwise first-person ramblings to declare: 'How art thou humbled in the dust, thou proud Clarissa Harlowe' (S. Richardson 891)—thereby moving the narration into the second person, if only briefly.

In the German novel *Die Blechtrommel*, translated into English as *The Tin Drum*, Günter Grass employs an unusual slant on pronoun shifting by moving the dialogue into dramatic form within a chapter of first-person narration. Oskar Matzerath, the clairaudient, drum-playing, growth-restricted protagonist, is the unreliable narrator of his own story, told from a mental hospital. He refers to himself in the second and third person and inserts a lengthy dramatic scene into the narrative as he becomes 'accustomed to the theatrical style' (Grass 322). For several pages the reader is treated to what is ostensibly a play. Oskar's insanity may be questionable since the novel is part political allegory and part magic realism, but his many slippages of perspective are undoubtedly there to indicate a volatile mental state.

The Yellow Wallpaper, by Charlotte Perkins Gilman—an influential text in the literature of madness—depicts a woman suffering from a 'nervous condition', one that nowadays is generally acknowledged to represent postnatal depression, who has been locked into a room with barred windows and denied all mental stimulation to the point where she loses her mind. 'I cry at nothing, and cry most of the time', she says, feeling bereft in spite of delivering 'such a dear baby' (Gilman 6, 3).

This text features an adaptation of the pronominal shift; for in spite of the fact that the protagonist persists with first-person narration, there is an unmistakable cognitive shift brought about through a skilful succession of substituted pronouns. The 'she' of the creeping woman behind the wallpaper—a manifest double of the narrator—becomes the 'they' of the many creeping women, and finally the 'I' of the creeping narrator, who, after tearing all the paper from the walls, announces: 'I've got out at last' (Gilman 15).

In Gilman's story, the fractured identity of the narrator is deliberately confused or conflated with an inorganic double, for madness is deflected from the protagonist on to the frenzied configurations of the wallpaper. This allows the narrative to remain coherent without losing a sense of authenticity. 'It is getting to be a great effort for me to think straight', the protagonist announces, and yet she continues to narrate her tale with the utmost lucidity, even when the patterns are 'torturing', and her observation of the 'lame uncertain curves' causes them to 'suddenly commit suicide' (Gilman 7, 9, 3). The wallpaper mirrors the narrator's psychosis, and even suggests the trajectory of her ultimate collapse, but the narrative voice does not falter in its description. The self-proclaimed confusion is relocated from the spoken word to the visual image, where the not-self mirrors the self and permits authentic incoherence. Interestingly, Günter Grass revisits Gilman's method in *The Tin Drum*, as his narrator Oskar surrenders himself to 'the madness of the wallpaper, the vertical, horizontal, diagonal madness' (Grass 478).

The place where the 'I' starts and the 'I' ends can be deliberately obscured in order to represent the fragmentation of mental processes. Frequently a variety of methods are employed together to enforce a sense of dislocation and identity confusion. These conceptual adaptations ultimately belong to the same thematic scheme—the notion that the self is not a stable, concrete entity and can be confused with the not-self or dissipate into a recognition of no-self. 'My mind is apart from my body', claims a patient with DPD, and this sort of psychic depersonalization is invaluable to the literatures of madness (Sass et al. 435). A character might express a sense of their own otherness, where mind and body seem to inhabit different realms of existence, as in Patrick McGrath's novel *Spider*, where the autodiegetic narrator relates his perception of a disintegrating subjectivity. 'I lose the easy, fluid sense of being-in-the-body that I once had', he claims, 'the linkage of brain and limb is a delicate mechanism, and often, now, for me, it becomes uncoupled' (McGrath 10).

Accurate fictional representations of the world as envisaged by the psychotic mind can be exceedingly perplexing to a reader, but the loss of being-in-the-body, as described by Spider, is a common accompaniment to fever and severe physical malaise. It is a readily coherent version of the alienated mind. Nevertheless, Spider's alienation and his sense of morphological change intensify as the novel progresses. He has fingers that seem 'not to belong' to him at all; and he acquires a 'two-head system', where the front of his head is 'what I used with other people in the house', the back 'was for when I was alone' (McGrath 13, 98). The protagonist, who we are told is named Dennis, adopts Spider as 'his real name'; it is the one he writes in faeces on the walls of the asylum. He also refers to himself in the third person, notably in times of extreme tension: 'will you stop your old Spider climbing onto a broken chair, with the loose end slipped through the ring to form a noose?' (McGrath 219).

Margaret Atwood's *Surfacing*

In terms of demonstrating the literary equivalence of some of the symptomatology recorded in the 2013 study by Sass and his colleagues, Margaret Atwood's novel *Surfacing* is paradigmatic. To reiterate, these included 'identity confusion', a 'distorted first-person perspective', 'ontological anxiety', 'morphological change', 'mirror-related phenomena', 'psychophysical misfit or incongruence', 'feelings of extraordinary creative power or insight', and a sense of 'bodily disintegration' (Sass et al. 435). *Surfacing* describes a state of breakdown and the descent into a mad state, and the autodiegetic narrator, a Canadian woman, a graphic artist, is in denial about the aborting of a child some years before: 'I'd carried that death around inside me, layering it over, a cyst, a tumour, a black pearl'; she distances herself from herself, because her feelings of culpability are too distressing: 'I couldn't accept it, that mutilation, ruin I'd made, I needed a different version' (Atwood 1972, 112, 111).

Part of this revisioning of her world is through language. 'I wanted to be whole', she says, but 'first I had to immerse myself in the other language'; and this disconnect from her known languages is a form of *identity confusion* at the most basic of levels, for she cannot recognize English or French, her native idioms, 'as any language I've ever heard' (Atwood 1972, 113, 122, 143). There is the sense that the words mean something—they are recognizable as language—but the conceit is that they no longer mean anything to the character, as if they belonged to another self entirely. Ferdinand de Saussure once wrote that 'without language, thought is a vague, uncharted nebula' (Saussure 112). A narrator articulating an inability to connect with words is uniquely self-contradictory; they may be lost in uncharted space, but they are still managing to communicate their predicament. Literary madness, even when it is alleged to involve a rupture with language and reason, must be portrayed both logically and linguistically.

One of the ways in which this is achieved in *Surfacing* is by suggesting a disrupt with language without actually disrupting the language to any great extent; so, for example, an abundance of commas fracture the grammatical flow to suggest a fragmented cognitive state. In her biography of Margaret Atwood, Nathalie Cooke relates the story of an industrious copy-editor who endeavoured to cull these commas. The author put them back. The overuse of punctuation was an intentional ploy, used to suggest an irrational 'state of mind' (Cooke 177). The narrator remonstrates with herself over the 'mirages raised by words', while reciting the nonsense mantra 'love conquers all, conquerors love all' (Atwood 1972, 128). These repetitions give a sense of disengagement between enunciation and association—a dislocation between sign and signified—without losing clarity. 'Language divides us into fragments', the narrator of *Surfacing* says, and indeed her fragmentation is swift and severe, but it is related with utmost coherence (Atwood 1972, 113). The disruption of language norms is another interpretation of the theme of confusion of self and not-self. The words are there—written, spoken—but there is a disconnect from the 'I' that comprehends them: the 'I' who is stable and concrete and known.

The pronominal shift is only fleetingly applied in this novel and never in the overt manner of Atwood's earlier work, *The Edible Woman*. 'I stay unmoving, don't give yourself away', the narrator says in one brief lapse into second person; and at another point the action moves from a focal 'I' to an objectifying 'it': 'My hand touched his arm. Hand touched arm', she says (Atwood 1972, 144, 113). The indications of *a distorted first-person perspective* are chiefly apparent in other forms. The narrator announces that she has come 'apart', was 'cut in two', and has discovered that 'the other half, the one locked away, was the only one that could live: I was the wrong half, detached, terminal' (Atwood 1972, 85). In a sense, she is living in her own double. This alternative manifestation of self appears to have certain advantages, notably *extraordinary insight*—'the power flowed into my eyes', she claims, 'I could see into him'—but it is, nevertheless, also acknowledged to be defective: 'from any rational point of view I am absurd', she proclaims, 'but there are no longer any rational points of view' (Atwood 1972, 118, 132). The sense of *psychophysical misfit* increases gradually, with the protagonist unable to connect with her own voice: 'it came from someone dressed as me, imitating me'; and dissociation escalates, until she appears completely alienated from her physical self: 'when I am clean', she says, 'I come up out of the lake, leaving my false body floated on the surface' (Atwood 1972, 84, 139). Physical metamorphosis is not only experienced by the narrator; it also infiltrates her worldview, for she describes the other characters 'turning to metal', while her partner unzips 'his human skin'; and her own sense of *bodily disintegration* and *morphological change* reaches a pitch when she states: 'I am not an animal or a tree, I am the thing in which the trees and animals move and grow, I am a place' (Atwood 1972, 123, 125, 141).

'I no longer have a name', the narrator of *Surfacing* says, from the depths of her psychological crisis, but in fact she has been unnamed from the start (Atwood 1972, 132). This, it could be argued, is an emblematic sign of depersonalization, particularly when it is explicitly signalled in the text. It suggests a perception of not so much not-self, as no-self. Names are often used as anchoring devices in first-person fiction, allowing the reader to engage with a character in a more compelling way. That is why a reader may feel wrong-footed by not knowing the protagonist's name; and the sense of a character's alienation is intensified by such an open acknowledgement of dissociation. An early, if momentary lapse into this state can be found in Richardson's *Clarissa*, where the eponymous heroine, at a low point, declares, 'my name is—I don't know what my name is' (S. Richardson 890). When used overtly, refusing to name a character, or otherwise distancing them from their name through aliases or amnesia, can imbue a sense of *ontological anxiety* and is a method noteworthy in several texts of madness.

Another common authorial anchoring tool is also reworked effectively in some of the literatures of madness. That is the delineation of the characters themselves. As a literary device a mirror is often used to deliver a description of a first-person protagonist, and it is a small step from there to becoming an apparatus for the psychotic mind to misrecognize itself, or even to recognize itself from a place where it feels it is not. 'I must stop being in the mirror', the narrator of *Surfacing* announces, suggesting a distortion of first-person perspective whereby the mirror image embodies her experiencing self (Atwood 1972, 137).

In the clinical phenomenon known as the *signe du miroir*—most often used in relation to schizophrenic patients—the subject may stare for hours at their own specular image as if compelled by what they see there. As Sass et al. have noted, 'the so-called mirror sign is also characteristic in DPD' (Sass et al. 435). Mirror-related experiences are just one of the many ways in which self and not-self can be confused in fictional madness. As I mentioned earlier, however, a misplaced or misrecognized sense of identity can be symbolized in numerous ways; not just through mirror images, but also doubles, and even inanimate objects such as the crazy wallpapers of Gilman and Grass. And when madness is displaced onto a *Doppelgänger*, a scapegoat character, or onto an object, the problem of the potential unintelligibility of the first-person voice can be conveniently circumvented. The self is often a tenuous concept in psychosis, as the empirical data shows, and this is why the confusion with the not-self provides so many popular, persistent, and widespread devices used in the literatures of madness.

Second-Person Narratives

A second-person narrative where the referent 'you' is a form of self-address is in effect a prolonged version of the pronominal shift; it is also easily locatable within the theme of the confusion of self with not-self, since there is a constant slippage between the stated 'you' and the not-stated, but intimated, 'I'. One of the best-known and most sustained examples of a deliberate misplacement of second person for first is Jay McInerney's novel *Bright Lights, Big City*. The protagonist is not so much psychotic as drug-crazed, or as he himself says, 'all messed up and no place to go' (McInerney 9). He describes his feeling of being dislocated: 'of always standing to one side of yourself, of watching yourself in the world even as you were being in the world, and wondering if this was how everyone felt' (McInerney 159). The narrator is alienated, traumatized from a failed relationship, and completely addicted to what he calls Bolivian Marching Powder—cocaine. Moreover, he has no name. Brian Richardson writes that the pronoun 'you' in this novel brings with it 'an element of instability' by virtue of its protean nature where various hypotheses of address/addresses remain plausible, 'while ensuring that none can be definitive' (B. Richardson 23). The prevailing effect is of 'defamiliarization' and this instability is magnified when the narrator moves to consider himself at a further remove, saying of himself at one point in the narrative, 'you thought of yourself in the third person' (B. Richardson 24).

The shifting of pronouns from first person to second is particularly conspicuous since it is a relatively uncommon form of narration; and as a result of its protean nature it can be disarming. It is a highly effective tool in the literature of madness because it plays with the multifunctionality of the second-person pronoun, creating, in Monika Fludernik's terms, 'a complex field of potential deistic significance to the reader' (Fludernik 450). 'You' can be narrator, protagonist, or narratee; it even reaches out to and encompasses the reader, and can draw them inside the mad world. It also suggests an acute level of detachment. 'You' as a substitute for 'I' not only implies emotional disconnection, but also, through its lack of familiarity, can be empowering in a dramatic sense. As Fludernik says, it sticks out. It attracts to itself an interest in its significance. In terms of the authenticity of using second-person speech as self-address, I refer back to Laing's recording of a patient who suffered 'a confusion of self with not-self', and spoke of herself 'in the first, second, or third person' (Laing 196).

Conclusion

Authenticity is an important consideration in literary representation because madness is, at least in part, a culturally constructed designation. It has a meaning that has fluctuated enormously over time and is still susceptible to expectations of locality, age, and gender. The fact that homosexuality was categorized as a sociopathic personality disturbance in the 1952 edition of the *Diagnostic and Statistical Manual of Mental Disorders* is one oft-cited instance of how the Western world's views on what is pathological and what is not have reformed even in recent times. Authors who write about madness are influenced by cultural perspectives, and medical reports, but fiction is also inexorably intertextual. Writers are also readers, and powerful motifs and mechanisms for representation are revisited, albeit in a transformed state. It is to be hoped that these mechanisms favour an authentic and empathetic illustration of what it is to suffer from mental distress.

A part of us longs for the mad to be different—other—because the fear and the reality is that they are just like us. For that reason, I have avoided the term 'mental illness'. It presupposes that there is such a thing as mental health, and my inclination is to adopt Darian Leader's view that 'there is simply no such thing' and that 'each of us faces problems that we tackle in our own unique ways'

(Leader 7). Literature is one way in which we can combat the sort of intolerance that is often shown towards people who suffer psychological aberrations, and because literary fiction is said to engage the empathy hub in the brain of both reader and writer, it is also one way in which we can potentially overcome the tyranny of our own prejudice (Kidd and Castano 474). Michel Foucault reminds us that in the Middle Ages 'madness borrowed its face from the mask of the beast' and was deemed unmanageable except 'by *discipline* and *brutalizing*' (Foucault 72, 75; italics in the original). While it is safe to say that the mad are no longer—or at least not often—portrayed as bestial, satanic, or divine, exceptional psychic states do often attract extremes of writing. And while the mad are less likely to be dismissed in fiction as apathetic brute creatures, psychosis continues to feature in genres that foreground elements of horror, allegory, or melodrama. Literature that focuses on madness, as Charley Baker has noted, can, in itself and in its transformations into film, theatre, and television, play 'a crucial role in shaping public perceptions of madness' (Baker et al. 2–3). Therefore the sensitivity of the signifying process—the way that creative writers write about madness—is of crucial significance. Mechanisms such as the pronominal shift and the confusion of self with not-self in its many manifestations can be used sensitively and compassionately. They accord with clinical evidence, in particular as related here to ipseity disturbances, and can be used in such a way that the coherence of the narrative style, particularly in first-person fictions, is not jeopardized.

If in fact you journey into madness, or as Atwood says, it comes to you, madness is a strange place to find yourself. The language and the customs may seem incomprehensible, and those suffering from madness may find themselves, like refugees, struggling to connect in a world in which they feel alienated. 'Now we're on my home ground, foreign territory', the narrator of *Surfacing* says (Atwood 1972, 11). Literary madness is capable of both clarity and plausibility. It is also, when it is written with sensitivity, able to nurture the sort of society that refugees of all categories need and deserve. It can offer them dignity, humanity, and respect.

References

Atwood, Margaret, *The Edible Woman* (London: Virago,1983 [1969]).
Atwood, Margaret, *Surfacing* (London: Little, Brown Book Group, 1972).
Atwood, Margaret, *Alias Grace* (London: Virago, 1997 [1996]).

Baker, Charley, Paul Crawford, Brian J. Brown, Maurice Lipsedge, and Ronald Carter, *Madness in Post-1945 British and American Fiction* (Basingstoke: Palgrave Macmillan, 2010). https://doi.org/10.1057/9780230290440

Blanchot, Maurice, *The Space of Literature* (Nebraska: University of Nebraska Press, 1982).

Cooke, Nathalie, *Margaret Atwood: A Biography* (Toronto: ECW Press, 1998).

Fludernik, Monika, 'Second-Person Narrative as a Test Case for Narratology: The Limits of Realism', *Style* 22.3 (1994): 445–79.

Foucault, Michel, *Madness and Civilization*, trans. by R. Howard (London: Routledge, 1997).

Genette, Gérard, *Narrative Discourse: An Essay in Method*, trans. by Jane E. Lewin (New York: Cornell University Press, 1980).

Gilman, Charlotte Perkins, 'The Yellow Wallpaper' in *The Yellow Wallpaper and Other Stories* (New York: Dover Publications, 1997 [1892]), 1–15.

Grass, Günter, *The Tin Drum*, trans. by Ralph Manheim (Harmondsworth, Penguin, 1985 [1959]).

Ingram, Allan (ed.), *Patterns of Madness in the Eighteenth Century* (Liverpool: Liverpool University Press, 1998).

Kidd, David C., and Emanuele Castano, 'Different Stories: How Levels of Familiarity with Literary and Genre Fiction Relate to Mentalizing', *Psychology of Aesthetics, Creativity, and the Arts* 11.4 (2017): 1–13. https://doi.org/10.1037/aca0000069

Laing, R.D., *The Divided Self* (London: Penguin, 1969 [1955]).

Leader, Darian, *What is Madness?* (London: Hamish Hamilton, 2011).

McGrath, Patrick, *Spider* (London: Penguin, 1992 [1990]).

McInerney, Jay, *Bright Lights, Big City* (London: Bloomsbury, 2007 [1984]).

Nünning, Ansgar, 'On the Perspective Structure of Narrative Texts' in Willie van Peer and Seymour Chatman (eds), *New Perspectives on Narrative Perspective* (Albany: State University of New York Press, 2001), 207–23.

Parnas, Josef, 'Self and Schizophrenia: A Phenomenological Perspective' in Tilo Kircher and Anthony David (eds), *The Self in Neuroscience and Psychiatry* (New York: Cambridge University Press, 2003), 217–40. https://doi.org/10.1017/CBO9780511543708.012

Porter, Roy, *Madmen: A Social History of Madhouses, Mad-Doctors & Lunatics* (Stroud: Tempus, 2004).

Richardson, Brian, *Unnatural Voices: Extreme Narration in Modern and Contemporary Fiction* (Columbus: Ohio State University Press, 2006).

Richardson, Samuel, *Clarissa, or, The History of a Young Lady* (London: Penguin, 2004 [1748]).

Sass, Louis, and Josef Parnas, 'Schizophrenia, Consciousness, and the Self', *Schizophrenia Bulletin* 29 (2003): 427–44. https://doi.org/10.1093/oxfordjournals.schbul.a007017

Sass, Louis, Elizabeth Pienkos, Barnaby Nelson, and Nick Medford, 'Anomalous Self-Experience in Depersonalization and Schizophrenia: A Comparative Investigation', *Consciousness and Cognition* 22 (2013): 430–41. https://doi.org/10.1016/j.concog.2013.01.009

Saussure, Ferdinand de, *Course in General Linguistics*, trans. by Wade Baskin (New York: Philosophical Library, 1959).

8 Rethinking Clinical and Critical Perspectives on Psychosis in Kathy Acker's Writing

Charley Baker

Kathy Acker's writing is widely recognized as being challenging, even alienating, for the reader through her destruction of linear narrative and coherent textual form, twisting of narrative time and place, and thematic concerns which emerge as sometimes violent, explicit, and boundary dismantling. It is this challenge that offers something novel to the way we understand and think about unusual or strange mental states formulated clinically as 'psychosis'. There are three key areas explored here: Acker's representation of sexual violence; Acker's textual constructions and how these might mirror the expression of unusual experiences; and Acker's core theme of a contemporary and inescapable instability of identity. The final part of this chapter explores how the uniqueness of each textual construction highlights the uniqueness of human experience—which concomitantly might not be fully realized through more homogenizing diagnostic frameworks and related treatment approaches common to contemporary psychiatric practice—offering insights into narratively supporting people experiencing what might be formulated as 'psychosis'.

The term 'psychosis' is used here to encompass states of mind that exist along a continuum of specific or unusual or strange thoughts and beliefs, from common perceptions of an external real to more individualized sensory or cognitive experiences. 'Psychosis' is an imperfect term to use—Acker's aim was not to resituate experiences as indicative of pathology or a particular psychiatric diagnosis. As she suggested, language can imprison and control, never quite representing the totality of bodily or mental experience. In Acker's work, 'psychosis' is a radically *individual* experience, drawing attention to the need to focus on the *person*. A focus in mental health practice on a paradigm shift from the homogenizing to the heterogenerative, to a view which privileges individual narrative content, meaning, and interpretation over the clinically discussed forms of symptoms that are grouped together as denoting a particular 'illness', is supported by narrative readings of radical texts (Leader). As Bracken and colleagues argued in 2012: 'Reductionist models fail to grasp what is most important in terms of recovery. The evidence base is telling us that we need a radical shift in our understanding of what is at the heart (and perhaps soul) of mental health practice' (Bracken et al. 432).

While it is outside the reach of this chapter to examine the range of approaches to mental illness and mental health, this chapter most closely aligns with more critically orientated mental health perspectives. Such perspectives do not deny that people have strange, unusual, or distressing experiences, but argue that current formulations are scientifically flawed, unhelpful for some, and specifically focus on pharmacological treatments in a disease- or drug-centric approach (Bentall 2004a and 2004b; Boyle; Davies; Whitaker 2003 and 2010; Lane 2007). It is now widely accepted that psychosis can be brought about and affected by psychological, biological, sociological, neurochemical, drug-induced, and even religious and cultural elements, following Zubin and Spring's oft-cited Stress-Vulnerability Model of 'schizophrenia' (Zubin and Spring 1977). Both the 2010 and 2013 UK National Institute for Health and Care Excellence (NICE) guidelines on the treatment of 'schizophrenia' and psychosis in adults and young people, respectively, suggest a range of biological, psychological, environmental, and social *possible* causes of psychosis (such as genetics, substance misuse, perinatal risk factors, and environmental and childhood adversity). While NICE acknowledge the possible benefits of psychological and social interventions, medication remains at the forefront of clinical treatment. Leader reiterates Whitaker's view, stating, 'due to the pervasive and crippling effects of long-term drug use, the idea of psychosis as a chronic and irreversible brain disease becomes a self-fulfilling prophecy' (Leader 2011, 329). More recently, longitudinal studies have emerged suggesting that people who stop medication sooner rather than later, and remain either off medication or on a small maintenance dose, have better outcomes in terms of general functioning, social engagement, and well-being (Harrow, Jobe, and

Faull; Wunderlink et al.). A recent British Psychological Society report promotes an individual and *normalizing* approach to unusual experiences. While not wholly *anti* medication or biomedically orientated treatment, the report was (unsurprisingly perhaps) received with quite some controversy in the UK from some psychiatrists (Cooke; Laws, Langford, and Huda; see also Moncrieff). Critically oriented movements such as Post-Psychiatry (Bracken and Thomas) and Open Dialogue (Seikkula and Olsen 2003; Seikkula et al. 2006) offer a range of interrogative views on current practice, humane ways of offering care and support, and belief in the power of hope and that people can recover from difficult or distressing times.

Acker's work breaks down binary oppositions of mad–sane, representing instead the fluidity of experiences that follow on a continuum of reason, without a clear point of rupture or departure from 'normal' to 'abnormal'.

Sexual Trauma in Acker's Writing

Acker's work has attracted attention crossing both humanities and healthcare disciplines, particularly from feminist perspectives and due to her frequent portrayals of sexual violence. Zaikowski (2010) notes that the literature of trauma traverses the terrain around 'how to navigate language when we are attempting to articulate not only the unsayable, but its very unsayableness', suggesting we 'confront the quandary of how to witness the unwitnessable through language' (Zaikowski 202–03). In Acker's *Blood and Guts in High School* (1978), which Zaikowski uses as her exemplar traumatized body of text, she suggests the central cohering features of post-traumatic stress disorder (hyperarousal, intrusion, and constriction) might be employed in reading Acker's disrupted and dissociated heroine Janey's narrative. Acker's textual methods reflect for Zaikowski 'not only the dissociation and confusion of identity; it also highlights the disruption of linear time and narrative so prominent in the minds of trauma survivors' (Zaikowski 206). Such a fractured text then, 'if examined through the lens of PTSD', offers 'invaluable information about language, society and healing', information that can lead to 'compassionate witnessing that will make real the possibility of healing, integration and, ultimately, a new world' (Zaikowski 217–18). Persevering through the radical dislocations of her works enables, in one sense, a witnessing of predominantly women's trauma and subjugation.

Dick suggests that Acker's depiction of sex 'works to bring the reader back to her body in a way no other literary strategy quite does' (Dick 113). Commenting on the arguments around pornography and pleasure that informed Acker's work, Dick highlights the 'paradoxical proposition that a specific body was always implicated in the construction of identity (and yet did not restrict the possible identifications and fantasies that that very body might enjoy)', suggesting that this 'was itself a feminist idea' (Dick 113). Dick's formulation of the interaction between the bodily and the intellectual is evident in the many forms that sex itself takes in Acker's work. The stark reality and endemic nature of sexual trauma *is set against* women's sexual pleasure in Acker's writing. Pitchford suggests that Acker's portrayals of 'acutely painful *bodily* desires' and the 'search for a language that can break free of existing codes to express those desires' have led to a range of work focusing on post-structural and psychoanalytic readings of such desire, which risk missing the '*historical* and *material* aspects of the reading practice Acker's novels might offer' (Pitchford 67, emphasis in original).

One historical and material aspect of Acker's writing is her portrayal of sexual violence and the impact this has on characters psychologically. Wollen notes Acker's presentation of sexuality is 'always bound up with issues of power, violence, and pain, whether explicitly through sadomasochism and rape or implicitly through a generalized oppression' (Wollen 8). Women in Acker's work are thus 'both sexually exploited and sexually voracious', creating for an 'antimony' which 'generates a cascade of complex discourses, crystallized in the figure of the outlaw heroine, both flaunting her independence, defying her oppressors and bolting in desperation, abject and humiliated' (Wollen 8). Wollen further suggests that this paradox has at its heart the *family*, with society acting as an external controller, a 'macro-family of powerful rulers and powerless subjects, terrorizing and terrorized, driving and driven mad—an extreme projection of the psychotic family, and its values, across the whole landscape of interpersonal relations' (Wollen 9). Acker's female characters are often in stasis, desiring sexual freedom and autonomy but constrained by societal and familial restrictions on sexuality and risks posed by sexual violence. Her portrayal of sex, sexual pleasure, and sexual violence does not always conform to the prevailing feminist discourse of her more radical feminist contemporaries, of whom she was critical (Jackson).

In Acker's *Empire of the Senseless* (*ES*, 1998), Abhor's ontological development occurs because *and* in spite of the gendered injustice she experiences. The 'society of disgust' (*ES* 227) that Abhor despises is the society that designates women as passive objects (to be done to) rather than desiring, active subjects (who do). Abhor's rape by the photographer in Paris is told in an unemotional, cold tone, as is her initial rape by her father which the reader first learns about through Thivai's retelling. This almost clinical recounting could be read as indicative of two interrelated responses—the 'everyday-ness' of rape for women in a patriarchal society, and the dissociative elements of the psychological response to trauma. Pitchford suggests that Abhor has 'learned young that she cannot rely on her body for any truth value', keeping 'ownership of her body unsettled' (Pitchford 98). Neither Abhor's body nor her mind are owned by Abhor—she is assigned multiple identities by others. As Pitchford suggests, this unsettling of bodily autonomy and ownership is 'an important strategy for women and other historically oppressed people' because it problematizes the notion that women can *ever* be free or autonomous, in body or mind, despite the 'concept of human freedom' that is 'so central to rationalism' (Pitchford 98). This novel can be seen as telling the story of Abhor's struggle to develop her own identity, outside of those that are given to her. Abhor's struggle for bodily *and* intellectual autonomy, which coexist, is threatened when another interrupts her bodily ownership through sexual violence. Abhor learns from a young age that bodily desire is tied up with intellectual desire, offering an example of how Acker offers a complex vision of 'I want', where desire holds multiple meanings. 'I want' is often removed, replaced by a powerless set of 'options'; Abhor has only one 'option' when raped as an adult—'I quickly chose a raped body over a mutilated or dead one' (*ES* 64). It is through Abhor's madness that what Schlichter (2003) perceives as Acker's contribution to the 'discourse of critical madness' emerges—to critically expose not only 'patriarchal concepts of femininity' but also the 'cultural conditions of their production' and to 'develop strategies for the reconfiguration of the representational order' (Schlichter 324).

In her early work *The Burning Bombing of America* (*BB*, 1972), published posthumously, Acker writes in a free-association stream-of-consciousness style, creating the first of her fragmented narratives with only fragile thematic strings holding the piece together. This segment shows how Acker combines literary strategies with a textually psychotic fragmentation in response to extreme fear:

> black kid sneaks in the door in back of me arms grab my arms just as I'm opening the elevator DON'T TOUCH ME WHY ARE YOU TOUCHING ME come into the elevator with me I won't hurt you race up stairs second floor going to race up back stairs elude rapist back stairs are less open stand by three doors doorbells protection look around black kid comes out of elevator I'm about to press three doorbells he disappears super's house there's a guy in the building somewhere he attacked me once a clack kid go away I don't want anything to do with anybody out comes my police whistle [...] Jerry's apartment a guy attacked me in the front hall he's somewhere in the building will you come down here don't have any clothes on go to hell after a while you learn the rules of the jungle you don't wear heels that click you're always ready to scream. (*BB* 152)

Acker here depicts the 'rules' women have to live by—to wear sexually chaste clothing, to be in a state of perpetual preparedness for attack. The fear of rape, instilled in women from a young age, is transmitted by the fractured and frenetic narrative tone here, reading like a stream of acute panic. There is also a lack of voice—imagination, fear, and vocalizations blur. Being female is a task, with its own male-defined rules, one that women have to work at rather than exist in, lived 'constantly on guard' yet 'as independent as possible', offering a double bind where women cannot 'win'. This early work is almost entirely written in stream-of-consciousness style and, despite its lack of narrative clarity, it offers a stark vision of patriarchal power and the anxiety and perplexity inherent in women's existence.

One impact of sexual violence on Acker's characters is their enacting of self-harm and feelings of suicidality, often via laceration of wrists. Self-harm is not always associated with clear mental health challenges involving psychosis or otherwise, but can be associated with traumatic experiences: this is a view that is borne out by narrative accounts of self-harm and suicidality expressed by people with lived experience (Baker, Crawford, and Biley 2013). For Acker's female characters, self-harm is a physical manifestation, a tangible bodily wound, of psychological trauma. Self-harm is enacted by Acker's characters following a repeated pattern of events: after sexual assault by, or due to the absence of, the father figure, and often involving an emotionally absent and cruel mother figure. For Red, in *Rip Off Red, Girl Detective* (1973) and Abhor in *Empire of the Senseless*, self-harm is induced following attempted rape by the father figure, and is treated dismissively by the mother figure. Red narrates a conversation with Mother: 'I'm selfish I'm insane I have to see a psychiatrist. I should be dead. I tell her to stop bugging me, I've been having a hard time: I show her my wrists which I've cut up rather badly with razors, trying to punish myself. She tells me not to talk about nasty things at the dinner table' (66). A near-identical silencing of the visible, outward manifestation of acute emotional pain is one which is not uncommonly seen in clinical reactions to self-harm, where approaches can vary from supportive and tender to more hostile and ignorant of what the visible wound may indicate, instead reacting to the 'behaviour' as 'attention seeking'.

It is in *Empire of the Senseless* that self-harm is most vividly written onto the body of Abhor and into the narrative:

> Then he [Father] taught me a final trick. He showed me how to insert a razor blade into my wrist just for fun. Not for any other reason. Thus, I learned how to approach and understand nature, how to make gargantuan red flowers, like roses, blooming, drops of blood, so full and dripping the earth under them, my body, shook for hours afterwards. During those afterhours, I fantasized my blood pouring outwards. This was my relief that there were no decisions left. (*ES* 9)

Here Abhor indicates a degree of *relief* at the bodily experience she experiences when translating her intangible emotional pain into an externally facing physiological trauma. Abhor's drive to hurt her body emanates from her relationship with her father, which induces acute anxiety, fear, and panic: 'Daddy left me no possibility of easiness. He forced me to live among nerves sharper than razor blades, to have no more certainties [...] Daddy taught me to live in pain, to know there's nothing else' (*ES* 9–10). In this way, for Abhor, self-harm translates inevitable emotional pain into physical pain. Self-harm might afford a degree of relief from tension but at the cost of accepting that there is 'nothing else' other than pain available to her in her existence. Acker here writes the physicality of pain, expressed as a self-inflicted bodily wound, as a *reasonable response* to different traumas, particularly sexual trauma. Her character's responses make manifest, in bodily exterior ways, the internal turmoil induced by trauma and by existence in the 'society of disgust' (*ES* 227) that Abhor inhabits.

Violence, child abuse, and sexual trauma are well documented as contributory and causal factors in experiences of distress, depression, psychosis, and a host of other mental health issues. Ussher exposes the ways in which depression, 'borderline personality disorder', post-traumatic stress disorder, and premenstrual syndrome are constructed by a patriarchal-orientated psychiatry to pathologize women's *understandable* responses to the violence and misogyny inflicted upon them. She suggests that the very act of labelling women through their various diagnoses 'acts to deny the social and discursive context of women's lives, as well as the gendered nature of science, which defines how women's madness is defined and studied' (Ussher 46; see also Chesler). The reality of women's experiences of oppression and trauma risks being ignored in formulations of female distress that pathologize their very *reasonable* responses to subjugation and the omnipresent risk of sexual and other violence. Ussher argues that the very real internal and external manifestations of women's distress in response to violence and abuse should not be pathologized as symptomatic of mental illness: distress is 'not about weakness, inherent vulnerability, or pathology in women' but is instead a 'reasonable response' to sexual violence: 'we need to understand the material conditions of women and girls' lives that facilitate such abuse—powerlessness, patriarchy, and absence of voice (or refusal of others to hear)' (Ussher 152). Acker makes evident in her texts the power structures which position and maintain women as 'victims' of men, providing a portrait of the external social conditions from which female experiences of distress and disorder emerge. It is these represented realities that allow Acker to demonstrate the causal and—crucially—*reasonable* development of unusual mental states in women. Unreason is often entirely reasonable for Acker's characters—particularly when unreason comes from the experience of trauma. Yet Ussher suggests that through a process of *subjectification*, 'truths about women's madness are reproduced and lived by women; the fictions framed as facts that serve to regulate women's experience of distress' (Ussher 7). Acker's portrayal of the effects of sexual violence shows the importance of recognizing the socio-political context of women's lives; the significance of personal content, meaning-making, storytelling, and interpretation; and the need to *believe* experiences of trauma.

Fragments and Fragmentation

Many of Acker's fragmented and challenging narratives offer a decentring effect on the reader, which gives insight into the experience of the chaotic, fragmentary, and confusing elements of psychosis. Fiction is one literary form that can tell madness via diegetic narrative—this process risks objectification, presenting madness as a spectacle of otherness where it remains something *outside* the reader, happening to *an other*. Acker, on the other hand, often *shows* madness at the level of the textual form, leaving the reader potentially disoriented and defamiliarized from the orienting features of linear and coherent narrative or narrative voice. Wollen notes Acker was a 'ceaseless explorer of the disorientating potential of language' (Wollen 2). Acker borrowed, appropriated, re-appropriated, and plagiarized an array of diverse sources while breaching boundaries of generic form and content, subverting orienting factors that the reader uses to situate themselves in the reading process.

Acker was aware of the disorientation that her work can effect on the reader. In one interview Acker noted, 'I want the reader to come right into the text because that's the only way you can take the journey', admitting this 'probably' makes her 'texts a bit unreadable' (Lotringer 15). The invitation to 'come right into' the narrative enables the reader to take something *clinically* useful away from the reading experience.

While there are multiple textual functions that Acker employs to produce a sense of immersion into fragmentation and psychological disintegration, the focus here is on her use of narrative fragment. This fragmentation of stable or coherent linear narrative, often with only a loosely connecting overall narrative framing, replicates textually elements commonly associated with 'psychosis'—such as thought disorder, loosening of associations, and tangential thinking. Acker's psychoticization of text through the cut-up/fold-in technique is especially apparent in *The Burning Bombing of America*. The below short fragment contains many of Acker's recurrent themes and tropes—gender roles, madness, capitalism, violence, and sex. There is a direct concern with notions of madness expressed, forming a typical example of Acker's fragmented narrative flow and depiction of interior consciousness:

> I'll just talk forget it inspiration gone energy high general feeling in the consciousness: can't get myself together what are you doing I'm flying into outer apace I'm going insane 25mg. Valium one seconal. 50mg. Benzedrine unknown chemicals in the food personality changes result. hospitals are for getting well. don't believe it don't believe anything you hear. Be as paranoid schizophrenic as possible. all sentences suspect. Stupid Man says the universities are in league with the evil magicians the so-called Death Wards

> Columbia deals arsenic-napalm DD3 welfare means lobotomy nurses are robotants. Allow people to do whatever they want allow the streets to be covered with silk people will dance wildly in the streets. (158)

The disjointed and tangential nature of this fragment offers a clear example of how people experiencing inner confusion and disjointedness might express such ideas. Themes of paranoia are also evident, a commonly depicted experience in Acker's work. Acker's use of triple spaces within the textual structure, between words and segments, is also interesting here. They indicate not a pause, as would be expected by a full stop, but have a curious reading impact, enhancing the sense of narrative flow (there is little actual pause) but also creating a sense of panic and franticness through frenetic condensing of multiple ideas into one segment of text, offering a thought stream rather than a storying written text. These spaces might also indicate a violent interruption, a literal fracture, in the stream-of-consciousness narrative flow. Acker here creates a new textual strategy that forms part of her development of a literary analogue of psychosis—the replication of what might clinically be considered 'psychotic' interior monologue, but where attention to the individual fragments and the overall segment might offer insights into the content (rather than the form) of concerns a person has.

In terms of the psychoticization of the text, Acker's short piece 'Politics' (1968) textually demonstrates various elements that are thought to be indicative of 'psychosis', such as thought disorder, tangential thinking, pressured speech, and disinhibited content:

> Lenny didn't leave me some dead tired Bob is disgusting a destroyer of human minds the second dream sequence written at 11.40 I'm feeling like shit get along with Hannah (I am) I can't cite down peacocks my nightmares all these invulnerable thoughts my great beauty I can try to talk to Hannah third dream tomorrow tell her Lenny says she's scared I should do everything to help her relax I want to be alone Greta Garbo Scylla and Charibdis I don't know how to return. (28)

The flow here is disjointed, chaotic, tangential, disordered. The reader (like the clinician) does not know who Lenny, Bob, or Hannah is, or why they should have such significance in the interior monologue, offering a distance from the story and a seduction into the flow. These 'others' crowd the narrator's world and expressed thoughts, but do not exist in any characterical sense. A reduction of a complex narrative expression to a series of symptoms would potentially deny the narrative function, content, and significance of this piece, however. The stream of incoherence that forms 'Politics' contains fragments of insight into the narrator's experience and existence, which might be missed if only searching for symptomatological examples of disorder, which correspond to a particular taxonomy. Lines such as 'my basic problem is I can't quite believe anything and cant react to anything similarly I never react to things when they happen but only later when they're less threatening' might, for example, be indicative of the wider existential concerns of postmodernity: loss of certainty, concerns about emotional flatness and superficiality, anhedonic response, loss of meaningful reaction to events (see also Woods). The final line of the piece screams out from the page: 'it doesn't mean what it should no one else thinks like this anymore I say angelic I'm sick of fucking not knowing who I am' (35), which might indicate problems with defining and securing an identity, a theme that Acker returns to frequently. Persevering through the anti-narrative of 'Politics' demonstrates the potential of fragments to both contribute to a sense of cohering a whole and to demonstrate the importance of meaningfully acknowledging the content, rather than concentrating on *only* identifying the form. A different reading here could have more clearly pinpointed different psychiatric symptoms in the two pieces noted above. Instead, I focus on how these narrative fragments might offer a sense for the reader of franticness, fear, anxiety, instability of belief, incoherence of thought.

The struggle towards coherent meaning making of fragments, then, offers for the reader one part of what Keitel (1989) termed 'reading psychosis'. The cumulative impact of the effect of immersion into incoherence might offer two potential responses that may aid a reformulation of how the experience of psychosis is considered, and how best to respond to dialogue that alienates the reader/listener from the content precisely through its apparent illogicality or confusion. Firstly, such fragments, while unfamiliar, might be paradoxically familiar to a clinical reader. That is, they replicate forms of expression that likely will have been heard elsewhere. Such fragments might mirror the way that people experiencing disruptions to their sense of self, belief, and cognition express those experiences. One possible response is to dismiss them as 'mad' writings. A different and more ethically minded response might, instead, take the time to consider the content of each fragment, to find the thread that ties the fragment to the whole, to consider the meaning of the individual element to the person. Secondly, and following this, the fragments might offer an opportunity to cohere different parts of a story together. Unpacking threads of importance amidst elements of intrusion or confusion might be challenging. The content of expression and the form through which it is presented might be alien to more common experience. This again opens a further space, a space between the literal ability to read words on a page and a broader understanding of the text itself. This space mirrors the lacuna Jaspers (1959) identifies between the understandable experience (neurosis) and the un-understandability of psychosis. Acker often leaves her readers suspended in the 'space between' the understandable and the un-understandable, with both plural and flexible interpretations available. Acker's texts open out, rather than closing down, interpretation. A binary framework of madness 'versus' sanity risks closing down, through the demarcation of 'mad' or 'sane', expression and experience.

I have referred elsewhere to Acker's writing as *writing psychosis*, an interpretation that takes Keitel's psychopathographical text beyond her initial theorization (see Baker et al. chapter 6). The effects on the reader of Acker's destruction of linear narrative into fragments, her use of repetition within narratives, and her depiction of the space in which experience resists conventional linguistic representation, are closely aligned to Keitel's analysis. The effect on the reader of reading psychopathographic narratives is clear for Keitel: 'Reading about psychosis becomes a reading psychosis' (Keitel 118). Acker does not write *about* psychosis: she provides a literary analogue *of* psychosis—she *writes psychosis*.

The reader does not recall Acker's 'stories' but the fragments contained within them. Defamiliarization with narrative coherence or, to paraphrase Keitel, the absence of the stabilizing mediating text, might leave the reader lost, excluded from content that is stable *and* simultaneously included into the disoriented experience of psychosis. Wheeler suggests that Acker 'sought to reveal the fact that familiar order and logic are much less native to our experience or the apparent order of nature and the "external" world', suggesting that sanity is 'arguably, merely the most familiar form of irrationality' (Wheeler). Acker textually creates irrationality in her 'irrational' texts. This offers readers a sense of confusion, insecurity, and dissociation from everyday experience or communication, fragmentation, fear, anxiety, joy, elation, and liminal experiences. This insight may be then further applied to clinical reflection on how such experiences might feel.

The Individual

Acker was fascinated with notions of identity, a theme that appears time and again in both her interviews and critical work. The sense of challenge in developing a coherent or coalesced centralized identity materializes as a regular issue through her narrative voices, often via interior monologue. Dissociated identities are written into the construction of Acker's texts; their expressions of experience are always bound up in notions of anxiety, fear, mistrust, ontological and existential insecurity, and the inherent instability of the language available to them to construct their 'selves'. Acker noted the radical disjunction that exists in the postmodern arena between the individual's view of reality and the world itself is 'insanity' incarnate, writing: 'Pretend that there is a distinct entity named *self* and a different entirety named *world* or *other*. Define *insanity* as the situation between the self's version of the world and the world. According to this definition, American culture is now insane' (Acker 1997, 2). Furthermore, the *expression* of this personally experienced and culturally demonstrated 'insanity' cannot be adequately demonstrated, for Acker, through '[w]ell-measured language, novels which structurally depend on Aristotelian continuities, on any formal continuities'; such works 'cannot describe, much less criticize, this culture' (Acker 1997, 2). This disparity, then, between the desired aim of a centralized identity and knowable real versus the reality of a fragmented sense of self and lack of ontological or existential certainty is best expressed, for Acker, through discordant narrative voices who have a limited sense of 'I am', 'I want', or 'I believe'.

Acker's characters are fragmented, unsure, insecure, paranoid, experiencing a fracturing between their perceptions and the perceptions of others. First-person narration sometimes involves multiple voices, a babbling of identities or elements of selfhood. Acker presents a plurality of identity alongside issues of plagiarism and blurring of autobiography, fiction, and critical writing in a complex fusion. Acker attributed this fusion as being born from her interest in 'schizophrenia', noting in an interview, 'I came to plagiarism from a different point of view, from exploring schizophrenia and identity' (Friedman). Again, in interview with Lotringer, she reiterates this view, stating, 'I became very interested in the model of schizophrenia. I wanted to explore the use of the word I' (Lotringer 7). The most viable identity in the postmodern world, Acker states, is formed of a splitting, a hyperreal merging of false/true, constructed and reproduced. In writing *The Childlike Life of the Black Tarantula by The Black Tarantula* (1973), Acker wrote that she wanted to explore:

> The idea that you don't need to have a central identity, that a split identity was a more viable way in the world. I was splitting the I into false and true I's and I just wanted to see if this false I was more or less real than the true I; what are the reality levels between false and true and how it worked. (Lotringer 7)

The most striking element of Acker's representation of a 'split' identity occurs through her decentring of a stable and secure narrative 'I' in her fragments and texts—as Schlichter notes in reference to Acker's *Don Quixote*, 'the destabilization of the point of view produces a variety of many small, local narrations that replace the master narrative' (Schlichter 321). Such a destabilization exposes the way identity fragmentation relates to issues of coherent self-narrative, but offers a narrative decentralization of the 'master narrative' of rationality as a masculine objective.

The curious use of 'I' and 'You' and 'We' in Acker distances both authorial 'I' and 'I-as-first-person narrator' because the 'I' (or 'I's) are inherently *unstable*. There is no coherent character identity created through the littered fragments of text that form the piece as a whole. The use of 'You' draws the reader directly into the text, appealing to them but simultaneously dissociating them from their expectations as a reader—for example:

> SWISH freaks maniacs Your schizophrenia SWISH Your giant hand covers our eyes pulls our fingers into long strands of light Your fingernails scrape the skin off our senses Your realm is not discussed there is no language for You […] You never rest You talk to me in the presence of other people I am alone I sit by myself I cry. (*BB* 179)

This section is accusatory in tone ('Your schizophrenia' / 'Your fingernails scrape the skin off our senses'), yet collective ('our'). In many respects, 'I' is every and any 'I'; 'You' is every and any 'Other'. The overt distancing, almost repelling, of the reader (both through the accusing of the narrative voice, and the literal fragments of text posing a challenge to coherent reading and sense-making) leaves a reader who is trying to navigate their way through the scattered fragments of a text that concomitantly depicts the scattered fragments of a desecrated America.

PERSPECTIVES ON PSYCHOSIS IN KATHY ACKER

Acker's narratives are often interrupted by different voices (including those of the author), making identification of a discrete 'I' challenging. In a 1990 piece, published initially in the journal *Postmodern Culture* as 'Dead Doll Humility' and reproduced in 1993 as 'Dead Doll Prophecy', Acker demonstrates these interruptive voices. This is a creative piece about the process of becoming a writer, creatively retelling the legal wrangling Acker experienced over plagiarism, and her feelings on the issue of plagiarism more generally. This fusion of creative and autobiographical writing is told in the third and first person (via Capitol's thoughts) but also signals concerns and influences that Acker discussed in interviews, for example the Black Mountain Poets. The text is often missing the subject pronoun 'she' or 'her', giving a curiously distant impression. Other capitalized sections put Capitol's thoughts into quotation marks, offering a further distance from the impression of Capitol speaking Acker's thoughts, ultimately leading to a doubling of Acker's voice. The different voices culminate and agree with one another. This is a feature throughout much of Acker's work, whereby 'I' becomes unstable through a multiplicity of narrators all speaking in the first person. Acker interjects explicitly autobiographical material, political commentary, seemingly irrelevant subplots that fail to become plots, and philosophical musings into many of her texts.

Hume suggests, writing on the destabilizing and deconstructing voices in Acker, that there *is* a consistent voice throughout Acker's work, one which 'projects itself through lyric lamentation, cries, the vocabularies of sex, pain and oppression' (Hume 509). Alongside the 'I' that speaks consistently of Acker's core concerns, in other ways the narrative 'I' in Acker's work is destabilized, autoscopically displaced and external to the self. The multiple points of view struggling for space within *The Childlike Life of the Black Tarantula by the Black Tarantula* are presented as a babble of voices. Within this text, there is no stable 'I' offering a discrete characterial identity—the first-person voices are multiple and undifferentiated by Acker: 'My name is Laura Lane. I'm born in Holly Springs, Mississippi, in 1837. My name is Adelaide Blanche de la Tremouille. I, K A, fall in love with D; D burns me' (17). The narrative here presents an authorial voice narrating contemporary events in a diary or self-analytical manner alongside the stories of female murderesses in the first and second chapters. The framing breaks down when Acker asserts that she is copying pornographic books, yet elements that Acker draws on (potentially) autobiographically ('I, K A' in the quote above) interject with the 'pornographic' tale of a relationship between two girls at a school. Where there is a babbling of 'I's speaking, the effect replicates the potential experience of auditory 'hallucination' for the reader, where thought is interrupted by more ethereal voices. Acker seems to directly appear in this text: 'Kathy also writes about this and her memory of it is the same as mine' (7). Acker explicitly links 'schizophrenia', identity, and the blurring of autobiography and fiction in discussion about the process of writing this text. In an interview with Lotringer she asserted that by the end of this text, 'I can't tell what's true or false, except for actual dates. If I say I was born in 1748, I know that's false' (Lotringer 7–8). This, then, implants the author into the narrative, further displacing authorial and characterial identities, closing the gap between author and text. Authorial identity is pluralized, like the 'schizophrenic' identities that Acker conveys, where the 'I's that multiply through this text describe an array of disturbing paranoia, unusual perceptions, and elements of confusion or distress.

Acker's work demonstrates the overwhelming sense of polyphony of personal meaning possible for cohering self-stories. It is the challenge of coherent self-awareness and self-expression that enables recognition of the uniqueness of human experience in dislocating or fracturing psychological experiences. It is these factors that offer clinical insights into the experience of fragmentation of self, disruptions in temporality, and the fear or anxiety that might be experienced by people in clinical settings. Here, it is not the *form of a symptom* but the *content of experience* that is crucial to understanding the individual subjective experience of psychosis.

Conclusion

Acker does not necessarily make 'psychosis' in its entirety 'understandable'. She highlights the external factors that both effect individual madness and contribute to the societal construction of madness. She demonstrates the complexity of how we construct ourselves, our experiences, our beliefs, and our emotions, through language—language that is far from benign and that does not offer uniformity of meaning and interpretation. Readings of Acker's work therefore offer the possibility of finding coherence in incoherence, method and resistance in madness, calm in chaos. One of Acker's key messages in writing through and from within the apparent incoherency of psychosis is to appeal to the reader to *attend to the content*, to deconstruct the destructive, to challenge accepted forms of logic, coherence, and understandability. This motif has a striking relevance for clinical practice, whereby the context and content of experiences remains secondary to the form and structure of 'symptoms' in terms of reaching a diagnosis of 'psychosis'—and particularly where women may be doubly pathologized.

Such readings of Acker's work may provide the basis of one form of resistance to marginalization that focuses less on the binary dualism between psychiatrist/patient or anti-psychiatry/biomedical psychiatry, and offers a way forward in the *spaces between* such positions. Health humanities offers one such liminal disciplinary space within which positive ways of working with people undergoing challenging or difficult experiences can emerge without resorting to binary positioning. Acker's work is situated in a liminal space, between fixed referents, political alignments, and belief systems. It is this space between that can interrogate and subvert, offer radically new visions of experience and emotion, and propose integrative ways of working with people that do not dismiss anyone's expertise, instead recognizing expertise as temporary, personal, and open to challenge and new knowledge. Thus, a health humanities-informed framework for approaching mental health via narratives can offer two core developments in practice and education where my readings of Acker may contribute. Firstly, in helping people to formulate and narrate their own experiences in a language and way that makes sense to them; secondly, in innovation in health education and the continuing professional development of clinical and support staff. Skills in narrative interpretation; close reading (or listening); learning to discover narrative threads through possible non-linear narration; appreciating the importance of socio-political context (social determinants of health and illness), characters (family members/friends), time and place (personal history), and personal meaning—all are vital in informing contemporary mental health. Literature that focuses on mental health has the potential to teach readers about how it might feel to experience unusual perceptions or beliefs, to feel acutely frightened or suspicious, to hear or see unfamiliar things in an unfamiliar way, or to feel the crushing bleakness of depression or the heightened sense of doom associated with acute anxiety.

Acker's narratives go a step further, immersing the reader in an experience that might be analogous to fragmentation and confusion. Acker may have begun her literary career with a focus on deconstruction and destruction, but later texts such as *Empire of the Senseless* offer more reconstructive proposals.

Her writing can offer something reconstructive from seeming fragmentation, chaos, randomness, and incomprehensibility. This reconstruction could lie in what is taken away from her novels in terms of how to clinically approach psychosis. Such a clinical-critical-literary reading of Acker offers a reconstruction—one which relies on a version of literary criticism which does not 'symptom spot' or interpret within the existing framing, but instead teases out the unknown and draws together the fragments to illuminate a way of working *with* a person—towards building, rebuilding, and maintaining the whole.

References

Acker, Kathy, 'From "Politics"', in *Hannibal Lecter, My Father*, ed. by Sylvère Lotringer (New York: Semiotext(e), 1991 [1968]), 25–36.

Acker, Kathy, *Rip Off Red, Girl Detective and The Burning Bombing of America* (New York: Grove Press, 2002 [1972/73]).

Acker, Kathy, 'The Childlike Life of the Black Tarantula by The Black Tarantula' in *Portrait of an Eye* (New York: Grove Press, 1998 [1973]), 1–90.

Acker, Kathy, *Blood and Guts in High School* (New York: Grove Press, 1978).

Acker, Kathy, *Empire of the Senseless* (London: Picador, 1988).

Acker, Kathy, 'Dead Doll Prophecy' in Carol Becker (ed.), *The Subversive Imagination: Artists, Society, and Social Responsibility* (New York: Routledge, 1994 [1993]), 20–35.

Acker, Kathy, 'William Burroughs's Realism' in *Bodies of Work* (London: Serpents Tail, 1997), 1–3.

Baker, Charley, Clare Shaw, and Fran Biley (eds), *Our Encounters with Self Harm* (Ross-on-Wye: PCCS Books, 2013).

Baker, Charley, Paul Crawford, B.J. Brown, Maurice Lipsedge, and Ronald Carter, *Madness in Post-1945 British and American Fiction* (Basingstoke: Palgrave, 2010). https://doi.org/10.1057/9780230290440

Bentall, Richard (ed.), *Reconstructing Schizophrenia* (Hove: Brunner-Routledge, 2004a [1990]).

Bentall, Richard, *Madness Explained: Psychosis and Human Nature* (London: Penguin, 2004b [2003]).

Boyle, Mary, *Schizophrenia: A Scientific Delusion?* (London: Routledge, 1997 [1990]).

Bracken, Patrick, and Philip Thomas, *Postpsychiatry: Mental Health in a Postmodern World* (Oxford: Oxford University Press, 2005). https://doi.org/10.1093/med/9780198526094.001.0001

Bracken, Pat, Philip Thomas, Sami Timimi, Eia Asen, Graham Behr, Carl Beuster, Seth Bhunnoo, Ivor Browne, Navjyoat Chhina, Duncan Double, Simon Downer,

Chris Evans, Suman Fernando, Malcolm R. Garland, William Hopkins, Rhodri Huws, Bob Johnson, Brian Martindale, Hugh Middleton, Daniel Moldavsky, Joanna Moncrieff, Simon Mullins, Julia Nelki, Matteo Pizzo, James Rodger, Marcellino Smyth, Derek Summerfield, Jeremy Wallace, and David Yeomans, 'Psychiatry Beyond the Current Paradigm', *British Journal of Psychiatry* 201.6 (2012): 430–34. https://doi.org/10.1192/bjp.bp.112.109447

Chesler, Phyllis, *Women and Madness: Revised and Updated* (New York: Palgrave Macmillan, 2005).

Cooke, Anne (ed.), *Understanding Psychosis and Schizophrenia: Why People Sometimes Hear Voices, Believe Things That Others Find Strange, or Appear Out of Touch with Reality, and What Can Help* (Leicester: British Psychological Society, 2014).

Davies, James, *Cracked: Why Psychiatry is Doing More Harm Than Good* (London: Icon Books, 2013). https://doi.org/10.1080/03060497.2013.11084326

Dick, Leslie, 'Seventeen Paragraphs on Kathy Acker' in Amy Scholder, Carla Harryman, and Avital Ronell (eds), *Lust for Life: On the Writings of Kathy Acker* (London: Verso, 2006), 110–16.

Friedman, Ellen G., 'A Conversation with Kathy Acker', *A Review of Contemporary Fiction* 9.3 (1989) http://www.centerforbookculture.org/interviews/interview_acker.html, accessed 9 June 2005.

Harrow, M., T.H. Jobe, and R.N. Faull, 'Do All Schizophrenia Patients Need Antipsychotic Treatment Continuously throughout their Lifetime? A 20-Year Longitudinal Study', *Psychological Medicine* 42.10 (2012): 2145–55. https://doi.org/10.1017/S0033291712000220

Hume, Katherine, 'Voice in Kathy Acker's Fiction', *Contemporary Literature* 43.3 (2001): 485–513. https://doi.org/10.2307/1208993

Jackson, Beth, 'Kathy Acker in conversation with Beth Jackson', *Eyeline* (Autumn/Winter 1996), http://www.acker.thehub.com.au/ackerjack.html, accessed 2 August 2005.

Jaspers, Karl, *General Psychopathology*, 2 volumes, trans. by J. Hoenig and M.W. Hamilton (Baltimore: John Hopkins University Press, 1997 [1959]).

Keitel, Evelyn, *Reading Psychosis: Readers, Texts and Psychoanalysis* (Oxford: Basil Blackwell, 1989).

Lane, Christopher, *Shyness: How Normal Behaviour Became a Sickness* (London: Yale University Press, 2007).

Laws, Keith, Alex Langford, and Samei Huda, 'Understanding Psychosis and Schizophrenia: A Critique by Laws, Langford and Huda', 27 November 2014, http://www.thementalelf.net/treatment-and-prevention/medicines/antipsychotics/understanding-psychosis-and-schizophrenia-a-critique-by-laws-langford-and-huda/, accessed 7 April 2015.

Leader, Darian, *What is Madness?* (London: Penguin, 2011).

Lotringer, Sylvère, 'Devoured, by Myths: An Interview with Sylvère Lotringer' in Kathy Acker, *Hannibal Lecter, My Father*, ed. by Sylvère Lotringer (New York: Semiotext(e), 1991), 1–24.

Moncrieff, Joanna, '"Psychiatric Prejudice": A New Way of Silencing Criticism', 23 June 2014, http://joannamoncrieff.com/2014/06/23/psychiatric-prejudice-a-new-way-of-silencing-criticism/, accessed 7 April 2015.

National Institute for Health and Care Excellence (NICE) and National Collaborating Centre for Mental Health, *CG88 Schizophrenia: Core Interventions on the Treatment and Management of Schizophrenia in Adults in Primary and Secondary Care (Updated Edition)* (London: The British Psychological Society and The Royal College of Psychiatrists, 2010).

National Institute for Health and Care Excellence (NICE) and National Collaborating Centre for Mental Health, *CG155 Psychosis and Schizophrenia in Children and Young People: Recognition and Management* (London: The British Psychological Society and The Royal College of Psychiatrists, 2013).

Pitchford, Nicola, *Tactical Readings: Feminist Postmodernism in the Novels of Kathy Acker and Angela Carter* (London: Associated University Presses, 2002).

Schlichter, Annette, 'Critical Madness, Enunciative Excess: The Figure of the Madwoman in Postmodern Feminist Texts', *Cultural Studies ↔ Critical Methodologies* 3.3 (2003): 308–29. https://doi.org/10.1177/1532708603254434

Seikkula, Jaakko, and Mary E. Olsen, 'The Open Dialogue Approach to Acute Psychosis: Its Poetics and Microplitics', *Family Process* 42.3 (2003): 403–18. https://doi.org/10.1111/j.1545-5300.2003.00403.x

Seikkula, Jaakko Jukka Aaltonen, Birgittu Alakare Kauko Haarakangas, Jyrki Keränen, and Klaus Lehtinen, 'Five-Year Experience of First-Episode Nonaffective Psychosis in Open-Dialogue Approach: Treatment Principles, Follow-Up Outcomes, and Two Case Studies', *Psychotherapy Research* 16.2 (2006): 214–28. https://doi.org/10.1080/10503300500268490

Ussher, Jane M., *The Madness of Women: Myth and Experience* (Oxon: Routledge, 2011). https://doi.org/10.4324/9780203806579

Wheeler, Kathleen, 'Reading Kathy Acker', *Context: A Forum For Literary Arts and Culture* [online edition] 9 (2001).

Whitaker, Robert, *Mad in America: Bad Science, Bad Medicine, and the Enduring Mistreatment of the Mentally Ill* ([n.p.] Perseus Books, 2003).

Whitaker, Robert, *Anatomy of an Epidemic* (New York: Broadway Books, 2010).

Wollen, Peter, 'Kathy Acker' in Amy Scholder, Carla Harryman, and Avitall Ronell (eds), *Lust for Life: On the Writings of Kathy Acker* (London: Verso, 2006), 1–11.

Woods, Angela, *The Sublime Object of Psychiatry: Schizophrenia in Clinical and Cultural Theory* (Oxford: Oxford University Press, 2011). https://doi.org/10.1093/med/9780199583959.001.0001

Wunderlink, Lex, Roeline M. Nieboer, Durk Wiersma, Sjoerd Sytema, and Fokko J. Nienhuis, 'Recovery in Remitted First-Episode Psychosis at 7 years of Follow-Up of an Early Dose Reduction/Discontinuation or Maintenance Treatment Strategy: Long-Term Follow-Up of a 2-Year Randomized Clinical Trial', *JAMA Psychiatry* 70.9 (2013): 913–20. https://doi.org/10.1001/jamapsychiatry.2013.19

Zaikowski, Carolyn, 'Reading Traumatized Bodies of Text: Kathy Acker's *Blood and Guts in High School* and Sarah Saterstrom's *The Pink Institution*', *Nebula* 7.1/7.2 (2010): 199–219.

Zubin, Joseph, and Bonnie Spring, 'Vulnerability: A New View on Schizophrenia', *Journal of Abnormal Psychology* 86 (1977): 103–26. https://doi.org/10.1037/0021-843X.86.2.103

Countering the DSM in Poetry about Bipolar Disorder

Lasse Raaby Gammelgaard

Since psychiatry conformed to the ideals of behaviorism in the 1960s (Nordgaard and Parnas 434), general psychiatry has been brought closer to general medicine with evidence-based practice, managed care, and standardized diagnosis (Scheurich 248), epitomized by the *Diagnostic and Statistical Manual of Mental Disorders*, developed by the American Psychiatry Association (the first one was published in 1952). The most recent updated edition is the DSM-5-TR from 2022. Its focus is on symptoms, diagnoses, and (often biomedical) treatment. This dominant psychiatric system has been criticized on several fronts. A prominent antagonistic group of the system is labeled 'mad studies'. In 'Carving Nature at its Joints? DSM and the Medicalization of Everyday Life' (the introductory chapter to the anthology entitled *De-Medicalizing Misery: Psychiatry, Psychology and the Human Condition*), the editors describe mental illness as:

> more or less understandable reactions to life's challenges de-contextualized and transformed into internal individual pathology—whether labelled as depression, psychosis or some other diagnosis. In other words, the relentless widening of the mythical net of 'mental disorder' is seriously corrosive of the sense that we can have, and make, of our selves and our circumstances. (Rapley, Moncrieff, and Dillon 4)

The goal of this chapter is not to endorse anti-psychiatric views of mental illness as a myth, as evidenced by my use of medicalized terminology such as 'bipolar disorder'. However, I am arguing that since psychiatric nosology has a very limited interest in the personal history of a patient and their unique context, it neglects the existential and phenomenological dimension of mental illness. Additionally, I argue that there is an affinity between mental illness and literary aesthetics in relation to a specific way of using language and producing meaning. To that end, I introduce and employ some of Virginia Woolf's observations from her seminal but slightly overlooked essay from 1925 entitled *On Being Ill*. Kimberly Engdahl Coates has highlighted this particular quality of *On Being Ill* in her article 'Exposing the Nerves of Language: Virginia Woolf, Charles Mauron, and the Affinity Between Aesthetics and Illness', in which she writes the following:

> 'On Being Ill' may thus also be read as a text that asks its readers to pay attention to the experience of being ill and the anomalies such an experience induces rather than to some diagnostic paradigm. In the essay, she counters diagnostic readings of her work and her illness with her own deeply phenomenological understanding of illness, thereby asking her readers to distinguish, as Kay Toombs puts it, between 'meaning which is grounded in lived experience and meaning which represents an abstraction from lived experience.' It is this phenomenological understanding of illness that in turn informs Woolf's use of illness to theorize her own aesthetic. (Coates 245)

I employ some central passages from *On Being Ill* to highlight how literature—especially poetry and lyrical modes of discourse—may offer a form of access to mental illness experiences that does more justice to the experience and the understanding thereof than the DSM. This is not to repudiate the truthfulness or relevance of the DSM, but is rather something I conceive as an attempt to show that literature (and in this case poetry) can supplement (not replace) a biomedical approach.

More specifically, I want to show how poetry about mood swings or bipolar disorder can counter the DSM by directly or indirectly playing off its discourse. Furthermore, I claim that the unique affordances of poetry (its potential to rhyme, arrange language in a particular way on a sheet of paper, etc.) play an instrumental role in countering the medicalized language and in offering an alternative way of understanding mental illness in general, and bipolar disorder in particular. I have selected three poems from the anthology *Living in Storms: Contemporary Poetry and the Moods of Manic-Depression*. One advantage of this is that all poets represented in the volume have agreed to having their poems included in a poetry anthology which is explicitly about 'manic-depression' (i.e. bipolar disorder). The three poems all use very different strategies for engaging with and countering the DSM. Peter Cooley's 'Returning from the Shopping Center to the Suburbs' exposes existential and poetic aspects of what might be termed a manic episode without making explicit reference to clinical psychopathology. Hence, the DSM is a silent other in this poem. Erica Dawson's 'Disorder', on the other hand, appropriates the medical language of the DSM by ironically quoting and inserting it in a parodic context. Finally, Chana Bloch's poem, 'Eclipse', completely disregards any clinical perspective; instead, it presents us with a cosmic vision of great existential abstraction. However, before engaging in the interpretations of my three cases, I want to introduce some theory and elaborate on the advantages of predominantly lyrical modes of poetry for countering a biomedical conception of bipolar disorder and of mental illness.

Poetry and Illness

Illness poses a challenge to narrative understanding and to narrative identity constructions. Illnesses are interrupting. They interrupt the flow of life. This has implications for narrative form. Shlomith Rimmon-Kenan has argued that illness narratives might lead us to rethink narrative theory in terms of 'contingency, randomness, and chaos rather than order and regularity' (Rimmon-Kenan 245), so that the teleological trajectory of narrative recedes into the background. Rimmon-Kenan even states that 'a disintegrating body may threaten the very possibility of narration' (Rimmon-Kenan 245). Her article is predominantly about somatic illness, but when the depicted illness is a mental one both the mind and the body sometimes seem to disintegrate. In some depictions of mental illnesses, this leads to fragmentary, incomplete, or incoherent narratives. However, a different way of approaching this issue is to turn to poetry, both subgenres foregrounding a lyrical mode of discourse and poems with brief narrative situations. In the article 'Narrative and Beyond', Geoffrey H. Hartman suggests that once the plot-oriented teleology of narrative is challenged, 'symbol and other strong poetic figures come into play as forceful condensations' (Hartman 343). Lyrical and poetic configurations offer an alternative route to narrative ones for depicting mental illnesses. Some poems retain degrees of narrativity, while other poems foreground nonnarrative gestures. Another aspect of the affordances of poetry, aside from figurative language, which Hartman mentioned, is the way in which poetry plays off the white paper it is written on. In poetry, language is organized in a way that gives privilege to certain places on the paper (e.g. the first and final word of a line of verse).

In *On Being Ill*, Virginia Woolf notes that a literature about illness would be received as one that lacked a plot, but, more importantly, Woolf dives further into the resources that might be released when one is experiencing illness. Woolf's essay is ostensibly about somatic illness, but it reveals itself to be at least as much about the mind. In the article 'Exposing the Nerves of Language: Virginia Woolf, Charles Mauron, and the Affinity Between Aesthetics and Illness', Kimberly Engdahl Coates writes that Woolf is '[k]eenly aware that illness can thwart creativity', but also that she 'nevertheless "mines" illness for its ability to expose "the nerves of language" [...] and to foreground a subjectivity of the body' (Coates 243). Coates emphasizes how Woolf in her essay foregrounds a 'state of hyperconsciousness capable of yielding great riches for the artist' (Coates 243). Coates explains how illness can lead to new visions:

> Woolf imagines illness and its attendant fevers, trembles, and hallucinations as an unexpected form of release from the commonplace. The essay is in part a fanciful study of the ways in which the hallucination of the senses, as induced by fever or illness, can serve the writer as a powerful strategy for re-vision. Its pain enables one to 'toy' with language and even to 'coin' new words. (Coates 243–44)

New words and a new language are needed when one attempts to describe illness in literature, according to Woolf. This is partly due to 'the poverty of the language' (Woolf 6). Someone in love, Woolf argues, has Shakespeare or Keats 'to speak her mind for her' (Woolf 7), but there are no authors to turn to, according to Woolf, if one needs to describe a headache. In that case, one is

> forced to coin words himself, and, taking his pain in one hand, and a lump of pure sound in the other (as perhaps the people of Babel did in the beginning), so to crush them together that a brand new word in the end drops out. (Woolf 7)

Such a new language is described as being 'more primitive, more sensual, more obscene' (Woolf 7). In illness, 'words seem to possess a mystic quality' (Woolf 21), and 'the words give out their scent and distil their flavor, and then, if at last we grasp the meaning, it is all the richer for having come to us sensually first, by way of the palate and the nostrils, like some queer odour' (Woolf 21–22).

Although venturing to suggest actual diagnoses for authors of the past will always be a precarious enterprise, the mental illness that Virginia Woolf suffered from has traditionally been considered to be bipolar disorder, and this is the illness that features in the three poems under scrutiny in this chapter. Despite the fact that bipolar disorder is a severe illness with a high suicide rate, many of the poems selected for *Living in Storms* are humorous. The humorous nature of the texts in spite of the seriousness of the affliction is also characteristic of Woolf's *On Being Ill*. In the opening sentence, which is more than a page long, readers encounter something approximating suicidal ideation ('how we go down into the pit of death and feel the waters of annihilation close above our heads'; Woolf 3) right next to funny descriptions of confusing the dentist telling his patient to rinse their mouth with 'the greeting of the Deity' (Woolf 3). In his 'Foreword', the editor of *Living in Storms*, David Wojahn, puts the tendency in the poems to invoke humor quite succinctly:

> The poets represented here are remarkably disinclined to confessional self-indulgence and self-pity; they confront their conditions with a harrowing lucidity, and sometimes with a self-mocking humor. (Wojahn xiv)

I argue that the humor is, among other purposes, employed to counter biomedical and diagnostic understandings of bipolar disorder. I will now turn to the first case, Peter Cooley's 'Returning from the Shopping Center to the Suburbs', which is the one among the three poems I have selected which possesses the highest degree of narrativity.

Symptoms Versus Poetic Figures in Peter Cooley's 'Returning from the Shopping Center to the Suburbs'

The first thing one notices when reading Cooley's poem is the stark contrast between the title's quotidian denotation and the remarkable, manic ride in the actual poem. I first want to highlight how the poem relates to bipolar disorder. Then, I will argue that it transcends a medicalized reading, employing poetic figures and humor. First, though, I want to quote the poem:

> I drive with the brights on
> like antlers to the dark. It's hard
> to get ahead these days; you know,

while your soul keeps panting up behind you,
licking your collar of its salt.

Tonight again I do it: drop the wheel
& pull my eyes into a fist: I see them,
God, I swear it, I can taste the roots,
that sweet bone marrow of the stars.

I start to die, right here & get reborn
before the car I'm facing now head-on
swerves on its horn out of the road.

Cooley, you're not even high & yet
you know it: I'm among the chosen. Like
those stars I'm going to live forever, listener,
not that you asked. And while we're at it:
how do you get through your life?

(Cooley 34)

Driving becomes a metaphor for the speaker's manic experience. It is quite easy to describe the poem using the language from manuals like the DSM or the ICD. The speaker clearly displays agitation and energetic behavior. There is an indication of a goal-directed activity (the speaker is trying to get ahead). It is not unreasonable to argue that closing your eyes and dropping the steering wheel would qualify as high-risk behavior caused by impaired judgment, something that could very well have painful consequences (indeed, another car driving in the opposite direction 'swerves on its horn out of the road' to avoid a car crash). Additionally, it is a recurring thing ('Tonight again I do it'), so it extends beyond just this one incident accounted for in the poem. The speaker seems to be easily distracted, and one could argue that his thoughts (and not just the car) are racing; he certainly does move quickly from one image, idea, or addressee to the next. Finally (though surely other clinical aspects could be highlighted), one could describe his thinking as grandiose and delusional. For instance, in stanza three, the speaker starts 'to die' and gets 'reborn', and in the final stanza, he believes that he is 'among the chosen', and that he is 'going to live forever'.

However, an interpretation of the poem that merely highlighted how the poem depicts a manic episode would be insufficient. The medicalized interpretation would miss the poetic aspects—and the oscillation between a poetic and a medical understanding—as well as the humor of the poem (reckless driving in real life is no laughing matter). Hartman writes that 'The literary shows its existential rather than conventional side and points to the link between symptom and symbolic action' (Hartman 343). Indeed, the images and the poetic strategy here transcend a medicalized reading and foreground the existential experience. The poem is replete with original metaphors, just as it moves rapidly from one image the next. In the first two lines, driving with the high-beam lights on is described as driving with 'antlers to the dark'. Deer use their antlers to fight for dominance, so it points towards a display of courage, defiance, and empowerment. Yet, how can antlers compete with, let alone beat, something as abstract as 'the dark'? The poem goes on to state that it is 'hard / to get ahead'. The enjambment emphasizes the difficulty, but it is left ambiguous whether the words 'It's hard' describe the attempt to attack the dark with antlers (with dark-hard being near rhymes), whether they constitute an intransitive sentence, or whether it is trying to 'get ahead' that is hard. Arguably, it is all three possibilities. The first stanza ends with a new metaphor for driving a car. The car or the drive is like a dog with a collar, and the speaker imagines that the 'soul' has the car/drive/dog on a leash and is trying to keep up, but is out of breath.

The poem ostensibly does not rhyme, or at least there are hardly any end rhymes ('reborn-head-on' being the exception). However, some of the most significant words in the poem rhyme or nearly rhyme, namely: dark, hard, stars, start, and car. Stanzas two and three narrate the reckless and possibly suicidal (and habitual?) decision to drop the steering wheel and close the eyes while driving. The speaker states that he 'pull[s] [his] eyes into a fist'—hence drawing attention to the visual likeness between the position of the index finger in a closed fist and your eyes if you squeeze them hard. This also means that the stars that the speaker can see and taste the roots and sweet bone marrow of in stanza two are the stars or sparkles one can see when one closes one's eyes—and perhaps is dazed and dizzy. The experience in stanza two corresponds well with the following quote from Woolf's *On Being Ill*: 'On the other hand, with responsibility shelved and reason in the abeyance [...] other tastes assert themselves; sudden, fitful, intense' (Woolf 20). In the final stanza, the speaker's association has suddenly made a leap from those sparkling stars a person sees when one pulls one's eyes into a fist to the actual stars in the night sky. The speaker's identification with the stars ('Like / those stars I'm going to live forever') is seen as part of his delusional grandiosity and self-exaltation, but, of course, there obviously is an ironic humorous aspect to that false conclusion: the stars in the night sky do not live forever. They die out, and many of the stars we see in the sky died out many years ago. The sun could be dead for all we know, since the sun we see from Earth is always some eight minutes and twenty seconds behind time. So, really, the comparison should be that just as the stars are not invincible, neither is the speaker.

Peter Cooley uses the line-by-line reading and the consequential potential for enjambment to mimic and sustain the rapid shifts and unpredictability of the racing thoughts. The reader has to follow the movement from the car as a deer with antlers, to the car as a dog on a leash; or from stars when the eyes are pulled into a fist, to the stars in the night sky. The final aspect of the poem to be addressed for the purposes of this chapter is the very question of the relationship—or, even, identity—of the poem's speaker and its addressee. Like the poem's images and narrative, the communicative setting is ambiguous and rapidly shifts between different levels. The poem uses an 'I' and a 'you', which is all very traditional. However, it is actually not clear who the 'I' and the 'you' refer to, and, in addition to those two personal pronouns, the poet 'Cooley' as well as the 'listener' are addressed in the final stanza.

The second personal pronoun, 'you', is highly ambiguous. It may signify an addressee in a conversation distinct from the first-person speaker. It may also be a form of self-address: 'You idiot', one might, for instance, exclaim or think, if you cannot remember where you parked your car. In the poem, one might see the 'I' and the 'you' as one and the same entity. One might even make the case that the 'I' represents the manic version of the speaker, i.e. the one who drives, drops the wheel, tastes the stars, is chosen, etc. The 'you', then, represents the version of the speaker who cannot keep up. 'You' may, of course, also refer to an unknown, universal or, at any rate, impersonal entity (like the 'you' one encounters in recipes in cookbooks). Whenever a literary text uses 'you', there is also an element of directly addressing the reader. This is, perhaps, what goes on towards the end of the poem, when 'you' is aligned with a 'listener'.

What, though, is the meaning of the poet's surname suddenly appearing in the final stanza? It could be interpreted as a form of self-address in the third person, which would be in line with both the self-exaltation and grandiosity expressed—perhaps it is even a manic psychosis—in that stanza. It would also fit with the interpretation of the 'you' as a form of self-address. It might, however, also be the case that something more complex is going on. Some readers might by default have assumed a correspondence between Peter Cooley and the speaker. Contrary to that position, one could argue that the speaker metaleptically addresses the poet. In that case, the speaker acknowledges that he was saved from the car crash, because the poet (who controls what is written) decided to have the other car veer off the road. Even as this would expose the fictitiousness of the event, the speaker nonetheless takes his existence seriously, stating that he is chosen, and that he is going to live forever like the stars. The metaleptic reading is supported by the fact that the speaker also abruptly addresses us, the listeners, in the final stanza, installing a metafictional element in the poem's conclusion.

Ironic Quotation in Erica Dawson's 'Disorder'

Erica Dawson's poem 'Disorder' counters the DSM in a more direct way, incorporating its vocabulary in an ironic context. The poem contains a motto, which is a quote taken from the DSM: 'For some diagnoses, the appropriate code depends on further specification' (Dawson 43). As an ironic citation, it suggests that there is an irreducible relativity to systems of standardized diagnoses for mental disorders. The poem itself engages in an elaborate play on the concept of a code and of coding as well as on the word 'episode'. It contains codes from the DSM in each of the four stanzas. It was published in 2007, so it is in dialogue with the DSM-IV from 1994 (or perhaps the revised version, the DSM-IV-TR from 2000), rather than the more recent DSM-V from 2013. The codes incorporated are related to bipolar disorder. The poem in full reads thus:

> I'm systematically deranged.
> Two. Nine. Six. Three. I've multiplied
> The digits, switched, then disarranged
> The code, prognoses side by side.
> And I begin. I'm certified,
> Depressed, no symptoms to decode—
> The signifier signified
> In this recurring episode.

And then the code is rearranged—
Two. Nine. Six. O, a manic ride.
It's me, sleeping all day exchanged
For vacuuming, a quickened stride.
With spasms, ticks, I'm bona fide
Fucked up, bipolar antipode
And looking at the small divide
In this recurring episode.

But wait, the code is interchanged—
Two. Six. Three. I can step beside
Myself and leave me there, estranged.
Delirium's like suicide
Without the mess, more dignified.
Now bury me in my abode
Twelve feet under. Pretend I've died
In this recurring episode.

Yet I wake up, always inside
This room, writing the palinode—
Two. Nine. Six. Three—identified
In this recurring episode.

(Dawson 43)

The code mentioned in stanza one and four, 296.3, is the code for major depressive disorder with recurrent episodes, so the speaker identifies with depressive moods in those two stanzas. The second line of verse in stanza two states 'Two. Nine. Six. O, a manic ride' and, indeed, this is the code for Bipolar I disorder with a single manic episode. Additionally, Dawson puns on the numeral 0, instead employing the poetic vocative exclamation 'O' (which audibly sounds and graphically looks the same). Stanza three suggests a manic episode with psychotic elements. The speaker experiences estrangement, delirium, and a feeling of being buried alive or of having died.

The poem revolves around the diagnosis of bipolar disorder. As the moods change, the codes change. The poem is circular while ironically punning on the words 'code' and 'episode'. Besides referring to the statistical code in the DSM, 'code' also describes the speaker as someone who is being coded. Dawson ironically and humorously reverses the normal order of steps in receiving a diagnosis. In the natural order, one is supposed to first account for a way of behaving and thinking, which can then be aligned with a set of symptoms that enables a doctor to propose a diagnostic code. However, in 'Disorder', it seems like the code—rather than being objectively descriptive—codes the speaker or prescribes/instigates the behavior. The word 'episode' is used as a refrain—'in this recurring episode'—ending each stanza. Both the meaning and the repetition of the line stress circularity.

The circularity and repetition are also inscribed in the poem's rhyme scheme. For a poem entitled 'Disorder', the stanzas are highly metric and orderly. The first three stanzas rhyme ababbcbc, while the final stanza rhymes bcbc. The stanza formation approximates several classical metric stanza forms. One may compare it to the ottava rima. This stanza also contains eight lines of verse, but the rhyme scheme is different in the final four verses: abababcc. The rhyme scheme is closer to Geoffrey Chaucer's rhyme royal—ababbcc—but this stanza form only has seven lines of verse. Perhaps the most similar stanza form is the Spenserian stanza (named after Edmund Spenser), which rhymes in the following way: ababbcbcc. The rhyme scheme is identical if the final line is deleted. The symmetrical order of Dawson's poem is further emphasized, because she uses the same rhymes in all the stanzas. Hence, there are only three different rhyme sounds in the poem's twenty-eight lines of verse. The rhymes in the a-spot only change slightly: deranged, disarranged, rearranged, exchanged, interchanged, estranged. That is, just like the code is only slightly adjusted—e.g. from 'Two. Nine. Six. Three' in stanza one to 'Two. Nine. Six. O' in stanza two—so are the sounds of the end rhymes.

In the final stanza, Dawson returns to the same code as in stanza one. The speaker in the poem has literally come full circle: 'Yet I wake up, always inside / This room, writing the palinode— / Two. Nine. Six. Three—identified / In this recurring episode'. A palinode is an ode from ancient Greece, in which an earlier statement is detracted (e.g. one could write an ode to the beauty of Helen, and then subsequently write a palinode taking it back). The speaker in 'Disorder' goes round in circles, constantly writing palinodes as the moods swing round the carousel of bipolar disorder.

The poem functions as a parody on a 'positivist psychiatric project of codifying human suffering into disease-like categories' (Rapley, Moncrieff, and Dillon 1) like the DSM. In a critique of the DSM-V, Line Joranger writes the following assessment, a message that resonates well with my understanding of the message in 'Disorder':

> Imagine that mental illnesses are a question of degree and a question of how meaningful connections are manifested, and imagine that anything really meaningful tends to have a unique, nonreferential form. Our medical and philosophical urge toward generalization will destroy these connections, and we should be concerned about how the new and revised manual of mental disorders, the DSM-V, is being used. (Joranger 520)

In opposition to that medical and philosophical urge, Joranger concludes that 'Meaningful connections are, as such, a matter of poetic expressions, not diagnostic and philosophical explanations' (Joranger 521). I would argue that the poems by Peter Cooley, Erica Dawson, and Chana Bloch, and other poems about bipolar disorder, help to establish such poetic and meaningful connections.

Existential Abstraction in Chana Bloch's 'Eclipse'

Chana Bloch's poem 'Eclipse' counters clinical perceptions of bipolar disorder in a way that distinguishes itself from Cooley's narrative poetry, as well as from Dawson's parodic and ironic treatment of medicalized ways of understanding the illness. 'Eclipse' is an abstract poem in which the meanings of central words and concepts are deliberately presented as an unresolved (maybe even unresolvable) ambiguity. It corresponds well with Virginia Woolf's notion of language in relation to illness, when she writes that:

> In illness words seem to possess a mystic quality. We grasp what is beyond their surface meaning, gather instinctively this, that, and the other—a sound, a colour, here a stress, there a pause—which the poet, knowing words to be meagre in comparison with ideas, has strewn about his page to evoke, when collected, a state of mind which neither words can express nor the reason explain. Incomprehensibility has an enormous power over us in illness. (Woolf 21)

When one reads 'Eclipse' as a poem about bipolar disorder (bearing in mind that it does appear in an anthology about that mental disorder), one might argue that Bloch attempts to create an existential and abstract vision that can help grasp the way that the two poles of bipolar disorder are both 'bi' (that is, divided into two moods) and interlocked as one illness. At the same time, the poem insists on not resolving the incomprehensible and ungraspable aspects of the illness. One way to read the poem is to see it as being about the two poles of bipolar disorder, their relation, and the meaning for one's self-perception. To contemplate this, Bloch plays with poetry's unique possibilities for organizing words on a white piece of paper. The poem consists of eight lines of verse, but there is more than one poem within that poem. Or rather, more than one way of reading it. Lines 1, 3, 5, and 7 start at the left margin, while lines 2, 4, 6, and 8 extend from the right margin. Additionally, the latter group distinguish themselves from the former by being italicized. Quoted in full, the poem goes as follows:

> There are two bodies floating above us:
> *They are one body*
> yours dark, a silence
> *tails of flame lashing the emptiness,*
> growing in space,
> *emptiness opening its mouth wide*
> mine a ring of fire clenched around it.
> *to swallow the fire.*
>
> (Bloch 12)

The two positions are both competing and in dialogue with each other while simultaneously inhabiting one poem. The situation described is one in which an 'I' and a 'you' lie down looking up at two 'bodies' that float above them. The bodies contain character traits from the 'I' and the 'you' respectively. The 'I' is associated with the left-centered lines, and the italic right-centered lines with the 'you'. The right-centered lines in italics seem to represent the depressive mood. Its 'body' is called 'dark, a silence', and 'emptiness'. The left-centered lines would then be associated with mania. The 'I' has a 'ring of fire', fire being a common image of mania (not least since Kay Redfield Jamison's seminal book, entitled *Touched with Fire: Manic-Depressive Illness and the Artistic Temperament*).

The two voices within one poem provide the reader with multiple reading options. One can read them as two independent poems that complement each other. The left-centered poem reads as follows: 'There are two bodies floating above us: / yours dark, a silence / growing in space, / mine a ring of fire clenched around it.' The right-centered poem would read: '*They are one body, / tails of flame lashing the emptiness, / emptiness opening its mouth wide / to swallow the fire.*' There are several disagreements between the two voices. In the left-centered text, the I's 'ring of fire' is dominating the dark body and the 'silence / growing in space'. The right-centered text in italics, however, comments on and even corrects what is uttered by the other voice. Thus, it puts forward a competing version of the state of affairs. Immediately after it is stated in the first line that there 'are two bodies floating above us', the right-centered text offers a correction in claiming they 'are one body'. The left-centered text ignores this correction as it continues to insist on 'yours' versus 'mine'. Whereas the left-centered text describes its ethereal body as 'a ring of fire', the right-centered text associates the other with 'tails of flame' that lash 'the emptiness'. The you-voice goes even further in asserting its own association with a circular shape, in that the 'emptiness' opens 'its mouth wide / to swallow the fire'. Not only is the 'I' described by means of tails of flame rather than a ring, but it is—according to the right-centered voice—the emptiness that has a circular shape. In the final three lines of the poem, two mutually exclusive options are presented. As the emptiness opens 'its mouth wide', the 'I' claims to be 'a ring of fire clenched around it', while the right-centered voice in italics gets the final say in stating that the mouth of emptiness attempts 'to swallow the fire'.

'Eclipse' is a deliberately disorienting poem with multiple reading options. Is it one, two, or more poems? Are there two bodies, or is it a duality within one body? Who has the upper hand? The fire or the emptiness? The spacing and visuality of the letters (normal versus italics, left-centered versus right-centered) contribute to making it an ambiguous text. For instance, it is difficult to work out if the lines refer to lines of their own kind (left-centered versus right-centered and italicized) or not. 'Eclipse' offers an abstract, visionary view of the two moods of bipolar disorder and their ways of being intertwined. Employing poetry's spacing of language and graphic visuality, Bloch has created a poem that insists on both the duality and internal struggle for dominance in an illness like bipolar disorder, depicting it as a kind of yin and yang. In the end, it is undecidable which one is the stronger. The left-centered text (the mania) posits to have a ring of fire clenched around the emptiness, whereas the right-centered text (the depression) claims that it opens its mouth wide to swallow the aforementioned ring of fire. And, of course, the title 'Eclipse' does not reveal whether readers are experiencing a solar or a lunar eclipse.

Conclusion

In this chapter, I have argued that the psychiatric system in place, represented primarily by the DSM, causes a neglect of the context and existential dimension of people experiencing mental distress. Hence, literary representations of mental illness become important resources for understanding existential dimensions of mental illness. To counter the DSM, then, means to critique and supplement it. Although a useful and necessary tool, clinical psychiatry's reduction of individual experiences into generalizable symptoms and symptom clusters leaves out important aspects of what it means to be in ill mental health.

Virginia Woolf's *On Being Ill* teaches us something about the connections between illness and the aesthetic mind. Coates writes that '[f]or Woolf, illness invokes the bodily awareness and the perceptual uniqueness necessary for reading a work of art. Illness, as she represents it in "On Being Ill," induces us to inhabit our bodies in a way that no other experience can' (Coates 247). Using some of the notions proposed in *On Being Ill*, I make the case that literature can, indeed, provide some of the perspectives and voices lacking in clinical psychiatry.

Furthermore, I discuss the benefits of writing (lyrical) poetry about mental illness (and in my cases, bipolar disorder more specifically). Although narrative understandings of illness proliferate, there is something deeply anti-narrative about illnesses. I have argued that poems about bipolar disorder are apt to incorporate, represent, and account for the interruptions that characterize illness narratives. Instead of trying to recuperate bipolar narratives within an Aristotelian conception of a teleological plot, they account for the subjective experiences by being cyclic, episodic, fragmentary, lyric, and abstract. In writing poetry, authors can experiment with the physical and material space of the poem (lines of verse cut off before the right margin, the interplay with and importance of the white paper, the rhymes, etc.). In the poems by Peter Cooley, Erica Dawson, and Chana Bloch this is employed to different ends and in distinct ways, displaying great creative resourcefulness.

References

American Psychiatric Association, *Diagnostic and Statistical Manual of Mental Disorder*, 5th edn, https://dsm-psychiatryonline-org.ez.statsbiblioteket.dk:12048/doi/book/10.1176/appi.books.9780890425596, accessed 20 September 2020.

Bloch, Chana, 'Eclipse' in Thom Schramm (ed.), *Living in Storms: Contemporary Poetry and the Moods of Manic-Depression* (Washington: Eastern Washington University Press, 2008), 12.

Coates, Kimberly Engdahl, 'Exposing the Nerves of Language: Virginia Woolf, Charles Mauron, and the Affinity Between Aesthetics and Illness', *Literature and Medicine* 21.2 (2002): 242–63. https://doi.org/10.1353/lm.2002.0018

Cooley, Peter, 'Returning from the Shopping Center to the Suburbs' in Thom Schramm (ed.), *Living in Storms: Contemporary Poetry and the Moods of Manic-Depression* (Washington: Eastern Washington University Press, 2008), 34.

Dawson, Erica, 'Disorder' in Thom Schramm (ed.), *Living in Storms: Contemporary Poetry and the Moods of Manic-Depression* (Washington: Eastern Washington University Press, 2008), 43.

Hartman, Geoffrey, 'Narrative and Beyond', *Literature and Medicine* 23.2 (2004): 334–45. https://doi.org/10.1353/lm.2005.0006

Jamison, Kay Redfield, *Touched with Fire: Manic-Depressive Illness and the Artistic Temperament* (New York: Free Press Paperbacks, 1993).

Joranger, Line, 'Mental Illness and Imagination in Philosophy, Literature, and Psychiatry', *Philosophy and Literature* 37.2 (2013): 507–23. https://doi.org/10.1353/phl.2013.0019

Nordgaard, Julie, and Josef Parnas, 'Editorial: A Haunting that Never Stops: Psychiatry's Problem of Description', *Acta Psychiatrica Scandinavica* 127 (2013): 434–35. https://doi.org/10.1111/acps.12092

Rapley, Mark, Joanna Moncrieff, and Jacqui Dillon, 'Carving Nature at its Joints? DSM and the Medicalization of Everyday Life' in Mark Rapley, Joanna Moncrieff, and Jacqui Dillon (eds), *De-Medicalizing Misery: Psychiatry, Psychology and the Human Condition* (New York: Palgrave Macmillan, 2011), 1–10. https://doi.org/10.1057/9780230342507_1

Rimmon-Kenan, Shlomith, 'What Can Narrative Theory Learn from Illness Narratives?', *Literature and Medicine* 25.2 (2006): 241–54. https://doi.org/10.1353/lm.2007.0019

Scheurich, Neil, 'Reading, Listening, and Other Beleaguered Practices in General Psychiatry' in R. Charon and P.L. Rudnytsky (eds), *Psychoanalysis and Narrative Medicine* (New York: New York State University Press, 2008), 511–41.

Wojahn, David, 'Foreword' in Thom Schramm (ed.), *Living in Storms: Contemporary Poetry and the Moods of Manic-Depression* (Washington: Eastern Washington University Press, 2008), xiii–xv.

Woolf, Virginia, *On Being Ill* (Ashfield, MA: Paris Press, 2002).

10

Seeing Feeling: Dissociation and Post-Traumatic Memory in the Graphic Novel *Perfect Hair*

Penni Russon

> The question to ask of the artwork is thus, not 'What does it mean?' or 'What trauma is depicted?' but 'How does it work?—how does it put insides and outsides into contact in order to establish a basis for empathy?' (Bennett 45)

In *Empathic Vision*, Jill Bennett writes of encountering artworks that 'evoked the processes of post-traumatic memory', locating this evocation neither in narrative content nor ostensible meaning, but rather a 'certain affective dynamic central to the work' (Bennett 1) in which the texts put 'insides' into contact with 'outsides' to generate empathy. I explore this affective dynamic in *Perfect Hair*, a graphic novel by Tommi Parrish, where 'feeling is both imagined and regenerated through an encounter with the artwork', a process Bennett calls 'seeing feeling' (Bennett 1). Parrish pushes the artistic qualities of the Figure, heightening embodied sensation and affect, while exploiting the disjunctive, asynchronous visual-verbal form of comics to simultaneously present inner and outer experience, including traumatic memory and dissociation. Parrish's isolation and foregrounding of the physical fact of the body is an essential part of the way narrative in *Perfect Hair* is mediated by the image. Narrative wants to subsume the image in its flow; however, Parrish's Figure, foregrounded, isolated, pulsing with feeling, resists the tug of narrative—like the traumatized self that stores the affective memory within the body, unlinking it from the mind.

Penni Russon, 'Chapter 10: Seeing Feeling: Dissociation and Post-Traumatic Memory in the Graphic Novel *Perfect Hair*' in: *Madness and Literature: What Fiction Can Do for the Understanding of Mental Illness*. University of Exeter Press (2022). © Penni Russon. DOI: 10.47788/WKFD8677

In this chapter I explore the ways in which Parrish uses the disjunctive, asynchronous visual-verbal form of comics to put insides and outsides into contact to evoke the processes of traumatic dissociation, representing a body that is at once present and absent. I will examine the ways in which the unsaid and unsayable, unknown and unknowable, unseen and unseeable act on graphic narratives. I propose that the inevitable 'narrative effect' of a sequence of images (Magnussen and Christiansen 199) draws attention to gaps or spaces in the narrative that must be negotiated by the body to 'feel' rather than 'think' the truth, something Jill Bennett calls 'the art of sense memory' (Bennett 26). I explore the way Parrish's use of different media and formal styles—moving from drawing to painting, black and white to colour—heightens sensation. Sensation is defined, to follow Deleuze, as the 'action of invisible forces on the body' (Deleuze 41), in which the unseen is rendered visible through a bodily exchange: between the body of the figure on the page, what Ronnie Scott calls 'the trace of the hand' (MacFarlane, Scott, and Caleo, unpaginated), or the residual body-traces of the comic's artist, and the body of the reader.

Parrish's *Perfect Hair* is a slim, seventy-two-page graphic novel; a complex comic that rewards close attention. *Perfect Hair* is a discontinuous narrative, told in a series of interrelated chapters, following a single day in the life of two characters, Nicola and Cleary. Nicola, a sex worker, arranges an appointment with a client, sorts through the proof sheets from a photo shoot, and later, as arranged, arrives at the suburban house of the client where they engage in domestic role-play. Cleary catches the train to a sex club, where they have an anxiety attack, then later rides their bike to the hospital to visit a dying, hallucinating grandmother. A closing scene depicts Cleary and Nicola together standing on the railing of a veranda. Nicola says, 'The days keep ending' and Cleary replies, 'I don't know where they go' (Parrish, unpaginated). The graphic novel is pieced together with fragments of these related stories progressing in a cumulative narrative, subtly wending towards this single point of narrative closure—implied more in the closing of the day than any sort of resolution or revelation.

Formal experimentation is a distinctive characteristic of Parrish's graphic style. Parrish switches between visual modes, sometimes on the same page, blending mediums, transitioning from pen to watercolour to pencil work, and mixing influences such as naturalism, impressionism, popular culture, and graphic design. Most immediately striking in the visual style of *Perfect Hair* are the proportions of Parrish's characters' large, exaggerated bodies and comparatively small, occasionally featureless, heads. There is a sculptural quality to these bodies; Sean Rogers notes: 'Parrish's art excels at worrying these boundaries between symbolic thinking and actual experience, endowing big, clayey bodies with rarefied grace' (Rogers), enhancing, as Dash Shaw comments, their 'sensorial' qualities (Parrish).

Psychological Trauma and Dissociation

Dissociation is defined by the American Psychiatric Association as 'disruption of and/or discontinuity in the normal integration of consciousness, memory, identity, emotion, perception, body representation, motor control, and behaviour' (American Psychiatric Association 291). Psychological trauma is generally understood to be the principal cause of dissociation. Psychological trauma can be directly linked to an experience, including war, the death or loss of a loved one, an accident, or childhood abuse; however, the underlying traumatic experiences can also be hidden 'early defining events' that are 'never brought into the light of consciousness', notes Steve Haines in his graphic non-fiction text, *Trauma is Very Strange* (Haines and Standing, unpaginated). 'Dissociation is a way of keeping overwhelming events, feelings, sensations, and thoughts away from the core self' (Wieland 6); however, while it is an adaptive mechanism aimed at protecting parts of the personality, this survival comes at a cost to the individual, problems arising 'when these coping strategies come into conflict with wider social expectations of the functioning adult' (Wastell 162). Haines describes the experience of dissociation—this fragmentation of the self—as 'an inherently confusing, frequently depressing, lost place' (Haines and Standing, unpaginated). Dissociation requires a 'constant alertness or vigilance of awareness', and the original traumatic experience is 'an affective memory held by the body' unavailable to the mind, elusive because that which 'was unbearable is relegated to a part of the self that is unlinked from what is preserved as a relatively intact "me"' (Sinason 164–65). In *The Body Keeps the Score*, Van der Kolk describes the toll this dual state of hypervigilance and numb protectedness has on daily life:

> Ordinary, day-to-day events become less and less compelling. Not being able to deeply take in what is going on around them makes it impossible to feel

fully alive. It becomes harder to feel the joys and aggravations of ordinary life, harder to concentrate on the tasks at hand. (Van der Kolk 67)

The narratives of original traumatic experiences may never be uncovered, but that which is unseen, unsaid, and unknown remains present in everyday life, taking its toll.

In *Trauma Fiction*, Anne Whitehead poses the question, 'if trauma comprises an event or experience which overwhelms the individual and resists language or representation, how then can it be narrativised in fiction?' (Whitehead 3). She further argues that the representation of trauma requires 'a literary form that departs from conventional linear sequence' (Whitehead 6), suggesting such fiction shares stylistic features with 'postmodern and postcolonial fiction' such as 'self-conscious modes of reflection or critique' (Whitehead 7). Goldsmith and Satterlee agree that writers 'employ narrative strategies to convey the fracturing of time, self and reality that often defines and accompanies traumatic episodes or recall' (Goldsmith and Satterlee 55), and in this chapter I will look at the narrative strategies Tommi Parrish uses to convey this sort of fracturing, but I also make the argument that the form of graphic narrative is particularly well suited to conveying experiences of trauma. Hillary Chute argues that comics' capacity to show and tell at the same time is key to the way comics represent disability and illness: 'Comics can make visible both external features of a condition, and internal, cognitive and emotional features that are otherwise hard to communicate accurately' (Chute 2017, 243). In particular, she notes the ways in which what usually occurs as a psychic state can be made physical on the page: '[D]rawing can offer a picture of a consciousness—a mental state or a psychic landscape—that is internal to an individual', rendering the 'mind's eye' into 'a visual form on the page that readers can encounter and understand' (Chute 2017, 258). In *Perfect Hair*, trauma and subsequent patterns of dissociation emerge in the reading-and-looking process, the nonsynchronous and 'disjunctive back-and-forth of *reading* and *looking* for meaning' (Chute 2008, 452; emphasis in the original) that characterizes the visual-verbal interplay within comics, and I will explore that in more detail below.

In their work comparing representations of trauma in clinical psychology and fiction, one of the particular strengths of fiction that Rachel E. Goldsmith and Michelle Satterlee identify is the capacity for fiction to situate trauma in 'a social context that complicates the experience' (Goldsmith and Satterlee 44).

Bennett also posits that 'trauma is not simply an interior condition', but also 'a transformative process that impacts on the world as much as on bodies' (Bennett 12). Goldsmith and Satterlee point to the capacity for literary representations of trauma to cross the private–public boundary; that is, while still allowing the presentation of highly personal, idiosyncratic experiences, fiction can reveal the social and cultural contexts of trauma and dissociation. Of particular interest to my reading of *Perfect Hair* is the notion that 'many emotions that accompany or define PTSD are not formed in isolation, but by and through connections with others' (Goldsmith and Satterlee 42); close examination of *Perfect Hair* reveals the social dynamics of dissociation.

In *Empathic Vision*, Jill Bennett writes of artworks she encountered that 'evoked the processes of post-traumatic memory without declaring themselves to be about trauma' (Bennett 1). *Perfect Hair* does not explicitly declare itself to be *about* trauma. I acknowledge here that there is a risk in labelling Parrish's work as being about trauma: 'To identify any art as "about" trauma […] potentially opens up new readings, but it also reduces work to a singular defining subject matter in a fashion that is often anathema to artists' (Bennett 2). However, following Bennett's line of thinking, it is in the ambiguity, the gaps, and spaces in the narrative that I locate the evocation of trauma, rather than in the 'narrative component' or the 'ostensible meaning' (Bennett 1). Bennett sees in the visual language of art 'an embodiment of sensation that stimulates thought' (Bennett 8), that neither merely illustrates or represents trauma, but generates 'a manner of thinking', drawing on Deleuze's conception of the *'encountered sign* […] the sign that is felt, rather than is recognised or perceived through cognition' (Bennett 7; italics in original). Feeling does not exist in opposition to thinking but instead precedes and prompts cognition. Rather than narrating the causes and consequences of trauma, *Perfect Hair* recreates the experience of living with the symptoms of trauma and the way traumatic memory permeates moments of being in the world.

Table of Contents and the Contents of the Body

If not trauma, what does *Perfect Hair* declare itself to be about? The function of a table of contents is to disclose what is to come, but Parrish's 'Table of Contents' offers disclosure in the confessional sense, foreshadowing the underlying emotional textures of the comic, while still remaining oblique about

SEEING FEELING

the relationship between text, image, and meaning. In a grid, Parrish displays words—*air, calm, anxiety, movement, saftey* [sic], *light (dappled), sex, exhaustion, stillness, breath (exhale)*—accompanied by simple expressive abstract shapes. The misspelling of the word 'safety', whether deliberate or not, resounds with human fallibility and vulnerability.

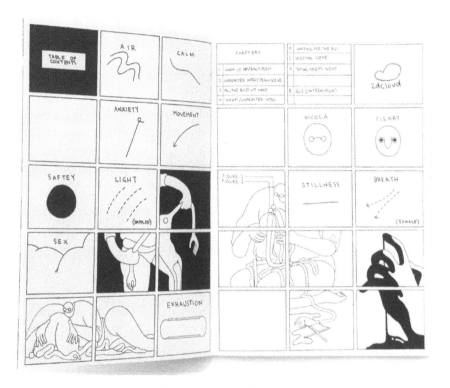

'Table of Contents' (Parrish)

The tension between concrete nouns and abstract shapes communicates that expressing the inner sensations of the body, and the ineffable qualities of the world the body perceives and encounters, is not straightforward. A small ball perches at the edge of a long drop to signify anxiety. Sex is represented by a simple outline that resembles the rumpled form of fleshy crevices that may be buttocks, but could also be a closed hand (as implied a few pages later in a series of images showing a fist opening and closing), or another part of the anatomy where the body curves and creases such as the knee or the arm. The image I see in the elongated form that accompanies 'exhaustion' is the outline of a menstrual pad. Breath and light mimic each other, and the orientation (breath,

185

movement, light) always points downwards. Stillness is a straight horizontal line. These images recur indirectly throughout the comic—for example, in one scene the reader shares Cleary's point of view at the top of a flight of stairs, recalling the steep descent of anxiety. The *contents* Parrish foreshadows are the contents of the body, its sensations as it encounters the environment through moments (Parrish uses the word 'scene') of movement and stillness, stasis and disruption.

The Fact of the Body

One effect of Parrish's painterly imagery is the foregrounding of the Figure and the subsequent intensifying of the sensorial, feeling body. Nicola particularly is often depicted alone, such as in the first image where she kneels naked by a stream wearing only her opaque glasses, a billowing sheet tied to a branch behind her. This juxtaposing of the body and a vivid, verdant landscape recurs throughout the comic, often in opposition to the city, though sometimes the city is depicted with the green encroaching on the urban environment, the conscious and unconscious worlds coming into contact. Deleuze, in *Francis Bacon: The Logic of Sensation*, relates the exaggerated, isolated Figure, pushed beyond illustrative or narrative function, to sensation. The Figure 'acts immediately upon the nervous system', as opposed to the abstract form which 'acts through the intermediary of the brain' (Deleuze 34). When the Figure is isolated it exists in addition to, or excluded from, '*figurative, illustrative* and *narrative* character' (Deleuze 2; italics in original). By sensation, Deleuze means a way of 'Being-in-the-World' (Deleuze 34), stating that 'sensation […] is in the body […] Color is in the body, sensation is in the body, and not in the air. Sensation is what is painted' (Deleuze 35). The Figure has a presence, signifying itself. In the composition of figures, Parrish, like Bacon and Deleuze, is particularly interested in the relationship between the head and the face:

> the Figure, being a body, is not the face, and does not even have a face. It does have a head, because the head is an integral part of the body. It can even be reduced to the head. […] the face is a structured, spatial organization that conceals the head, whereas the head is dependent upon the body, even if it is the point of the body, its culmination. It is not that the head lacks spirit; but it is a spirit in bodily form, a corporeal and vital breath, an animal spirit. (Deleuze 20)

Like Francis Bacon, Parrish 'dismantle[s] the face' and 'rediscover[s] the head'. In images in which the body appears for its sensory, affective properties, the face often vanishes—it comes and goes over the sequences of panels to highlight interiority and exteriority. The overall impression is always one of heightened sensation but also distance from the 'thinking' self. The body is engulfed by its own physical form. In times of extreme dissociation when the boundaries between inner and outer fail, all distinctive physical features—form and flesh—vanish and the body is represented as a simple outline.

Parrish's isolation and foregrounding of the physical fact of the body is an essential part of the way narrative in *Perfect Hair* is mediated by the image. In comics, narrative wants to subsume the image in its flow. Scott McCloud emphasizes what happens between panels: 'Comics ask the mind to work as a sort of in-betweener—filling in the gaps between panels as an animator might' (McCloud 88); so, presumably, no image signifies without the context of other images, and the image is always in a state of transition, flowing from one moment into the next. But Parrish's Figure resists the narrative pull, further emphasized in the comic as it departs from the square and rectangular panels into the use of full-page portraits, panel-less pages, inset panels, and the recurring use of circular panels. Deleuze is fascinated by the 'round area' and the way it relates temporally to narrative:

> Within the round area, the Figure is sitting on the chair, lying on the bed, and sometimes it even seems to be waiting for what is about to happen. But what is happening, or is about to happen, or has already happened, is not a spectacle or a representation. (Deleuze 12–13)

That is, that which occurs in the circular panel, following Deleuze's line of reasoning, has its weight in the present moment and exists in isolation from narrative. In a double-page spread, Parrish has drawn eight circular panels. At the top of the page reads the words: 'It feels like' and each panel is labelled with an implied narrative, juxtaposed against an image or object that seems to exist in relation to the sensorial body on the previous pages. For example: 'It's like writing "easy going and casual" in menstrual blood across your forehead' sits under a panel depicting a pool of blue fluid in the shower, recalling the coy advertising convention of using blue fluid to represent the capacity of menstrual pads to absorb blood. In another: 'It feels just like $1 7Eleven café latte's [*sic*]' is juxtaposed against an image of a torso, depicted in the tight circle, topped with the characteristic small, round, featureless head (Parrish). There is a patina of narrative, but the irony, arbitrariness, or discordance in the relationships between text and image only heighten the status of the Figure—in which the narrative and the non-narrative, the illustrative and the non-illustrative, simultaneously occur: 'Sensation has one face turned toward the subject (the nervous system, vital movement, "instinct," "temperament" [...]) and one face turned toward the object (the "fact," the place, the event)' (Deleuze 34). While the reader might be prompted to assemble a narrative by puzzling out the relationship between the panels and to the overall story, Parrish's deliberate ambiguity and irony appeals directly to resonances in the body to make sense of the metaphors.

The Figure resists narrative. In terms of Parrish's treatment of trauma, whereby Nicola and Cleary routinely withdraw inward from social contexts and appear to suffer pain, anxiety and distress, or dissociation and denial, the Figure reiterates the irretrievability of the past. Parrish gives no hints as to what underlying stories might exist to inform Nicola and Cleary's experiences of anxiety, trauma, and dissociation. One way the Figure resists narrative is through the isolating of the Figure, as explored above. However, on the same continuum is the repetition of the Figure. Another visual motif Parrish employs is that of a pile of anonymous bodies, contorted in strange shapes, suffering and comforting, intruding on each other but also providing support for each other as they crowd together in the same confined space. This motif calls into question the integrity of the body as a structural container for the self, but also troubles the notion of the body as a discrete unit that operates in predictable ways within a social structure.

The Meaning of Colour and the Line

In 'Character Intro/Train Scene', Cleary sits at the train station, apparently waiting for a train. On the verso page, this scene is in full colour; the straight grey lines of the train station and railway lines are contrasted against the rounded form of Cleary in pink top and blue jeans, and against the brightly coloured autumn trees first shown in the distance, and then inset close up as a panel in the bottom right corner. On the opposite page, the background disappears, the colours are eliminated, and Cleary is presented as a faint pencil sketch. The effect of the switch from colour to light grey pencil lines suggests a switch from surfaces and appearance to sensation. The reader transitions from being outside Cleary's body, in the realm of the visual, to a heightened awareness of Cleary's embodied sensory experience—in the pencil sketch, faint motion lines convey the sensations of breeze, light, and warmth on her body. Overleaf, the train arrives, over a few coloured panels. Briefly, Parrish re-enters the realm of sensation, switching back to Cleary as a faint pencil sketch, with directional lines that indicate the wind of the train's arrival. In a coloured panel, the silhouettes of the passengers are shown in the train and the doors open and people begin to exit. The platform is filled with diverse characters, a crowd scene in which each figure is distinct, many with some particular detail of characterization: a backpack, a headscarf, holding a baby, clearly defined bottom cheeks. Another passenger lies on their back in the middle of the crowd, which suggests surrealism, subverting reasonable expectations of the way bodies operate in this space. Cleary continues to sit as the people gradually disperse. The train departs and Cleary remains as the last passengers move away. The viewer zooms out to a high-angle long shot that takes in Cleary, the train station, and the last few passengers. There are few verbal cues; this is a largely textless comic.

The chronology of events is deceptively simple. Cleary waits at a train station: the train arrives, passengers disembark, Cleary interacts with no one, and does not board the train. The train leaves and Cleary remains at the station. The narrative threatens to fail as a narrative if narratives are predicated on moments of change, choice, or confrontation (Bal). What evokes a response in the reader is that *nothing happens*. Parrish utilizes a series of formal transitions—from colour to black and white, painterly flow to sketched lines, stylized and abstract to representational and illustrative, stillness to movement—in lieu of language. The reader traces these shifts—surface to sensation, exterior world to interior self—to assemble a narrative, but the shifts are traced in part through an affective response that comes when the reader apprehends a chasm in the narrative, unaided by verbal cues. This comic exemplifies the way Parrish brings insides into contact with outsides, 'yielding information to the body' (Bennett 41).

Cleary's heightened awareness and subsequent failure to act expresses the cycle of vigilance and detachment of psychological dissociation. The palpable absence of change, choice, or confrontation takes on narrative tension. Cleary defies the regular expectations or 'logic of events' (Bal 7) set up by the train station setting by not boarding the train. 'If art registers the shock of trauma (the flashback that one involuntarily revisits), it maintains this in tension with an experience of the present, an encounter with the "outside"' (Bennett 11). As readers we have access to Cleary's bodily sensations, but not the content of their thoughts. To follow Bennett, Parrish is 'concerned less with the integrity of subjective expression than with the complex dynamic of speaking from an "inside" position to an "outside"' (Bennett 12). In this comic, 'feeling is both imagined and regenerated through an encounter with the artwork' (Bennett 41), a process Bennett calls 'seeing feeling'.

The Violence of Discourse

In *Perfect Hair*, the narrative-resisting body retreats from the violence of discourse. In '"Haha"/Character Intro', Nicola is in the bedroom, sitting on her bed in her underwear, paper strewn on the floor around the bed. As the panels 'zoom in', the papers are revealed to be panels—each uniform in size and shape: photo proof sheets, though they also bear uncanny resemblance to the comic book panel. The disembodied monologue is the photographer: 'You are so fucking hot. Such a pretty girl. You know that, right?' As Nicola disrobes, the voice continues: 'Yeah, / I can see that you do' (Parrish). The disembodied voice performs the 'determining male gaze' (Mulvey 837), as it continues to appraise her: 'I love those little tits … / You must work out a lot / because you look like you'd fuck like you're training for the Olympics, haha' (Parrish). The tone is aggressively objectifying and self-gratifying: 'A lot of guys don't like little tits, but I'm different … /And well let's just say I'm not too bad myself' (Parrish). The relentlessness of the monologue is contrasted against the visual narrative, as Nicola removes her clothes, and then her breasts—'twist/pop'—and finally her yellowy-brown painterly skin, stepping out as a black-and-white hand-drawn outline, walking through the empty terrain of the blank page outside the panels, away from the final syllables of the crushing monologue: 'Ha / ha / ha'. The chapter closes with a single square of wilderness, recalling the pastoral scene and the Figure from the beginning of the novel. The reader is left with a sense of relief, witnessing Nicola's liberation from her codified body, the escape from narrative and context into blank space, the hints of the reprieve of the pastoral fantasy. However, there is a lingering impression of dissociation, of a retreat from a lonely urban existence and the social production of the body, into an inner world where Nicola is severed from narrative ... but at what cost?

In these panels we witness the social triggering of Nicola's dissociation. The internal gaze of Nicola is refracted through the Other. The disembodied gaze of the male photographer forms a violent discourse of looking and appraisal that also conjures the generalized male gaze as it manifests in culture. Nicola is prompted to dissociate through a process of rejection and withdrawal from his relentless gaze, but is also forced to withdraw from her own internal monologue, which repeats and amplifies the intrusive discourse of the other. Underneath this involuntary memory—the automatic 'playback' of the violent discourse—lurk deeper memories, memories hidden within the history of the body, unavailable to the mind that severs itself from the body; equally unavailable to the viewer or reader of the comic. Bennett's two understandings of traumatic memory come to mind here: *common memory*, which describes 'a social or properly understood discursive framework, designated as the site where history is written' (Bennett 25), and *sense memory*, which presents 'the physical imprint of the ordeal of violence', or to put it another way: 'Francis Bacon paints the scream, not what causes the scream' (Bennett 39). If introduced as backstory, the dissociation would become secondary to the narrative of the past. Parrish keeps us in the moment of dissociation, the contemporaneous muted horror of the unsayable, unseeable, and unspeakable as it acts upon the body. The project of the reader is not the forensic uncovering of an originating trauma, or its restoration to *common memory* (and therefore language), though such a trauma may be in part dramatized or reconstituted through the discourse of the aggressive male gaze. Rather the reader accesses the *sense memory*, through apprehension of the Figure, the sensorial body that resists its positioning in relation to time and memory, and denies language and narrative.

Empathy and the Gaze

In *Perfect Hair* the affective dynamics of dissociation are closely related to the affective dynamics of empathy and self-compassion. In 'Hospital Scene', communication is shown to be a fraught process with many moments of connection and disconnection. Cleary greets Grandma, glancing out the window and making an awkward comment about the weather, which serves to emphasize the artificial, enclosed space of the hospital: even small talk in *Perfect Hair* is never straightforward or neutral. This is further illustrated by the doctor who enters the room in the following panels, whose speech is punctuated by emoji symbols. 'Ours is an increasingly symbol-oriented culture', writes Scott McCloud, predicting: 'As the twenty-first century approaches, visual iconography may finally help us to realise a form of universal communication' (McCloud 58). The use of emoji in *Perfect Hair* is darkly humorous, but comedy borders on horror in the context of the hospital and the patient–physician relationship. 'How are we feeling today [smiling face with open mouth]?' asks the doctor; Grandma looks him in the eye and says, 'I'm 89. All I have the energy to do is watch TV and wait to die', and the doctor replies 'LMAO!' (Parrish). McCloud's idealized vision of a universal language is countered by the way Parrish plays with the non-verbal iconography of communication by placing it within the icon of the speech bubble. The doctor's relentless cheeriness is a deflective mechanism that protects him from seeing the grandmother's pain, and effectively renders her words, her pain, and her experience meaningless. The doctor mistakes Cleary for a grandson: 'OMG! Your grandson's visiting, cute!' he declares, with the word 'cute' written in childish bubble writing.

> *Grandma:* He called you my 'grandson'. I keep telling you that you look like a boy when you dress like that.
> *Cleary:* I don't mind.
> *Grandma:* Well I do. Everyone will think you're a lesbian if you don't put a dress on every now and then.
> *Cleary:* This is just how I feel comfortable.
> *Grandma:* That's a shame. (Parrish)

In the panels during this exchange, Cleary diminishes, receding while the grandmother is foregrounded. The grandmother transforms, losing her facial features and becoming just a head with a mouth to talk and drink with. After the exchange, Cleary leans on the bed and looks at Grandma, whose features are restored here, and in the next panel, Cleary's head is oriented in the other direction, and Cleary's own facial features have disappeared. Grandma also looks away, as if dismayed by the exchange. Again the experience here is one of estrangement and alienation from the other and dissociation from the self.

However, when Grandma asks Cleary about her breathing exercises, and Cleary in turn asks Grandma about her hallucinations, this process is disrupted, and connection is re-established:

> *Grandma:* Today it's flowers. / Everything's covered in flowers.
> *Cleary:* That sounds nice. So, the children are gone now?
> *Grandma:* More or less. Now I only see the tops of their little heads just before I fall asleep. (Parrish)

Grandma's hallucination, 'the tops of their little heads', recalls the first panel of this chapter: an image of the top of Cleary's head, as Cleary rides to the hospital. Grandma and Cleary are able to overcome the experience of detachment and disconnection. The final panel, the interior green world of Grandma's hallucinations, becomes a territory both can imaginatively enter.

Nicola also references Grandma's ghosts in the next chapter, 'Young Spirits Scene':

> *Nicola:* My friend's Grandma has ghosts that follow her around. / Young children mostly.
> *Chris:* Mmm. Powerful Spirits …
> *Nicola:* She says they want to impregnate her so they can be born back into the world. / She can feel them tugging at her sleeves. (Parrish)

This further reinforces a sense of social connectedness through empathy. The recounting of Grandma's story is a shared (if brief) moment of identification between Nicola and Chris. In the comic, while we visually look upon Nicola's and Chris's bodies as they recount this story, another body exists in the imaginative space of the panel, the discursive body of Cleary's Grandma. The same social dynamic that triggers dissociation in *Perfect Hair*, that of the internal gaze refracted through the other, is at play; however, in this case, moments of connection and identification recast the other as a non-object.

In another double-page spread, 'Waiting for the bus', Nicola takes out a packet of cigarettes and lights one. She stands on the footpath, looking up at the top storey of the building opposite in which a ballroom dancing class is taking place. The comic draws us into the dance class, panel after panel zooming in closer and closer, and for a moment—for the extent of one panel—the viewer is inside the room. Nicola smiles, extinguishes her cigarette, the bus arrives, and she gets on. In the last panel, we are left with the empty street. Without discourse, without the pitfalls of language, the comic communicates empathy as an embodied state, but also the ways in which empathy and connection with others implies connection with the self. Empathy and self-empathy, in this paradigm, are creative, imaginative acts. Intriguingly, this paradigm helps demonstrate how self-empathy is intersubjective, requiring not one mind or body, but in fact a conception of two embodied minds.

This model of self-empathy may give clues to the reading of comics. 'I've never felt so connected to detachment', writes R.J. Casey in a review of *Perfect Hair* in *The Comics Journal* (Casey, unpaginated). *Perfect Hair* holds the reader at arm's length. The Figure, foregrounded, isolated, pulsing with feeling, resists the tug of narrative. However, as the attentive reader experiences themself reading the comics, encountering narrative gaps generated from the tension between the narrative effect of sequential art and the unnarratable (the unseen/unseeable, unsaid/unsayable, unknown/unknowable), perhaps the key to navigating these gaps is an act of self-empathy. The Figure is always not-the-self, but the horror of the figure (Bacon's scream) is multiplied in the body of the reader, who negotiates what can never be seen, known or said, the affective memories held in their own bodies. The green worlds into which the characters retreat, Grandma's visions, Nicola's dissociative state, encase the physical text, spreading from the cover into the endpages, so that the whole comic seems to become a shared hallucination in which the reader is also implicated.

The gaze connects the inner and the outer world, the invisible line between what is outside the body and what occurs inside the body. The language of seeing—the articulated gaze—can dissemble, destroy, and fragment: subjects are made objects under the objectifying gaze. But the gaze turned inwards can also prompt moments of connection, empathy, and self-compassion, when insides and outsides, subjects and objects, come into contact in forgiving, yielding ways.

Art as Dissociation

Parrish implies that art itself (including, perhaps, the comic we are reading) is dissociative:

> Figure 1 is an artist of mounting acclaim. At 36 Figure 1 will say to their therapist that they have always used art to dissociate from life. The therapist will nod gently and ask how this makes Figure 1 feel. 'It makes me feel nothing' Figure 1 will say in annoyance 'Thats [*sic*] obviously the whole point'. (Parrish)

An image of Nicola operating two flesh-coloured puppets on the front cover of *Perfect Hair* signals a recurring image and narrative thread in the comic that ties into themes about art, and themes about dissociation. The puppets, like comics, straddle the divide between the material world and the poetics of the unconscious. In the chapter from which the above quote is drawn, 'Generic Love Story', the plot is played out between the two puppets, called Figure 1 and Figure 2. There are enough clues in the story to equate Figure 1 with Nicola and Figure 2 with Cleary, and the preceding set of images suggests this story is told in a solitary enactment by Nicola, the 'artist of mounting acclaim'.

People experiencing a trauma response can report feeling like puppets (McGilchrist), where the puppet represents 'a figure of human passivity' (Cappalletto 325). 'The puppet's apparent autonomy suggests free will, while its manipulation evokes determinism, the issue of "who controls whom" is one of the many recurrent paradoxes in puppet theory' (Williams 122). In *Perfect Hair*, the body of the puppeteer and the body of the puppet are depicted in a yielding sort of dance where one shapes the other. The puppet represents the exteriority of the body, residing as it does outside the body, an object with surfaces; it also stands in for the interior self, a performance of which would otherwise remain hidden.

The puppet is Deleuze's 'encountered sign, the sign that is felt rather than recognised or perceived through cognition' (Bennett 7). We feel *for* the puppets, but we also feel *with* the puppets—they are instruments of feeling and as Bennett tells us, feeling precedes cognition. 'Bodily response [...] precedes the inscription of narrative, of moral emotion or empathy' (Bennett 36). The figure of the puppet brings insides and outsides into contact while remaining oblique enough to not insist on meaning one particular thing. The idea of art-making being a type of dissociation is unsettling, bringing to mind the embodiment of form in the wobbliness of the hand in comics-making and the vulnerability of the misspelt word—the traces of the body in the comic itself. As Bennett writes, the embodiment of trauma in art 'orchestrates a set of transactions between bodies', registering 'pain's call for acknowledgment' (Bennett 50). As readers we become implicated in Nicola's experience of trauma and in Parrish's expression of it; pain is not hidden or contained within subjects, but inhabits a world. Parrish invests both the experience and the responsibility of pain into the reader.

Conclusion

In this chapter I have explored ways in which Tommi Parrish uses the form of comics to put insides and outsides into contact, conveying processes of traumatic memory in *Perfect Hair*, including the unseen symptom of mental ill health, dissociation. Parrish exploits the narrative effect of a sequence of images to create gaps of not-knowing that the reader negotiates via the body's affective response. Parrish's sensorial Figure holds the reader in the space of a single panel, resisting the narrative pull which threatens always to submerge the individual image in the flow of narrative—the movie in your head Scott McCloud conjures when he talks of the reader's role in animating the gaps. Parrish draws attention to the conflict between the image that wants to be seen and the narrative that wants to be told through her use of circular images, full-page portraits and figures who step out of the panels and into the blank space of the page.

Parrish's Australian contemporaries in the comics scene—artists such as Eloise Grills, Lee Lai, Marc Pearson, and Rachel Ang—are conducting similar experiments with form and the figure, using painterly techniques to foreground a body that becomes its own character: sensorial, lumbering, responsive, calling on the body of the reader to feel their way through the gaps in the narrative. Eloise Grills uses this painterly technique to represent the dissonance between the social construct of the fat body and the fact of the body itself in her experimental non-fiction 'Big Beautiful Female Theory'. In 'Notes on Diversity', Lee Lai transitions between black-and-white line drawing and painterly textures of colour to emphasize her thoughts on the cultural pervasiveness of whiteness, as she explores the problem of intersectional representation versus tokenistic inclusion of diverse bodies in comics practice. Marc Pearson's character Mr Ray interrogates the dynamics of the gaze in depicting the vulnerable nudity of an elderly white man. Rachel Ang's dream diaries trouble the boundaries between waking and sleeping life as lived through the figure of the body. Trauma and traumatic dissociation may not be present, but nor is the possibility of it ever absent, as characters—and readers—navigate the contact points between insides and outsides.

Seeing is feeling, something that is never more apparent in *Perfect Hair* than when Gran and Cleary are envisaging the same hallucination, along with the reader, the hallucination manifesting itself on the page, but also on the endpapers, suggesting something about the nature of comics reading and the shared dream of creator and reader. Language can contain and convey images, such as Nicola sharing the story of Gran's ghosts with Chris, but language and the violence of discourse threatens the safety of the body and the cohesion of the self when the body retreats from its own image. While the narrative effect of a series of images leads us to make sense of the way the images are arranged, it is our bodies and the way the images make us feel that we use to navigate the gaps. This affective dynamic seems to be particularly an effect of Parrish's painterly, abstract style, her big bodies and blank faces, the way she switches between mediums, and her experiments in form. Seeing is feeling: in the art of the image and the sensorial form of the body—the hyperbolic Figure—all is sensation.

References

American Psychiatric Association, *Diagnostic and Statistical Manual of Mental Disorders*, 5th edn (Arlington, TX: American Psychiatric Publishing, 2013). https://doi.org/10.1176/appi.books.9780890425596

Ang, Rachel, *Dream Diaries* (Melbourne: Glom Press, 2018).

Bal, Mieke, *Narratology*, 3rd edn (Toronto: University of Toronto Press, 2009).

Bennett, Jill, *Empathic Vision: Affect, Trauma, and Contemporary Art* (Stanford, CA: Stanford University Press, 2005). https://doi.org/10.1515/9781503625006

Cappelletto, Chiara, 'The Puppet's Paradox: An Organic Prosthesis', *Res: Anthropology and aesthetics* 59–60 (2011): 325–36. https://doi.org/10.1086/RESvn1ms23647798

Casey, R.J., 'Reviews: Perfect Hair', *The Comics Journal*, https://www.tcj.com/, accessed 18 January 2019.

Chute, Hillary, 'Comics as Literature? Reading Graphic Narrative', *PMLA* 123.2 (2008): 452–65. https://doi.org/10.1632/pmla.2008.123.2.452

Chute, Hillary, *Why Comics? From Underground to Everywhere* (New York: Harper, 2017).

Deleuze, Gilles, *Francis Bacon: The Logic of Sensation* (London: Continuum, 2003).

Goldsmith, Rachel E., and Michelle Satterlee, 'Representations of Trauma in Clinical Psychology and Fiction', *Journal of Trauma & Dissociation* 5.2 (2004): 35–59. https://doi.org/10.1300/J229v05n02_03

Grills, Eloise, 'Big Beautiful Female Theory', *The Lifted Brow* 39 (September 2018): 36–49.

Haines, Steve, and Sophie Standing, *Trauma Is Really Strange* (London: Singing Dragon, 2016; unpaginated).

Lai, Lee, 'Lee Lai', *The Lifted Brow* 39 (2018): 90.

MacFarlane, Elizabeth, Ronnie Scott, and Bernard Caleo, 'Into the Third Space', *Axon: Creative Explorations* 8.1, https://axonjournal.com.au/issues/8-1/third-space, accessed 9 May 2022.

Magnussen, Anne, and Hans-Christian Christiansen, *Comics & Culture: Analytical and Theoretical Approaches to Comics* (Copenhagen: Museum Tusculanum Press, University of Copenhagen, 2000).

McCloud, Scott, *Understanding Comics: The Invisible Art* (New York: Harper Perennial, 1994).

McGilchrist, Iain, *The Master and His Emissary: The Divided Brain and the Making of the Western World* (New Haven: Yale University Press, 2009).

Mulvey, Laura, 'Visual Pleasure and Narrative Cinema' in Leo Braudy and Marshall Cohen (ed.), *Film Theory and Criticism: Introductory Readings*, 5th edn (New York: Oxford University Press, 1999), 833–44.

Parrish, Tommi, *Perfect Hair* (Minnesota: 2dcloud, 2016; unpaginated).

Pearson, Marc, *The Claw: The Terrible, Beautiful Claw* (Melbourne: Glom Press, 2018).

Rogers, Sean, 'Review: New Comics from Alan Moore, Tommi Parrish, François Schuiten and Benoît Peeters', *The Globe and Mail* (2017), https://www.theglobeandmail.com/, accessed 18 January 2019.

Sinason, Valerie, *Trauma, Dissociation and Multiplicity: Working on Identity and Selves* (London: Routledge, 2011).

Van der Kolk, Bessel A., *The Body Keeps the Score: Brain, Mind, and Body in the Healing of Trauma* (New York: Viking Penguin, 2014).

Wastell, Colin, *Understanding Trauma and Emotion* (Crow's Nest: Allen & Unwin, 2005).

Whitehead, Anne, *Trauma Fiction* (Edinburgh: Edinburgh University Press, 2011).

Wieland, Sandra, 'Dissociation in Children and Adolescents' in Sandra Wieland (ed.), *Dissociation in Traumatized Children and Adolescents: Theory and Clinical Interventions* (New York: Taylor & Francis, 2011). https://doi.org/10.4324/9780203855447

Williams, Margaret, 'Including the Audience: The Idea of "The Puppet" and the Real Spectator', *Australasian Drama Studies* 51 (2007): 119–32.

Part III
Literary Instrumentality and Clinical Psychopathology

11 Writing Therapy, Writing Data: Therapeutic Writing as a Methodological and Ethical Approach in Researching Digital Sexual Assault

Signe Uldbjerg

Digital sexual assault (DSA) is the practice of non-consensual sharing of intimate images on digital media, often also referred to as non-consensual sexting, revenge porn or image-based sexual exploitation (Maddocks). It has become a hot topic in Denmark recently. In January 2018, it became known to the Danish public that more than a thousand people had been charged with distributing child pornography after spreading a non-consensually produced sex video of two teenagers (Quass), and since then, several other cases have gained public attention. The cases have sparked intense debate about DSA and the rights and wrongs of both aggressors and victims. This is not the first time, however, that DSA has been discussed in Denmark. In 2014, Emma Holten published an essay called 'Samtykke' ('Consent') describing how she had become a victim of DSA (Holten), along with a series of new consensually produced nude pictures called 'A New Story of My Body' (Bødker). Holten's radical reclaiming of her body made DSA (or revenge porn, as it was called at the time) a well-known phenomenon. Subsequently, other victims have come forward with their stories (Stubbe and Mærsk; Thisgaard, Tolberg, and Andersen; Aagaard and Mahmoud).

Despite the subject being so broadly discussed and despite surveys suggesting that 0.5% of Danes (Heinskou et al.) and between 3-6% of young people in Denmark (Crawley and Møller; Childnet et al.) have experienced DSA, there is limited knowledge about the phenomenon to this day, and especially about the consequences that victims face. In my PhD, I investigated the experiences of victim-survivors, and particularly their relation to social media. Some of the most commonly reported psychological consequences of DSA against children and adolescents are self-hate, anxiety, depression, PTSD, and shame and trauma reactions such as nightmares, flashbacks, and insomnia (Sørensen et al.; Bates). In the group of young women that I have worked with, several of these reactions and diagnoses were experienced. However, little has been said about the role of social and digital media in shaping these experiences, and studies interested in mediated sexuality and violence seem to currently be moving focus away from victim experiences (see Thorhauge et al.).

To conduct research that involves people who are vulnerable obviously calls for extra ethical precautions; and maybe even more so when based on creative production, since sharing personal writing puts you in a vulnerable situation in itself. In the following, I will argue that principles from therapeutic writing can be brought into this work and can serve as ethical guidelines. The aim is to protect the research participants from potential harm, and to work in a way that will support and empower them in their recovery, e.g. by finding new ways of expression and by developing new ways of understanding the assault experience beyond the narrow perception of DSA victims often seen in the public discourse. Furthermore, I will suggest that insights from the therapeutic writing tradition provide a starting point for understanding how participants' writing might develop over time, a process which is embedded in the design of the therapeutic writing tasks and which obviously influences the data.

Therapeutic Writing

Before moving on, I will give a quick overview of the field of therapeutic writing and some of its tensions. Therapeutic writing is a tradition that sees writing, and creative writing in particular, as a tool in clinical psychology. The field is related to areas like narrative medicine, where reading and writing are used to enable doctors to better understand the narratives and thereby the illnesses of their patients (Rasmussen 2017a; Rasmussen and Goyal; Rasmussen and Maagaard;

Charon 2001 and 2012; Remen). Therapeutic writing, however, focuses on the writing activities of the patients and the benefits that they might gain.

In the following, I will present four different arguments for why engaging with texts through the act of reading or writing may have a positive effect. The arguments vary depending on whether the field is seen from the perspective of medical or literary practitioners or from that of psychologists.

The first claim is that literature and writing offer a different kind of language which makes it easier to express things that might otherwise be difficult to talk about (Bolton, Field, and Thompson; Bolton; Rasmussen and Goyal; Llambías 2017). Practitioners from various backgrounds generally support this argument. Pablo Llambías, an author who teaches writing, emphasizes how literary writing helps people move beyond the platitudes that we often use to describe emotions. He defines literary language, as opposed to everyday language, as more 'precise, emotional, beautiful, uplifting, oppressively revealing together through unheard precision, unheard beauty' (Llambías 2017, 52; my translation). In short, he presents it as a more fully rounded way of describing and exploring human emotions.

The second claim is that the therapeutic benefits of reading and writing come from engaging with art. In particular Mette Steenberg, who comes from a literary tradition, supports this claim (Steenberg; Steenberg and Ladegaard). Steenberg and Ladegaard (2017), who work with reading rather than writing, distinguish between three different ways of reading literary texts: the expressive, the autobiographic, and the aesthetic way. The expressive way involves a special bodily engagement with the text where the readers exchange emotions and experiences with the characters, as well as developing and modifying their own emotions in the meeting with something new or different offered by the text. The autobiographic readers recognize themselves in the text. Unlike the expressive readers, they do not meet new and different emotions, but instead they mainly meet themselves. Finally, the aesthetic readers focus on the formal qualities of the text. Unlike the other two, they have little emotional engagement. An individual reader can of course switch between the different modes when reading a text, but according to Steenberg, it is the readers who engage in the most expressive way who benefit most from reading workshops. The reason for this, she suggests, is that the mode of reading facilitates an investment by the reader in the text to such a degree that thoughts and emotions are modified. In other words, expressive reading works because engaging with a text helps readers to change their emotions and thought patterns through learning new and different ways of being and thinking from the text. Steenberg describes this as a cognitive process that enhances empathy and the understanding of oneself through emotional engagement with fictive others (Steenberg 838). This claim shares some similarities with findings from narrative medicine, which show how reading, and especially engaging with narratives, also encourages empathy (Charon 2001). Unlike most practitioners of narrative medicine, however, Steenberg emphasizes literary texts and the mode of reading, which moves focus away from the reader or the patient and towards the text. In the same way, Llambías sees literary writing as having therapeutic potential in itself. Thus, they both belong to a branch of the therapeutic writing field that emphasizes the literary quality of the text rather than its ability to describe or resonate with the reader. While this approach shows promising results in the health sector (Steenberg and Ladegaard; Rasmussen 2017b), it can hardly be used as a method in social and literary research, because the rejection of autobiographic reading or writing makes it difficult to use texts or text conversations as data on a specific subject. Put differently, how would I be able to use writing as a methodology in researching digital sexual assault if the participants do not write about the traumatic experience of the assault? Thus, some level of modification of this principle is necessary if therapeutic writing is to be incorporated into a research design that is not meant to investigate therapeutic writing in itself.

The third claim is mainly supported by practitioners with a background in psychology. It posits that writing about oneself and one's life and traumas can have therapeutic benefits because it encourages and facilitates conscious self-reflection (Pennebaker; Wright; McNichol) and helps reshape one's self-narrative after a tragic event (McNichol; Bolton). Unlike the previously mentioned positions, this tradition puts the writer rather than the text in focus. Bolton explains the difference between literary and therapeutic writing in terms of audience: in literary writing, the audience is imagined, while in therapeutic writing, the audience is a professional whose main interest is the writer and not the written text. Furthermore, she states that they differ in that literary or creative writing has rules and conventions for what makes a good text, while therapeutic writing does not (Bolton 42). This means that text quality in this approach is about how well the text is able to describe and re-scribe the writer, while text quality in the above approach is about how well the text facilitates engagement and presents something new and different to the reader. The challenge, if this approach is to be used by non-psychologists, is that the qualification and motivation to continue a therapeutic conversation based on the text is most likely not there. However, with this approach, the trauma is central, making it possible to investigate it rather than analysing the text for its literary quality.

What this approach also offers is a description of the risks that might be associated with asking people to write about their traumas. This is described in detail by McNichol (2016). She explains how writing about trauma in some cases might do more harm than good if it causes the writer to get stuck in retelling the same story. Thus, what must come after describing one's experiences is what she calls 'a conscious effort of self-reflection' (McNichol 37). This means that the writer must reflect on their first text, and then move on from writing about the trauma to writing about the 'why' and 'how' of the experience. Following these reflections, it is possible for the writer to reconstruct the original story in a more reflective way that leaves room for the traumatic event, but where it is framed and understood, giving space to other aspects of the self as well. The process that McNichol describes here is worth taking into account when planning writing workshops, because it might help minimize the risk of the participants being re-traumatized or caught in the recalling of their memories.

Each of the claims described here thus relate to different therapeutic writing traditions that present different challenges and benefits if they are to be used as methodological approaches in social research. The literary writing and reading approach seeks to engage the reader and make people write nuanced texts that are interesting in themselves, instead of writing directly about traumas. Basing a methodology for researching a specific experience on this approach is problematic, because practitioners are opposed to reading or writing directly about traumatic experiences. The other approach encourages self-reflection through writing about trauma. It offers tools to protect research participants in a writing process where they do write about their traumatic experiences, but on the other hand, it also focuses on producing texts that are probably more interesting to the writer's therapist than to anyone else. The oppositions at play can be described as a matter of engagement versus communication and otherness versus familiarity. The literary approach wants to create engagement, while the psychologist approach wants the text to communicate the patient's feelings; the literary approach wants the reader or writer to find something different and new in the text, while the psychologist approach wants the writers or readers to find and reflect upon themselves in the texts. Despite these differences, I will argue that they can still be combined in an effective way. First, for therapeutic writing to work as a methodological approach, focus needs to be on communication rather than engagement to actually create data on the subject. This, however, does not mean that participants cannot still effectively and interestingly convey their experiences in the text. Secondly, the focus on otherness and finding new ways of expression can make the data more generally interesting. In fact, when looking at it in practice, the difference between what McNichol calls self-reflection and what Steenberg considers being confronted with something new might not be that big. Both emphasize the change and reflections that the participants must go through. This means that the possibility of combining the two approaches in fact lies in holding on to otherness, while also making the otherness about self-reflection and having a new perspective on oneself. Importantly, however, this means that some teaching and practice in creative writing is necessary as part of the data construction process. Furthermore, McNichol believes that the progress of the creative writing process has ethical implications and can help protect and empower the participants.

The fourth and final claim is that if the reading or writing is done in a group setting, the group itself can have a positive influence on the participants' experiences (Steenberg and Ladegaard). This is not in conflict with any of the first three claims, so at this point, I will not elaborate further on it. Instead, I will turn to discuss the practical implications of these principles.

Planning Writing Workshops for DSA Victims

Now, I will describe how I used the above principles in the planning of four writing workshops. In doing this, I combined therapeutic writing with other approaches to writing that have different focus areas. These are:

1. Creative writing (Llambías 2015; Zola Christensen; Donelly and Harper, Fenza) as a tradition that offers practical tools for planning and executing writing workshops, and in particular for teaching participants how to become better writers and create interesting texts.
2. Writing as a creative research practice (Gauntlett 2005 and 2007; Kara). This approach focuses on data production and is the basis for applying

writing as a research method in the first place, in order to produce a kind of data that describes certain aspects of an experience that differ from those accessed through other more traditional methods.

3. Writing workshops as a participatory research approach (Bergold and Thomas; Reestorff et al.). Including the participants in the decision-making and analysis is one way to make their perspective the dominant one, as well as holding on to the claim that they are experts on their own experiences. It is also an ethical approach because it offers participants a better chance to understand what they are taking part in and to protest against potential misinterpretations and misrepresentations along the way.

The different approaches have different purposes. The purpose of therapeutic writing is to elicit therapeutic effects; the purpose of creative writing is mainly education; writing as a research method is a means of data production; and, finally, the purpose of writing as a participatory research practice is both education and data production. All three purposes are relevant in relation to writing workshops as a methodology. Data production is, of course, the main goal, while therapy is an ethical goal, and education is a necessity to create interesting data and is an ethical goal in itself. Much more could be said about each of these approaches, but here I will narrow my focus to the therapeutic approach and how I integrated the principles described in the former section into the workshop format.

In practice, I organized four workshops for three young women who had experienced DSA. The first workshop was spent on discussing the project and the participants' expectations and on doing some initial writing exercises. The next two workshops started with the participants reading aloud the texts that they had worked on at home after the former workshop. These texts focused on DSA and were based on a writing task that I had given them. After the reading (and a lunch break), we would practise writing and give feedback on each other's texts based on basic creative writing principles. Finally, the participants would be given a new writing task centred on DSA to complete at home. The fourth and final workshop also started with a collective reading of the writing tasks, but then moved on to collective data coding and discussions on where to go with the analysis from there.

As described, the two primary activities of the writing workshops were writing practice (which did not involve writing about DSA) and collective reading and analysis of the texts that did focus on DSA. The writing practice was important in relation to the therapeutic principles, because it was a way of encouraging participants to seek new meanings through writing and trying to express themselves in different ways, as Steenberg and Llambías describe. The fact that participants had the chance to practise their writing also eventually meant that they were producing more experimental and varied texts when writing about their experiences with DSA. This, in other words, gave more nuanced data. The collective readings of the DSA-focused texts, on the other hand, meant that data was actually being produced about DSA specifically.

While these were considerations concerning the structure and planning of each workshop, I also applied McNichol's principles for progression of therapeutic writing into the planning of the workshop series as a whole. Thus, the first DSA-focused writing task was to describe immediate thoughts and feelings, the second was to reflect on the experience in relation to identity and social media, and the last was to imagine and reconstruct a sense of identity and future where it was possible to deal with the assault in a better way. In incorporating this progression into the writing tasks, I was trying to minimize the risk of re-traumatization.

To sum up the above, there were three mutually dependent interests at play in the planning related to the principles of therapeutic writing. One was to produce data on DSA and thus to write directly about DSA, one was to protect participants from harm, and one was to increase the chance of them benefitting personally from their participation. The connection between them is 1) that protecting participants through therapeutic principles was mainly necessary because of the need to write directly about the assault due to the interest in data production; 2) that the usefulness of the data depended on the participants' ability to write nuanced and interesting texts; and 3) that the literary approach, which was useful for nuanced data production, can, according to Steenberg, assist recovery as well.

Now I will focus on how these purposes were implemented in the specific writing tasks. To do so, I will take the third writing workshop as an example. The programme for this workshop was as follows:

12:00–12:45 Collective readings of home writings
12:45–13:15 Lunch
13:15–13:45 Writing practice I: Flow writing and 'describe a food'

13:45–14:30 Writing practice II: Writing around the traumatic event
14:30–15:00 Presentation of home writing task

Generally, the reading of home writings would develop and the conversation would gradually move further away from the text and become a general conversation about DSA experiences, which continued over lunch. When the participants had read their texts, I would usually ask a few questions about what the text meant to them and why they had made certain choices. Examples of such questions could be 'What does that element mean to you?' or 'Why did you decide to take this perspective?' At other times, the texts would resonate so strongly with the other participants that it immediately triggered a conversation, and they started sharing similar experiences. Their conversations and their own interpretations of the texts gave deep insights into their worlds and life experiences. All these conversations were recorded and the participants had the chance to read the transcriptions and elaborate on them in the final workshop.

The writing practice always started with flow writing as a way to get them to put pen to paper. In the workshop exemplified here, the focus of the next writing exercise was to practise writing using all senses. The exercise is borrowed from Zola Christensen (Zola Christensen 21), and it basically entails giving the participants five minutes to write a text that describes the sensations of eating a specific food, including all the senses and without using adjectives. Afterwards, the participants would read their texts to each other, and we would talk about their strengths and weaknesses as aesthetic texts. Usually, I would point to a couple of things that the participants had done well, e.g. a good image to describe a taste or an untraditional combination of words that had a strong affective effect, and encourage them to incorporate the same techniques or styles into their home writing task.

In the second part of the writing practice, they would write a longer text (ten or fifteen minutes instead of five) that was closely related to DSA but was not supposed to be directly about it. In the third workshop, the task was to describe the moment they first realized the assault, such as the room or the context. The feedback on these exercises focused on how well the principles they learned in the former exercise were incorporated (in this case describing sensations), and on pointing out some of the clichés about DSA that would sometimes work their way into the texts. We would then talk about whether these were actually good descriptions that had a place in the text, or if there were better ways to describe each individual's experience. We would finish off by talking about the home writing task and brainstorming on what to write. To illustrate what kind of material this process resulted in, I will now give an example of a writing task.

A Text Example

The writing task in the third workshop was as follows:

> Think about the person you have described in the former writing tasks. How is she today? What has changed? Answer this with a short fictive story describing a situation that shows (doesn't tell) how and who she is now. [translated]

This is obviously from the last step of McNichol's process of therapeutic writing: retelling your story. The participants found this task challenging and chose to solve it in different ways. One did not get around to writing it, but she wrote down some points instead that she shared with the group at the next workshop. The other two participants' texts were very different. One participant chose to describe a tough day in her life struggling with PTSD and loneliness. Her text was about accepting that some days were bad and that she could do things in life despite sometimes having to pull the plug and stay at home. The other based her story on a specific challenge in her life: that of overcoming her fear of meeting young men in public who she thought could have seen the pictures of her. Her text describes an empowering situation where she manages to overcome her anxiety:

> The sun has come out early this year. The winter coats have been packed away at the back of the closet. She can no longer hide behind dark coats and scarfs. The folds of the green flowered dress are dancing in the light wind. The determined steps of the high heels are echoing between the tall old buildings. Her back is straight and her eyes a little distant. The city is vibrant. Young men and women with red and blue hats [high school graduates]. They are happy. When she sees a group of young men all wearing red hats, she straightens up, more than what seems possible, while passing them. She looks straight ahead. Cool, with a rigid glance. [translated]

Apart from describing a specific important situation, she is playing with contrasts: lightness, heaviness, colours and darkness. The change in her clothing symbolizes a change in her state of mind, and the sound of her steps and her body posture become a shield against the heaviness of the city and the playfulness of the high school graduates inhabiting it. Both the darkness of the winter and the uncontrollable lightness of the joyful cityscape in spring around graduation time are perceived as threats by her, but with her coolness and colourfulness she manages to overcome them both. The pace of the text is also noticeable; with the use of short sentences, she mimics the rhythm of her steps, moving fast through the city, suppressing the feeling of anxiety and showing her determination to do so. The strength of this text as data lies in its ability to convey an affective experience. For her, the text was a tool to live out what she had described in fiction.

Therapeutic Writing as Ethics

Before returning to the outcome of the workshops, I will describe in more detail on what ground I base my understanding of ethics in relation to therapeutic writing. This mainly concerns media ethics, because many of the relevant ethical challenges relate to the subject being part of a digital context. The participants are more vulnerable to being identified, because this might result in increased harassment and exposure on social media. Their need to be heard is partly a need for acknowledgement of their digital existence and sexuality—for example, that people accept that they cannot just 'turn it off'.

As might already have become clear, I am dividing my ethical assessment into two parts: one is protection or 'minimisation of harm' and the other is 'maximisation of benefits' (Markham and Buchanan). Benefit in this understanding covers both the immediate benefits for the participants and the more long-term benefits that the research can have. These two might sometimes be in conflict, or as Staunæs and Kofoed refer to it: 'the sometimes almost absurd contradiction between long-term contributions and doing good in the here and now' (Staunæs and Kofoed 26). The therapeutic aspect of my methodology has the here-and-now benefits as its primary focus. As described, the conflicts that arise in relation to the interest in data production can be viewed as taking place between the here-and-now interest of the participants—both their protection and their personal benefits—and the long-term benefits of the research, which means prioritizing data construction. Thus, in balancing the two therapeutic approaches and the data regards, I am trying to balance the two ethical regards as well.

The next questions are: Did it work? Did we produce interesting data? Did the participants feel safe in the process? Did they benefit from participating? First, I will try to answer the last two questions, and the most straightforward way to do that is to ask the participants, which I did in the final workshop. When asked about how the writing had been, one said:

> It is hard to pull yourself together to do it, because you know you will feel bad afterwards. It is like you're really too exhausted to re-enter it

What she describes here is the exhaustion of always having to go back and re-experience the same things every time the topic of conversation is the assault. This is what the writing form, according to the above, should help overcome, because it gives people the ability to move beyond everyday language and reflect on their experience in a different way. The same participant continued: 'But it has been more beneficial than it has been hard', indicating that something different than the usual retelling of the same story did come out of the workshops.

Generally, the participants were happy with the process even though they experienced the writing in different ways. One participant was particularly positive regarding the outcome of the writing, and she had also been at all the workshops and had always finished the writing tasks on time. It is therefore no surprise that she was happier with the outcome of the writing than the other participants were. They did all agree, however, that the writing had, to some extent, been a good tool. But what they emphasized even more was the influence of the group and getting to meet others in the same situation.

In the final workshop where we discussed the outcome of the work, the participants agreed that loneliness was one of the central aspects of the experience of DSA and one of the things that the project had particularly helped them overcome. This turns our attention towards the group format of the workshops. However, it is important to notice that the group conversations were largely facilitated by the texts. Thus, it is impossible to separate the outcome of the writing and reading from the outcome of being in a group setting. The conversations the participants had during the workshops probably would have been different if they had not been catalysed by the writing tasks and texts. In particular, the work done on finding metaphors to explain complicated aspects of the DSA experience started in the writing and resonated through the conversations.

Therapeutic Writing and the Problem of Data Production

Now I will turn to the question of whether the method did produce interesting data and how this was influenced by the therapeutic writing approach. McNichol's description of the therapeutic writing process in particular had a very direct influence on the kind of texts the participants were asked to write. These texts, however, also had to help the participants produce knowledge on the experience of DSA and its relation to digital media. In the same way as each of the three main writing tasks was to comply with a step in the therapeutic process, they also had to relate to a specific part of the research questions.

For the first writing task, this was relatively simple. Concerning the therapeutic goal, the task had to be a concretization or description of the experience. Concerning the data aim, I wanted this task to give an initial description of what the participants found most important in relation to their experience. Therefore, I asked them to write an open text on whatever they felt the greatest need to share and give a reason for their participation. This produced texts that gave an overview of their cases and where they stood, and it was a good starting point for them to share their experiences in more detail during the following conversation.

The second task had to reflect the participants' own experiences and be about their relations to digital media. Here I asked the participants to describe a social media platform as a room. This, I hoped, would both give an insight into their attitude to and experience of being on social media, and cause them to reflect on how the assault had changed that aspect of their reality. To make the reflection on change clearer, they were also asked to describe the same social media before the assault and compare the two texts.

In the final writing task, which was also described earlier, the participants were asked to imagine a better version of their lives as DSA victims, and to produce more data on the affective experiences of the assault. In relation to data production, this task was similar to the first one, but now their experience was no longer described in a standardized way but evaluated through conversation and communicated with a better level of writing skills.

Thus, the therapeutic principles of McNichol shaped the focus of the writing tasks and the mode of writing, so that the writings about digital attitudes were mainly reflective, while the writings about the experience of DSA were mainly descriptive or speculative. This meant that the process that brought onto the participants by the ethical guidelines influenced the modes of expression in the data. In the analysis, this is important because it would be a mistake to view this process or these modes of writing as part of the participants' own choice of expression. How is their process of thought then reflected in the data? Generally, I would say that it is reflected in the way they decided to interpret the writing tasks. As explained earlier, the focus of the final writing task was to show which problems each person was struggling to overcome at the time of the writing—whether this was overcoming anxiety, for example, or accepting vulnerability. This, however, also worked because the participants had the chance to nuance their perspectives in the less organized conversations during the workshops.

What kind of data do I have, then? I have data that is rich in affective descriptions and reflections, but I also have data that is produced within a very specific framework. The central point here is that ethical precaution and the need for data production are linked, and prioritizing between these two was an ongoing task during the planning and execution of the workshops.

Apart from McNichol's guidelines, there were other influences on the data connected to the therapeutic writing approach—especially the assessment of what constitutes a good text. In Steenberg's work, good literature encourages expressive reading and confronts the reader with something new and different. In other words, it is not constructed in the same way as everyday speech and is not dominated by well-known standard expressions and reflections. To get closer to this ideal of good writing in the workshops, I drew on tools for teaching writing based on work by the authors Llambías (2015) and Zola Christensen (2005). They both, but Llambías in particular, have a very specific understanding of what good writing is and how to teach it. Their main advice, which was heeded in the workshops, is to make sensible descriptions; to show (describe) what is happening rather than just telling it, and to avoid clichés and prioritize different ways of perception and communication. Of course, other aesthetic and literary traditions have different parameters of quality, e.g. the development of narratives (Brooks), which could have been another concept to base the workshops on, were affective expressions here and not the main interest.

The standard that I have been teaching the participants is thus a specific one from a relatively narrow Scandinavian tradition. The strength of this tradition, in comparison to international and American-dominated approaches to creative writing (Donnelly and Harper; Fenza), however, is that it is not primarily practised at universities and is therefore generally more accessible to non-academics. This accessibility is crucial in a project like this. Furthermore, this standard is suited for affective descriptions because it prioritizes sensibility and the bodily feeling of the text—rather than, for example, the reflective and narrative qualities.

Conclusion

With this chapter, I set out to do three things: 1) describe the differences between approaches to therapeutic writing and reading, and show how they can be combined in a methodology for researching DSA; 2) evaluate the ethical strengths of this methodology; and 3) reflect on how therapeutic writing and reading can be combined with approaches to data production, and how the data is influenced by ethical and therapeutic principles.

In the first part, I described the differences between literary approaches to therapeutic writing and reading, and psychological approaches. One contradiction concerns the purpose of the text; is it supposed to emotionally engage the reader or communicate the experiences of the writer? Another contradiction is found in relation to what the text gives to the reader or writer; does it present new ways of thinking or does it encourage self-reflection? While these are in some ways opposites, I argued that they could be combined as a method for data construction by drawing on the text's ability to communicate the emotions of the writer, but in a different and reflective way. This meant that the writing practice became an important part of the method because it helped the participants create texts that did not only communicate their experience, but also gave room for playful and experimental ways of doing so.

The ethics of the methodology were evaluated on two parameters. Did the participants feel safe in the project and did it minimize the risk of harm, such as re-traumatization? And did the method maximize the chance of benefits, both for the participants and in producing useful and interesting data beneficial to the project as a whole? To minimize the risk of harm, I drew on McNichol's recommendations regarding the therapeutic writing process model.

This involved moving the mode of writing from description to reflection and finally (re)construction of a new perspective. Implementing this process in practice was, of course, not as simple as it sounds. The distinction between writing and talking about writing, especially, was not clear. When asked, the participants found writing beneficial, but they emphasized the group format of the workshops as the strongest benefit. The unanswered question here is whether the group talks would have had the same effects if they were not based on the writing. It is important to note that the writing catalysed the conversations in a way that makes the two hard to separate. It would be interesting to investigate the differences between conversations based on writing and for example traditional group therapy. However, it is my impression that the mode of writing did bring alternative perspectives to the conversations, e.g. when exploring metaphors for understanding different experiences.

The final subject was data production. Did the method produce useful data, and how were the occasional conflicts with regard to ethics and data production negotiated? I described how each of the writing tasks was designed to comply with both a step in McNichol's process for therapeutic writing and an aspect of the research topic. The greatest dilemma in relation to data production was that most literary practitioners of therapeutic writing or reading do not recommend writing about traumas, but in order to produce data, I had to ask the participants to do so. This is where the ethical precautions mentioned above became particularly important, but also where much current research on writing and health falls short; what does the process of writing about trauma actually do (Pennebaker)?

The study referenced here is relatively long-term, and it only included three participants. Working with a small group of people over a long time obviously provides certain advantages in terms of building a confident atmosphere and encouraging participation, which means that writing and sharing texts becomes less vulnerable. If writing is to be used as a research method, and especially if the subject is as personal as this one, the vulnerability of sharing creative emotional texts is something that needs to be addressed and met with precaution. The discussion of vulnerability in a group setting is what I see as the biggest lack in the writing approaches described here. In combining them, I have tried to overcome this, but it is an ethical and a practical discussion that should be addressed in the future.

Note: The research participants have approved this chapter.

References

Aagaard, Mads, and Abdel Aziz Mahmoud, 'Hævnporno' *Shitstorm*, *DR P1*, 19 May 2018.

Bates, Samantha, 'Revenge Porn and Mental Health: A Qualitative Analysis of the Mental Health Effects of Revenge Porn on Female Survivors', *Feminist Criminology* 12 (2017): 22–42. https://doi.org/10.1177/1557085116654565

Bergold, Jarg, and Stefan Thomas, 'Participatory Research Methods: A Methodological Approach in Motion', *Historical Social Research / Historische Sozialforschung* 37 (2012): 191–222.

Bødker, Cecilie, 'En ny historie om min krop', *Friktion: Magazin for køn, krop og kultur*, 1 September 2014.

Bolton, Gillie, '"Writing is a Way of Saying Things I Can't Say": Therapeutic Creative Writing: A Qualitative Study of its Value to People with Cancer Cared for in Cancer and Palliative Healthcare', *Medical Humanities* 34 (2008): 40–46. https://doi.org/10.1136/jmh.2007.000255

Bolton, Gillie, Victoria Field, and Kate Thompson, *Writing Works: A Ressource Handbook for Therapeutic Writing Workshops and Activities* (UK: Jessica Kingsley Publishing, 2006).

Brooks, Peter, *Reading for the Plot: Design and Intention in Narrative* (Cambridge: Harvard University Press, 1984).

Charon, Rita, 'Narrative Medicine: A Model for Empathy, Reflection, Profession, and Trust', *Journal of the American Medical Association* 286 (2001): 1897–902. https://doi.org/10.1001/jama.286.15.1897

Charon, Rita, 'At the Membranes of Care: Stories in Narrative Medicine', *Academic Medicine: Journal of the Association of American Medical Colleges* 87 (2012): 342–47. https://doi.org/10.1097/ACM.0b013e3182446fbb

Childnet, KekVonal, SaveTheChildren and UCLan, 'Young people's experiences of online sexual harassment' (report), Institution: European Commission, P. deSHAME (2017)

Crawley, Susanne, and Steen Møller, 'Ungeprofilundersøgelsen 2016', *SSP Odense, Udannelsesforum, Odense Kommune* (2016).

Donnelly, Dianne, and Graeme Harper, *Key Issues in Creative Writing* (Bristol/Buffalo: Multilingual Matters, 2012). https://doi.org/10.21832/9781847698483

Fenza, David, 'The Centre Has Not Held: Creative Writing & Pluralism', *New Writing* 8 (2011): 206–14. https://doi.org/10.1080/14790726.2011.615399

Gauntlett, David, 'Using Creative Visual Research Methods to Understand Media Audiences' *MedienPädagogik* (2005): 1–32. https://doi.org/10.21240/mpaed/09/2005.03.29.X

Gauntlett, David, *Creative Explorations: New Approaches to Identities and Audiences* (London: Routledge, 2007). https://doi.org/10.4324/9780203961407

Heinskou, Marie Bruvik, Laura Marie Schierff, Peter Ejbye-Ernst, Camilla Bank Friis, and Lasse Suonperä Liebst, 'Seksuelle Krænkelser: Omfang og karakter', *Det Kriminalpræventive Råd* (2017).

Holten, Emma, 'SAMTYKKE' *Friktion: Magazin for køn, krop og kultur*, 1 September 2014.

Kara, Helen, *Creative Research Methods in the Social Sciences: A Practical Guide* (Bristol: Policy Press, 2015). https://doi.org/10.2307/j.ctt1t88xn4

Llambías, Pablo, *Skrivning for begyndere: Om skønlitterær skrivekunst for begyndere: en personlig refleksion* (København: Gyldendal, 2015).

Llambías, Pablo, 'Der er ingen forskel på at undervise mennesker med kræft og mennesker uden kræft i skrivekunst' in Anders Juhl Rasmussen (ed.), *Læse, skrive og hele: Perspektiver på narrativ medicin* (Odense: Syddansk Universitetsforlag, 2017).

Maddocks, Sophie, 'From Non-consensual Pornography to Image-based Sexual Abuse: Charting the Course of a Problem with Many Names', *Australian Feminist Studies* 33 (2018): 345–61. https://doi.org/10.1080/08164649.2018.1542592

Markham, Annette, and Elizabeth Buchanan, *Ethical Decision-Making and Internet Research: Recommendations from the AoIR Ethics Working Committee (version 2.0)* (n.p.: AoIR, 2015).

McNichol, Kathleen, 'Who Am I? Writing to Find Myself', *Journal of Arts and Humanities* 5 (2016): 36–40. https://doi.org/10.18533/journal.v5i9.990

Pennebaker, James W., 'Telling Stories: The Health Benefits of Narrative', *Literature and Medicine* 19 (2000): 3–18. https://doi.org/10.1353/lm.2000.0011

Quass, Lisbeth, 'Over 1.000 unge sigtes for at have delt børneporno på nettet', *DR Nyheder*, 15 January 2018.

Rasmussen, Anders Juhl, 'Indledning' in Anders Juhl Rasmussen (ed.), *Læse, skrive og hele: Perspektiver på narrativ medicin* (Odense: Syddansk Universitetsforlag, 2017a).

Rasmussen, Anders Juhl (ed.), *Læse, skrive og hele: Perspektiver på narrativ medicin* (Odense: Syddansk Universitetsforlag, 2017b).

Rasmussen, Anders Juhl, and Rishi Goyal, 'Hvad vil det sige at lytte til patienter, og hvordan kan det læres?' in Anders Juhl Rasmussen (ed.), *Læse, skrive og hele: Perspektiver på narrativ medicin* (Odense: Syddansk Universitetsforlag, 2017).

Rasmussen, Anders Juhl, and Cindie Maagaard, 'Narrativer i medicin' in Anne-Marie Mai and Peter Simonsen (eds), *Syg Litteratur* (København: Munksgaard, 2018).

Reestorff, Camilla Møhring, Louise Fabian, Jonas Fritsch, Carsten Stage, and Jan Løhmann Stephensen, 'Conjunctions: Introducing Cultural Participation as a Transdisciplinary Project', *Conjunctions: Transdisciplinary Journal of Cultural Participation* 1 (2014): 3–25. https://doi.org/10.7146/tjcp.v1i1.18601

Remen, Rachel Naomi, 'The Power of Words: How the Labels We give Patients can Limit their Lives (West of the Rockies)', *Western Journal of Medicine* 175 (2001): 353. https://doi.org/10.1136/ewjm.175.5.353

Sørensen, Kuno, Gitte F. Jakobsen, Henrik Gundorff, and Helene Almind Jansen, *Hvor slemt ka' det være? En antologi om it-relaterede seksuelle overgreb på børn og unge* (København: NC3, 2015).

Staunæs, Dorthe, and Jette Kofoed, 'Hesitancy as Ethics', *Reconceptualizing Educational Research Methodology* 6 (2015): 24–39. https://doi.org/10.7577/rerm.1559

Steenberg, Mette, 'Litteratur som behandling eller æstetisk praksis?', *Månedsskrift for almen praksis* 91 (2013): 836–42.

Steenberg, Mette, and Nicolai Ladegaard, 'Guidet fælleslæsning: Litterær-æstetisk sundhedsfremme' in Anita Jensen (ed.), *Kultur og sundhed: En antologi* (Aarhus: Turbine, 2017).

Stubbe, Ida Kirstine, and Kamilla Mærsk, 'Jeg vidste godt, at da først videoerne var blevet delt på nettet, ville ingen kunne gøre noget ved det', *Information*, 31 March 2016.

Thisgaard, Julie Kragh, Camilla Tolberg, and Maria Andersen, '13-årig pige blev filmet topløs—og så blev hun sexafpresset i to år', *TV2*, 13 May 2018.

Thorhauge, Anne Mette, Jakoc Demant and Stinne Krogager (eds.), 'Intimacy and visual communication in social media' (SI), *MedieKultur: Journal of Media and Communication Research* 36 (2020): 67, 1–5. https://doi.org/10.7146/mediekultur.v36i67.118198

Uldbjerg, Signe, *Rewriting Victimhood: Stories of digital sexual assault* (PhD dissertation, Aarhus University, 2021). https://doi.org/10.7146/kkf.v29i2.124893

Wright, Jeannie K., 'Autoethnography and Therapy Writing on the Move', *Qualitative Inquiry* 15 (2009): 623–40. https://doi.org/10.1177/1077800408329239

Zola Christensen, Robert, *Manual til skrivekunsten* (København: Gyldendal, 2005).

12. A Question of Context: Sites for Cultural Negotiation in Narratives of Manic Depression

Megan Milota

During our six-week undergraduate course in Medical Humanities at the University Medical Center Utrecht, we devote an entire week to the study of scientific philosophy; in addition to four lectures on the topic, our students read a variety of texts by scholars such as Karl Popper, Thomas Kuhn, Thomas Merton, Hans Jonas, and Bruno Latour.[1] The goal of the reading exercises and corresponding small group discussions is not to frustrate our students, although this invariably occurs, but to challenge their overwhelmingly positivist positions regarding the purpose and goals of scientific research. One of the issues that consistently challenges our students' preconceived notions about scientific progress is the role that intuition, tacit knowledge, and *Fingerspitzengefühl* [instinct] often play in important scientific discoveries.

I mention this example for two reasons: first, this chapter will attempt to expose and examine some hidden norms and preconceived notions about the purpose of and potential uses for illness narratives about manic depression. Second, my own 'discovery' of the three narrative cases I intend to discuss in this chapter was the result of a series of provident interactions and a certain degree of *Fingerspitzengefühl*. Together with a small interdisciplinary team of teachers and researchers that call ourselves the New Utrecht School,[2] I helped organize a series of public dialogues at our university in the spring of 2018. Each of the four dialogues broached a topic related to health and intersubjective experience and showcased a specific art form: literature, dance, painting, sculpture, and theater. For our first lecture, 'Literature, Narrativity and Psychiatry', we invited three guests to explain the relevance of illness narratives in their work: Femke Schavemaker, whose debut novel *Karkas* (2017) had received critical praise for its depiction of manic depression; clinical psychiatrist and founder of the Story Bank for Psychiatry (*Verhalenbank Psychiatrie*) Floortje Scheepers; and Gaston Franssen, a professor of literature and expert in celebrity pathographies. Two weeks later, I had the pleasure of meeting Jim van Os, professor of psychiatric epidemiology, advocate for mental healthcare reform (see, for example, Os et al.), and co-founder of PsychoseNet, an online support platform with chat rooms and blogs for specific mental health issues, including manic depression. Having encountered four very different perspectives on the uses, forms, and functions of illness narratives in such a short period of time, I decided to interpret this series of events as an invitation to explore some ways in which contemporary Dutch stories about mental illness—both factual and fictional— are circulated, consumed, and appraised. Like Jerome Bruner, I contend that 'narrative, including fictional narrative, gives shape to things in the real world and often bestows on them a title to reality' (Bruner 8). My approach, which I will outline below, is thus an attempt to model a narrative analysis that can simultaneously constitute a form of cultural analysis (Bal 12).

A Theoretical Approach to Cultural Negotiation

My medical students' idealized view of their own profession certainly derives, in part, from their evidence-based, methodologically rigorous training. In other words, their opinions about and practice of science are both shaped and reinforced by the environment in which they learn and work. Similarly, I contend that our perceptions about mental illness, such as manic depression, are molded by the norms, practices, habits, and dominant discourses we encounter in our personal and professional lives. The theoretical foundation for my assertion draws from Pierre Bourdieu's field theory, which states that individuals act according to a system of dispositions, or habitus: 'a durable and transposable set of principles of perception, appreciation, and action capable of generating practices and representations that are (usually) adapted to the situation, to the immanent demands of the world, without being the product of an intentional search for adaptation' (Bourdieu 1991, 29).

Bourdieu's field theory can thus give us a broad theoretical framework from which to approach narratives about mental illness. We can use it, for instance, to explain dominant trends in appraisal and to identify patterns in the types of narratives being circulated. But field theory is perhaps too blunt a theoretical tool to be applied to individual appraisals of unique narratives. As David Hesmondhalgh admits, 'it is remarkable how little we know about why and how people value the texts that they like and dislike' (Hesmondhalgh 509). Admittedly, Bourdieu made some remarks about how consumers assess the *aesthetic* elements of a text based on a hierarchically ordered, static conception of the field. Bourdieu implied that the higher the class of reviewer and corresponding readership, the more distanced and neutral the review.[3] According to Bourdieu, those with more cultural capital will approach a work of art from a 'distance, a gap—the measure of this distant distinction' and will avoid discussions of personal relevance or textual aspects of the text, such as the characters or plot. Instead, Bourdieu argues, they will focus on the text's form or style and compare it to similar works (Bourdieu 1994, 34). This may be true for the appraisal of some kinds of narratives—such as highbrow or literary fiction—but other factors surely play a role in readers' appraisals, depending on the type of text and the readers' expectations, tastes, and purposes for consuming a given narrative. Pathographies are a case in point; on the one hand, we can logically presume that the consumption of and appraisal of these illness narratives would favor precisely the personal connections and affective impact of the text. On the other hand, we cannot simply assume that factors like style and form are less important or irrelevant for those who read such illness narratives.

Bourdieu's lack of attention to individual preferences has also been noted by Nicholas Garnham, who argues that 'by focusing on shifting tastes and regimes of value [field theory] avoids the question of what makes types of symbolic form or cultural practice special and why humans invest time and effort in either their production or consumption' (Garnham 153). One rather obvious answer is that people produce and consume art—including narratives—because it is fun. Janet Wolff's contribution to the field of narrative theory and cultural analysis adds the needed nuance to the theoretical conceptions of field theory by addressing the role of pleasure in narrative interest; Wolff asserts, for example, that one can, and should, explore 'the particular kind of pleasure involved in past and present appreciation of the works themselves' (Wolff 106). But what about the consumption of illness narratives? One could assume that the act of reading itself could constitute a pleasurable activity, but certainly other motivations play a role in a reader's decision to read such narratives, besides pleasure or amusement. Wolff proffers an additional means of approaching reader appraisal in her assertion that:

> the reader is guided by the structure of the text, which means the range of possible readings is not infinite. More importantly, the way in which the reader engages with the text and constructs meaning is a function of his or her place in ideology and in society. In other words, the role of the reader is *creative* but is at the same time *situated*. (Wolff 115, original emphasis)

Wolff thus acknowledges that the consumption and appraisal of a given narrative occurs in a non-arbitrary historical context that imposes a limited number of possibilities in the reading of a text (Wolff 116). This, in turn, harkens back to Bourdieu's habitus; and according to Judith Butler 'the *habitus* is formed, but it is also *formative*' (Butler 116).[4] In other words, the habitus can be considered the reproduction of a society's opinions, preferences, and beliefs. At the same time, it is also the site where an individual's dispositions are generated and disseminated. Butler does not see the potentially transformative process of interaction between habitus and field; instead, she views Bourdieu's construction as a troubling feedback loop where 'the dispositions are thus generated by the *habitus*, but the *habitus* is itself formed through the mimetic and participatory acting in accord with the objective field' (Butler 117, original emphasis).

While these theories all contribute to our understanding of either broad social fields of consumption and practice or individual readers' negotiations of narratives, I personally see Luc Herman and Bart Vervaeck's (2009) analysis of narrative interest as a process of cultural negotiation as a way out of the theoretical bind I've briefly sketched, for their approach combines field theory and narrative theory into one applicable framework for examining both literature and readers. The authors begin by stating that narrative interest occurs when the material being circulated coincides with 'the reader's disposition as it derives from his or her cultural embeddedness' (Herman and Vervaeck 112). In other words, they contend that a reader's assessment of a text is directly influenced by the impact of the materials being presented in the text. Herman and Vervaeck focus on three 'sites for cultural negotiation': the topic, the perceived strengths and weaknesses of the text (assets and liabilities), and the genre conventions or domains of communicative activity (fields). By focusing on these three sites for cultural negotiation, Herman and Vervaeck argue, we can arrive at a better understanding of how a 'narrative presented to the reader is transformed into something worthwhile' during and after the act of reading (Herman and Vervaeck 112). Furthermore, their theoretical model accounts for textual features such as the author's writing style and the themes, as well as readers' reactions to these elements. For as the authors state: 'if interest is construed, it emanates from the interplay between the various elements and parties entering the negotiation. No single element or party is ultimately responsible for narrative interest' (Herman and Vervaeck 113).

Using Herman and Vervaeck's analysis of narrative interest as a guide, this chapter will analyze three Dutch cases where narratives about manic depression are told, dispersed, consumed, and appraised: the Story Bank for Psychiatry, PsychoseNet, and the novel *Karkas*. My contention is that the three cases that I have chosen will each reveal a different set of parties and elements engaging in the negotiation of illness narratives. Although the topic, or subject of negotiation, in each of these cases is presumably the same, I expect that the perceived assets and liabilities of the narratives, or 'the elements that convince the reader of the story's value' (Herman and Vervaeck 118), will differ between sites, as will the genre conventions determined by the site of production and the readership consuming the narratives. The goal of this exercise is twofold: first, I aim to gain a deeper insight into the ways in which readers' understanding of mental illness is informed and shaped by the presentation and content of illness narratives; second, I want to consider whether or not the three narrative cases I have selected serve as examples of epistemic (in)justice as defined by Miranda Fricker (2007) and appropriated by Stephanie LeBlanc and Elizabeth Anne Kinsella (2016).

Case 1: Story Bank for Psychiatry

During her oration on 21 March 2018 in honor of her appointment as chair of Innovation in Mental Health Care at the University of Utrecht, Professor Floortje Scheepers outlined her vision for a new approach to mental healthcare, called 'blended psychiatry'. The blended approach, according to Scheepers, would combine the lived knowledge and experience shared by patients during the telling of their individual illness narratives, the clinical knowledge of experienced healthcare providers, and the accumulated insights gained from large-scale applied data analytics in an attempt to address and ultimately overcome the 'destructive standstill' that patients with complex psychological conditions often experience in the current healthcare system (Maasen).

The Story Bank for Psychiatry (*Verhalenbank Psychiatrie*) constitutes Scheepers' first step toward the practical implementation of her blended approach. This growing database of patient narratives—collected by trained volunteers—is meant to serve as a source for both small-scale qualitative analyses of patients' illness experiences, and large-scale computer-generated analyses meant to identify overarching patterns and themes in the corpus. The purpose of the Story Bank, according to the research team, is not to find more effective 'cures' for those suffering from a mental illness. Instead, the aim is to find better and more effective ways to help patients recover or restore a meaningful and productive life (personal communication with former Story Bank coordinator, 12 December 2018).

These underlying goals are reflected in the following message on the homepage of the Story Bank's website:

> A story gives meaning to an experience. This can be a source of comfort, strength, and empowerment. True stories can also provide a starting point for improving care and recovery support. We want to scientifically analyze stories with the aim of helping medical professionals to better connect with the life world of people with psychiatric illnesses. Are you an (ex-)patient, family member, or professional: we'd love to hear your story![5]

This statement also provides valuable information about the genre or type of story valued in this particular field of narrative production and dissemination. Narratives are of interest to the Story Bank if they provide a true or accurate depiction of a lived experience or 'life world' of the teller. As explicitly stated in this quote, such narratives must be worthy of and relevant to scientific study and should help medical professionals gain new insights into the lived experiences of the patient population they treat.

When I accessed the website,[6] there were only three narratives by (ex-)patients that addressed the topic of bipolar disorder. I chose the narrative with the title 'During my psychosis I felt alone and totally isolated' for this case analysis. 'Stephan's' narrative about his diagnosis of depression in his late thirties is told in chronological order and predominantly in the first person, switching to second person only during general descriptions of his illness and corresponding symptoms. Stephan provides a clear trigger for his first depression, the death of his father, and adds that his initial diagnosis came as a relief as it helped clarify and explain his symptoms. The majority of the narrative consists of Stephan's description of his third depression, which ends in a manic-psychotic episode and with Stephan being shot in the leg by police agents in an attempt to subdue him. In the clear description of the events leading up to his being shot, Stephan explains what he was thinking and experiencing during his psychotic break and why this led him to exhibit aggressive behavior. Stephan's narrative concludes with the pragmatic admission that while his current state of health is stable, he realizes that another depressive episode is a likely possibility. Nevertheless, his outlook is positive and hopeful:

> Maybe it sounds crazy, but my experiences have also enriched me. I've become more empathetic and know my strength. I have a better understanding for people who've gone through something similar. Hopefully, I can cultivate that understanding in others with *my* story. And that my story can help others endure their lot and recover.

As the Story Bank website doesn't currently allow readers to post responses to the narratives, we can only make conjectures about reader reception and the corresponding perceived assets and liabilities based on the information provided on the website itself. As the landing page excerpt explicitly states, a 'good' or 'worthy' narrative has an instrumental function: it helps both the teller and the online reader make a step toward recovery. For this reason, such narratives cannot just describe events that have occurred; they must also attempt to make sense of the experienced events. Stephan's narrative is exemplary in this respect. He narrates his illness experience from a rational and distanced perspective, concisely pinpointing triggers for the onset of his illness and his manic episode, and reflecting upon his behavior and its effect on those around him. For example, when describing the events leading up to his being shot, he says: 'I think they tried to ask me to come with them. That had no effect because I wasn't capable of normal contact at that moment. In the little entrance hallway in my house I started to verbally attack the relatively small police agents—me a guy who is nearly two meters tall.' Stephan's self-reflective capacity signals that he has 'recovered' from this manic state, as do his attempts to draw lessons from his own suffering and his desire to serve as a source of inspiration or comfort for his presumed readership.

After a volunteer donates their story to the Story Bank, they are asked if their narrative may be edited for the Story Bank website. If the participant agrees, a member of the Story Bank research team writes an abridged narrative based on the transcript of the interview. The completed narrative is then given back to the participant for approval before it is placed on the website (pers. comm. with former Story Bank coordinator, 12 December 2018). We can assume that the version of Stephan's story on the website bears some resemblance to the original, as he had to read and approve it before it was posted. Still, it's unclear to what extent the original material was manipulated to make it align with the site administrators' own criteria for an appropriate narrative. Furthermore, we have no concrete information about readers' motivations for accessing the Story bank narratives, nor do we know whether or not their ideas of an 'appropriate' or 'good' narrative align with the preferences of the website's administrators.

Case 2: PsychoseNet

As the homepage of PsychoseNet proclaims:

> Medical professionals, researchers, patients, and experience experts [*ervaringsdeskundige*] all work for our organization PsychoseNet at the same level and together to offer plain and hopeful information about psychosis, mania, and depression. Our website provides a concrete starting point for recovery […]. In a time where people want to actively look themselves for solutions to their symptoms, PsychoseNet can provide a valuable contribution.

The website, which is funded by both private and public grants, offers online appointments with healthcare providers as well as the opportunity to 'chat with an expert' during regular office hours. Users can also report relevant upcoming events, sign up for a weekly newsletter, and submit their own blog entries.[7] These entries, according to the website, 'must be interesting for the target audience' of persons with a psychosensitivity and/or mood disorder, their care providers, and other 'experience experts'. The website also clearly states that accepted blogs will be copyedited and that changes may be made to increase the readability of the submission. Still, the author of the blog must approve of the changes made by the editorial team.

When I was drafting this chapter, PsychoseNet included twenty-six blog posts about manic depression;[8] I chose the post entitled 'My recovery from manic-depression'. In this narrative a male 'guest blogger' describes his first manic psychosis as an undergraduate medical student. His narrative follows a clear chronological order and attempts to establish a causal relationship between events in his life and the onset of his first manic episode. The blogger also describes for his readership what he thought and felt during his psychotic break:

> I thought I was the new savior. I became very sensitive and could feel what was 'wrong' with other people. I understood how the world worked, a sort of divine omniscience. Every now and then I even had a beautiful experience of connection. I understood that people wouldn't understand and that they'd find me crazy and would want to have me locked up. But in my opinion I wasn't crazy, just special.

For reasons that are not entirely clear in the narrative, the blogger is involuntarily admitted to a psychiatric hospital where he is 'drugged stupid'; as readers we are told that a fellow medical student manages to get him released and personally cares for him until he stabilizes. This 'traumatic' experience behind him, the narrator briefly summarizes a series of long depressions with brief intervening hypomanic episodes. He writes that after unsuccessfully trying traditional treatment methods, like psychotherapy and medication, he discovered an alternative treatment that worked. His narrative concludes with the following statement: 'my two years of intensive therapy freed me from my bipolar disorder. Apparently it's not possible to recover from a bipolar disorder, but nevertheless I was able to do it.'

Unlike the Story Bank website, readers can post responses to the blogs on PsychoseNet. This can help us gain a more nuanced picture of the preferences of the PsychoseNet readership and the habitus from which they make their appraisals. Four users responded to this blogger's post, and they all praised him for sharing his experiences. All of the respondents also commented positively on the blogger's claim that he was able to discontinue his medication and, with hard work, recover from his mental illness. For example, one respondent wrote that 'we really need stories like this, ones that describe the possibility of a life without medication. This possibility was never openly discussed by treating medical professionals, medication was invariably the only remedy.' Two of the respondents briefly compared the blogger's narrative with their own experiences with manic depression and struggles to find appropriate and sustainable treatment. Only one of the four respondents was critical of the narrative, but softened his critique with the assertion that 'the reality is probably much more complex than the truth in this article'.

What emerges from this case is a slightly different set of perceived assets and liabilities for 'appropriate' illness narratives about manic depression. As the PsychoseNet website clearly states, the editors value plain and hopeful narratives that describe clear paths to recovery; but unlike the Story Bank, there doesn't appear to be an explicit prerequisite that the narratives be 'true'. Like the Story Bank, narratives that are selected for the PsychoseNet website must nevertheless have an instrumental therapeutic function; they should be self-reflective and self-empowering for the teller, and informative and interesting for the target reading audience. Although the PsychoseNet website administrators admit that they may 'clean up' or edit the narrative submissions, they do not seem to be editing out content that is critical of standard treatment protocols or that touts the benefits of alternative medicine or treatment. As the site information makes clear, the administrators want PsychoseNet to serve as a space where people can seek solutions for their symptoms without their healthcare providers acting as gatekeepers to such information.

Case 3: *Karkas*

In contrast to the previous two 'factual' illness narratives, one could assume that Femke Schavemaker's novel *Karkas* (2017) would provide a more nuanced and uncompromised depiction of manic depression for two reasons. First, the fact that *Karkas* is a novel and not a short blog post means that there's simply more room for an expansive narrative. Second, as Crawford et al. contend, 'literatures of madness both *tell* madness in their narrative themes but also *show* madness textually through deconstructed and destructed form, structure, internal dialogue, and narration' (Crawford et al. 43, original emphasis).

The chapters of *Karkas*, rather than being numbered chronologically, are numbered to denote the age of the narrator, Nora van Middelaar, at the time the events being described occur. Nora's language fluency, vernacular choices, mental preoccupations, and degree of self-awareness change with each chapter to mark her development from a fourteen-year-old girl to a thirty-year-old woman. In addition to essentially having to adjust to a different iteration of

Nora with each chapter, the reader must try to make sense of the italicized second-person vignettes interspersed throughout the novel, which are not anchored to the surrounding temporal situations. As the events in the storyworld are told in the first person present, the reader must simultaneously interpret the narrated events with Nora through the filter of her own consciousness. For example, the reader follows Nora's increasingly erratic reasoning as she writes her master's thesis on the philosophical concept of Nothingness and slips into her first hypermanic state, where everything is connected and has metaphysical significance:

> Jesus said: 'Whoever has come to know the world has discovered a carcass, and whoever has discovered a carcass, of that person the world is not worthy.' I see the carcass. The world is as flat as can be. But with impossibly complex structures. Through which everything flows which we cannot grasp. It's rushing through me. I can't see it. (Schavemaker 119)

Similarly, the reader shares Nora's shock when she realizes that the person she has been talking to in a café does not actually exist. In the aftermath of this psychotic break, the reader has to make sense of Nora's lithium-addled ruminations, such as the following: 'I sink with my entire weight onto the mattress. I have no thoughts to prick like balloons. No grumbling. No rattling. I think that I should try not to think. But I forget why. I am nowhere. Lost in a now where there is nothing to do' (Schavemaker 148–49).

After three years, Nora decides to stop taking lithium because it has made her lethargic, overweight, and numb to the world around her. Her therapists refuse to continue to see her if she quits taking medication, so she decides to manage her mood swings on her own. She adheres to a regulated diet and exercise regime and develops an extensive list of 'life rules' that vary from the practical—'never spend more than 100 Euros on one thing. With a margin of 10%' (Schavemaker 248)—to the existential—'it's important that you never ask yourself how you feel. Especially not at 7AM. Then you'll always feel something. Somewhere' (Schavemaker 210). The novel concludes with a second-person vignette, presumably Nora's consciousness or internal life coach trying to cajole her to follow her 'life rules' during a bout of depression. This sobering vignette complicates the reader's impression in the final chapter of the novel that Nora's successful career in advertising proves that her self-management strategies have worked and that she has reached a stable state of recovery.

Although *Karkas* is marketed as a novel—this word is even prominently printed under the title on the book cover—it has been overwhelmingly positioned as a memoir or pathography in both professional and amateur reviews. The following book review from a popular Dutch newspaper provides a fitting example of this propensity to elide the narrator in the novel with the writer of the novel:

> Now, with fiction you should never identify the main character as the author, but in this case the similarities are undeniable. The lonely child, the smart philosophy student who received a 9 [out of 10] for her master's thesis on 'Nothing,' the working woman with a tangle of self-conceived life rules to help her control her moods. It is all Femke herself. (Koelewijn)

In spite of the author's insistence that her work is a piece of fiction, Dutch readers seem to want to believe that Femke and the fictional Nora are the same person. For this reason, I think *Karkas* fits Evelyne Keitel's description of *psychopathographies*: texts that 'first appeal to but then undermine and ultimately frustrate the reading habits acquired from consuming contemporary literature' (Keitel 14, cited in Crawford et al. 46). A review of the novel in another prominent Dutch newspaper, the *Volkskrant*, adds another item to the list of frustrating elements in *Karkas*: 'you long for a plot, for a lively dialogue, for a joke. It's all so sad that you want to put down *Karkas*. Until you realize that this is precisely what Nora feels. This book describes her disorder so well that it's almost unbearable' (Houwelingen). One could conclude from these reviews that the novel's strengths, or assets, are its ability to immerse the reader in the mind of the narrator, the realistic depiction of manic depression, and even the similarity between the fictive narrator and the writer. These strengths presumably compensate for its perceived weaknesses, such as a lack of a clear plot or a conclusive, affirmative ending.

Dutch Illness Narratives and Epistemic (In)justice

As the brief studies of Story Bank, PsychoseNet, and *Karkas* hopefully made clear, the context and perceived purpose of contemporary narratives about manic depression can have a profound impact on the content of the narratives themselves. This, I have argued, is due in part to the habitus of the readers. But it is also a result of the expectations determined by the field in and for which the narratives are produced. In the final part of this chapter, I would like to consider the impact that constraints on the relational production of illness narratives can have on those who suffer from the illnesses being described.

In their essay on 'sanist' versus 'Mad' discourses, Stephanie LeBlanc and Elizabeth Anne Kinsella (2016) extrapolate upon Miranda Fricker's (2007) concept of epistemic injustice as a means of describing the various ways in which persons with a mental illness are often marginalized, exploited, and silenced by dominant psychological discourses and practices. According to LeBlanc and Kinsella, 'a failure to recognize the epistemic value of the perspectives of those living with madness is so entrenched in Western social practices and discourses [...] that epistemic injustice is often perpetuated without consideration of potential social harm' (LeBlanc and Kinsella 61). This failure to acknowledge or honor individuals' illness narratives manifests itself in two interrelated forms: via testimonial and hermeneutical injustices.

Testimonial injustice occurs 'when a speaker is undermined in their capacity as a giver of knowledge, owing to an identity prejudice held by the hearer, impacting the hearer's judgement of the speaker's credibility' (Fricker, cited in LeBlanc and Kinsella 62). This can take a variety of forms. For instance, the mentally ill may be subjected to negative or prejudicial stereotypes, such as the assumption that they are violent or that their account of events is unreliable or untrustworthy. A more subtle and pervasive form of testimonial injustice resides in the 'deep-seated social assumptions that mad persons are unable to exercise their full citizenship, and are therefore incapable of fully participating as *knowers*' (LeBlanc and Kinsella 64, original emphasis). Testimonial injustice can also entail silencing, which the authors explain is 'enacted through exclusion from participation in communicative exchange, where knowledge, judgments and opinions of marginalized groups are simply not solicited' (LeBlanc and Kinsella 66). Finally, testimonial injustice can manifest itself as epistemic objectification, in which case 'Mad persons' are allowed to participate in the sharing of knowledge about their illness but are made the object of study rather than the empowered agent or subject (LeBlanc and Kinsella 66).

The second of Fricker's categories that LeBlanc and Kinsella expand upon, hermeneutical injustice, relates to individuals' ability to be understood or to express themselves, and is linked to the availability of outlets for persons with mental illnesses to share their stories. As the authors explain, 'hermeneutical injustices are revealed in the lack of opportunities for Mad persons to participate in the generation of interpretive resources for making sense of madness' (LeBlanc and Kinsella 67). LeBlanc and Kinsella warn that 'Mad persons', even when given the opportunity to interpret their own illnesses, are often forced to adhere to dominant psychological discourses in order to be taken seriously (LeBlanc and Kinsella 69).

In my opinion, of the three cases treated in this chapter, Story Bank is the most at risk of perpetrating a form of testimonial injustice by treating illness narratives primarily as objects of study. In addition, by editing the oral narratives before posting them on the Story Bank website, one could argue that the researchers are merely picking and choosing aspects of the narrative that best fit their 'recovery-based' approach to symptom management. The researchers working for Story Bank are clearly acting with the best of intentions and have made a concerted effort to stress the importance of considering each individual's illness narrative rather than merely running through DSM checklists. I think they are also sincere when they claim that they want patients to become more equal and active partners in their treatment and care. Nevertheless, the Story Bank's preference for 'true' and coherent narratives results in a form of testimonial injustice by excluding those who cannot make sense of their experiences or cannot articulate them. While PsychoseNet appears to have a broader definition of acceptable narrative than Story Bank, it still favors a certain type of testimonial, one with a clear structure and positive or 'hopeful' message. Again, such prerequisites run the risk of alienating those who are experiencing a psychosis, cannot articulate their experiences, or who have not experienced a feeling of recovery or restoration.

One might assume that a creative work of fiction like *Karkas* would not be as likely to be subjected to forms of epistemic injustice, as there are hypothetically far fewer constraints imposed upon literary works—yet the fact that the novel is so frequently read and appraised as if it is a memoir serves as an example of testimonial injustice. One could argue that the author is not taken seriously as a fictional writer simply because she, too, has the same mental illness as the character in her novel. In other words, readers commit the mistake of assuming that the author's own experience with manic depression must be the same as the experiences of the fictional character she created. During her lecture at the New Utrecht School event, Schavemaker told an anecdote about a conversation with her publisher, who asked her to add references to compulsive shopping and sex in order to conform to potential readers' image of manic depression.

This can be seen as an example of hermeneutic injustice as it confirms the power dominant discourses can have over the shape and content of individual illness narratives. This also reveals something about readers' preferences in this particular field of consumption: the editor's suggestions were meant to make the novel into a more easily recognizable, and therefore more profitable, product for consumption.

Conclusion: Shaping the Habitus, Changing the Field

The aim of this case study of three Dutch narratives about manic depression was to gain a clearer picture of both the habitus of the readers of such narratives and the various sites in which such narratives are produced and consumed. This chapter looked at both factual and fictional narratives about manic depression as a means of modeling one approach to a critical engagement with the narratives, as outlined by Herman and Vervaeck and framed by Bourdieuian field theory.

While this analysis pointed out some potential testimonial and hermeneutical blind spots on PsychoseNet and Story Bank, I do not wish to imply that they be summarily dismissed as sites of epistemic injustice. On the contrary, I think these websites—as well as Schavemaker's novel—have an important role to play in increasing awareness about mental illness. These websites are trying from the ground up to enrich and broaden the public's perception of those with chronic mental illnesses. More importantly, they serve as public and easily accessible platforms where 'Mad' individuals can share their knowledge and experiences, seek and find solace, and hopefully augment the dominant discourses about mental illness.

Although it is clear that more can be done to expand the variety of narratives about manic depression in circulation, I think it is important to commend websites like PsychoseNet and Story Bank, and to reflect upon the cultural significance of the critical success of a novel about manic depression. For as Valeria Williams has argued,

> it is essential that society becomes aware of their own assumptions about human behaviours, values, biases, preconceived notions, personal limitations, and that they try to actively understand the different world view of a person experiencing mental illness, without negative judgment. (Williams 451–52, cited in LeBlanc and Kinsella 72)

Antoine Hennion calls appraisal, or taste-making, a developmental and communicative process governed by collective techniques (Hennion 98). In other words, 'taste is not an attribute, it is not a property (of a thing or of a person), it is an activity. You have to do something in order to listen to music, drink a wine, appreciate an object' (Hennion 101). Hennion uses the image of wine tasting, and highlights the 'tiny ongoing adjustments' in opinion and expertise that occur with each tasting. The same can be said for readers' assessments of fictional and factual narratives about mental illness. A reader has a general idea about what type of narrative they like, and makes a choice based on their predispositions. But adding a new type of narrative to their mental repertoire results in a minor adjustment of their preferences. Following this line of reasoning, both online narratives on Story Bank and PsychoseNet and offline narratives like *Karkas* can arguably provide a forum for amateurs to take stock of their taste and to clarify and amend their views. This, Hennion adds, is also a collective process as 'amateurs characterize their own tastes by taking stock of them. For this to occur amateurs have to form some sort of a community for [...] our taste is the taste of others. We rely on others in a reflexive way to constitute our tastes' (Hennion 102–03). If Judith Butler is correct, and an individual's habitus impacts and is impacted by the broader field, then a more nuanced and more accurate public perception of mental illness must happen at both the individual and societal level. Only when more narratives about mental illness are in circulation, and when more platforms are available for the dissemination of such narratives, can such awareness truly begin.

To return to my anecdote at the beginning of this chapter about my medical students, I contend that one means of expanding future medical practitioners' knowledge about individual illness experiences is to expose them to a wide variety of illness narratives and to simultaneously guide them in a critically reflective reading and discussion of these narratives, which would ideally include a querying of their own underlying assumptions and biases. In other words, I contend that illness narratives can and should be utilized instrumentally in the process of training future medical practitioners. As Crawford et al. point out, the use of literature in clinical education serves two important pedagogic functions. First, 'literature—particularly first person accounts of illness, but also fiction, poetry, prose, and reflective pieces from others—promotes the consideration of the individual's *experience*' (Crawford et al. 50, original emphasis). And 'a second core function is the enablement and promotion of reflection through narratives on a student's own values, life experience, expectations, assumptions and knowledge' (Crawford et al. 51).

In the spirit of self-reflection, I think it is appropriate to end this chapter with a critical analysis of my own position as researcher and reader of illness narratives. I selected and analyzed these three cases for the purpose of contributing to this academic edited volume, and my strategies for engaging with these narratives risks committing its own set of epistemic injustices. My reading, just like everyone else's, is an act of interpretation. I have inevitably approached these stories about manic depression with my own set of presumptions and judgments about the people writing, publishing, consuming, and assessing the narratives. In other words, even the most well-meaning use of another's narrative is bound to be colored by the habitus and interpretive lens of the individual reader. Rather than seeing this as a source of reprobation, I believe it is a good starting point for further conversation and contemplation.

Notes

1. As the primary philosophical texts are often overwhelming for our medical students, we read them together with the exemplary volume of explanatory essays, *What is Research?* (Koster).
2. The original Utrecht School was an interdisciplinary research group active from 1945 to 1960 at the University of Utrecht, and included scholars from the fields of medicine, psychiatry, psychology, and education. In 2017, we launched an interdisciplinary educational and research platform based on the same underlying vision as the original Utrecht School members, namely that the humanities should play an intrinsic role in the training of future healthcare professionals.
3. Bourdieu uses phrases like 'ironic antiphrasis', 'poised between endorsement and distance', 'neutralized, by ambiguity and negation' and 'ostentatiously neutral discourse' to summarize reviews from *L'Aurore*, *Le Figaro*, *L'Express*, and *Le Monde*. Judging from his brief qualitative study, it seems that distanced, neutral reviews are indicative of a higher social class and more social capital (Bourdieu 1986, 143–46).
4. Bourdieu has offered as many definitions for the terms 'field' and 'habitus' as studies about them; Butler succinctly defines habitus as 'those embodied rituals of everydayness by which a given culture produces and sustains belief in its own "obviousness"' (Butler 113–14). Although, to my knowledge, Bourdieu never explicitly links his use of the term habitus to Aristotle, his definition and use of the word is closely related to the Greek philosopher's discussion of *schesis*. In *Categories*, Aristotle

defines *schesis* as different relationships and, according to Saba Mahmood, the word is meant to capture 'a sense of embodied habitation and intimate proximity that imbues such a relation [...] both suggesting a bodily condition or temperament that undergirds a particular modality or relation' (Mahmood 847).
5. The primary source materials for the three case studies in this chapter are all written in Dutch. The translations are my own.
6. This narrative was accessed on the Story Bank website, http://psychiatrieverhalenbank.nl, on 7 August 2018, when this chapter was initially drafted. Some of the content of the websites may have been altered or changed in the intervening period.
7. The blog entries on PsychoseNet are subdivided into the following thematic groupings: psychosis, schizophrenia, manic depression, treatment, medication, family, and help/recovery.
8. The website, https://www.psychosenet.nl, was accessed on 7 August 2018.

References

Bal, Mieke, *Narratology: Introduction to the Theory of Narrative* (Toronto: University of Toronto Press, 2009).

Bourdieu, Pierre, 'The Production of Belief: Contribution to an Economy of Symbolic Goods' in R. Collins (ed.), *Media, Culture, and Society: A Critical Reader* (London: Sage, 1986), 131–63.

Bourdieu, Pierre, 'Questions of Method' in E. Ibsch, D. Schram, and G. Steen (eds), *Empirical Studies of Literature: Proceedings of the Second IGEL-Conference, Amsterdam 1989* (Amsterdam/Atlanta: Rodopi, 1991), 19–36.

Bourdieu, Pierre, *Distinction: A Social Critique of the Judgment of Taste*, trans. by Richard Nice (London: Routledge and Kegan Paul, 1994).

Bruner, Jerome, *Making Stories: Law, Literature, Life* (Cambridge: Harvard University Press, 2002).

Butler, J., 'Performativity's Social Magic' in R. Shusterman (ed.), *Bourdieu: A Critical Reader* (Oxford: Blackwell, 1999), 113–28.

Crawford, Paul, Brian Brown, Charley Baker, Victoria Tischler, and Brian Abrams, *Health Humanities* (Houndsmills: Palgrave, 2015). https://doi.org/10.1177/1749975510368471

Fricker, Miranda, *Epistemic Injustice: Power and the Ethics of Knowing* (Oxford: Oxford University Press, 2007). https://doi.org/10.1093/acprof:oso/9780198237907.001.0001

Garnham, Nicholas, *Emancipation, the Media, and Modernity: Arguments about the Media and Social Theory* (Oxford: Oxford University Press, 2000). https://doi.org/10.1093/acprof:oso/9780198742258.001.0001

Hennion, Antoine, 'Those Things that Hold us Together: Taste and Sociology', *Cultural Sociology* 1.1 (2007): 97–114. https://doi.org/10.1177/1749975507073923

Herman, Luc, and Bart Vervaeck, 'Narrative Interest as Cultural Negotiation', *Narrative* 17.1 (2009): 111–29. https://doi.org/10.1353/nar.0.0012

Hesmondhalgh, David, 'Audiences and Everyday Aesthetics: Talking About Good and Bad Music', *European Journal of Cultural Studies* 10.4 (2007): 507–27.

Houwelingen, Bo van, 'Mooi: Schavemaker is een debutant die geen allemansvriend wil zijn', *Volkskrant*, 27 May 2017.

Keitel, Evelyne, *Reading Psychosis: Readers, Texts and Psychoanalysis* (Oxford: Basel Blackwell, 1989).

Koelewijn, Rinskje, 'Femke Schavemaker: "Ik ben een neppersoon"', *NRC*, 28 April 2017.

Koster, Edwin (ed.), *Wat is wetenschap? Een filosofische inleiding voor levenswetenschappers en medici* (Amsterdam: VU University Press, 2010).

LeBlanc-Omstead, Stephanie, and Elizabeth Anne Kinsella, 'Toward Epistemic Justice: A Critically Reflexive Examination of "Sanism" and Implications for Knowledge Generation', *Studies in Social Justice* 10.1 (2016): 57–78. https://doi.org/10.26522/ssj.v10i1.1324

Maasen, Henk, 'Pleidooi voor "blended psychiatrie"', *Medisch Contact*, 26 March 2018.

Mahmood, Saba, 'Religious Reason and Secular Affect: An Incommensurable Divide?', *Critical Inquiry* 35.4 (2009): 836–62. https://doi.org/10.1086/599592

Os, Jim van et al., 'The Experience Sampling Method as an mHealth Tool to Support Self-Monitoring, Self-Insight, and Personalized Health Care in Clinical Practice', *Depression and Anxiety* 34.6 (2017): 481–93. https://doi.org/10.1002/da.22647

Schavemaker, Femke, *Karkas* (Amsterdam: Nijgh & van Ditmar, 2017).

Williams, Valerie, *'Sanism', a Socially Acceptable Prejudice: Addressing the Prejudice Associated with Mental Illness in the Legal System* (Hobart: University of Tasmania, 2014; unpublished doctoral dissertation).

Wolff, Janet, *Aesthetics and the Sociology of Art*, 2nd edn (Ann Arbor: University of Michigan Press, 1993). https://doi.org/10.1007/978-1-349-13262-1

13 Conscripting Dante: History, Anachronism, and the Uses of Literary Precedents in the 'New' Diagnosis of Hoarding Disorder

David Orr

While other chapters in this section focus on 'literary instrumentality' with the purpose of direct clinical application, this chapter considers the uses made of a literary work to stabilize and give authority to a 'new' diagnostic category. Here, literature is used to contribute to the nosological framework through which psychiatry—and by extension, much clinical care and mental health law—operates. The chapter therefore considers a sociological and historico-literary question with very practical implications: what does it mean to co-opt historical literary works to make the case that a recently formulated disorder has roots that go back centuries? How should we evaluate such a claim, and what effects might it have on the people diagnosed and the people doing the diagnosing?

Diagnoses are 'the classification tools of medicine' (Jutel 2009, 278) and, like all classifications, each one has a history. Hoarding Disorder (HD) is a diagnosis that officially came into existence in 2013, the year in which it was adopted in the fifth edition of the American Psychiatric Association (APA)'s *Diagnostic and Statistical Manual of Mental Disorders* (DSM). The move followed many years of amassing arguments and evidence which ultimately led the APA to take this step. As a disorder 'in formation', HD presents opportunities to study the different dimensions along which a diagnostic category coalesces. Here I consider one of these: the historical record, and the widespread claim that evidence for HD appears in Dante Alighieri's *Divine Comedy*, suggesting that hoarding dates back at least to early fourteenth-century Florence. I first set out the ontological and theoretical approach informing the analysis. I then outline the history of clinical hoarding, before exploring the literary prehistory that has been claimed for it. Through a contextualized reading of the relevant passages in the *Comedy*, I argue that this prehistory is somewhat distorted and suggest that HD has a rather shorter history than is commonly believed. This leaves us finally to ask why HD's ancestry should matter, and what modern-day sociological work Dante's masterpiece is being enlisted to do.

Diagnosis and History

Sociologists, anthropologists, philosophers, and historians have mapped the pathways, pressures, and events through which several specific diagnoses have over time achieved official status, and shown the significant social, cultural, and/or political 'work' that must be done in the process in order to stabilize them. To acknowledge this is not to reduce the conditions indexed by such diagnoses to nothing more than such 'work' by writing biological and material factors out of the picture; rather, it is to attempt to scrutinize the influences globally, without *a priori* affording superiority to any of them.

For psychiatric disorders, socio-cultural influences are explicitly recognized in no less a resource than the DSM-5 itself, which states in its introduction that

> Mental disorders are defined in relation to cultural, social, and familial norms and values. Culture provides interpretive frameworks that *shape the experience and expression* of the symptoms, signs, and behaviors that are criteria for diagnosis. (APA 2013, 14; emphasis mine)

Despite this awareness that culture determines not just recognition and validation of 'disorder', but also the very ways in which it manifests and is lived, historical accounts of how a diagnostic category developed often become an arena for confrontation. Claims to reality based primarily on universal biology confront claims that the diagnosis's reality is the product of a particular set of historical circumstances (Hacking). In identifying and advocating for a novel diagnosis to be accepted, its proponents may put forward an account of how the problems it indexes appeared in the past and seek to explain why they have not already become part of the reigning nosology, usually attributing lack of understanding to earlier societies and their medical practitioners. Sometimes such accounts nominate particular historical figures as possible sufferers from the condition *avant la lettre*.[1] They provide legitimacy to the diagnosis by highlighting evidence to suggest that the condition has afflicted humanity for some time, which is often taken to mean that it has a biological basis—all too often seen as the acid test for legitimacy in modern matters of illness (Easter). The fact that a condition may be biologically based but nonetheless only emerge under certain social conditions is rarely enough to unsettle this assumption.

Critical historians, by contrast, tend to emphasize discontinuities and transitions in experiences, symptoms, or interpretations, challenging whether a direct lineage can be traced from apparent 'past sufferers' to the present-day phenomenon. They rarely fail to offer disclaimers that they do 'not deny the pain that is suffered by people diagnosed or diagnosable' (Young 10) or that, for instance, 'hoarding can hurt' (Herring x). Yet their interventions may be received with hostility by advocates of the legitimizing genealogy if they are seen to be destabilizing the credibility of the suffering involved. Such historical controversies have been seen with post-traumatic stress disorder, claimed by some to be a transhistorical experience found in the seventeenth-century writings of Londoner Samuel Pepys or even in the *Epic of Gilgamesh*, and by others as a condition that only coalesced into its present form in the twentieth century (Young 3; McNally). Similarly, anorexia nervosa has seen debate over whether historical extreme fasting practices, found among young women in holy orders such as Catherine of Siena, correspond meaningfully to present-day self-starvation (Brumberg).

Why do these questions provoke controversy? What is at stake in the recognition of a new diagnosis? While studies addressing this question have a long history, they were given renewed coherence and impetus by a handful of key works that laid out an agenda for the 'sociology of diagnosis' (Jutel 2009 and 2011; McGann and Hutson). Among the contributions of this school was to explore systematically the range of social functions performed by establishment and maintenance of a diagnostic framework (Jutel 2009). These include, most obviously, that a diagnostic framework facilitates prediction and maps out a course for appropriate therapeutic management of a condition. It affords the person diagnosed a social role, entitling them to particular consideration such as sick leave or disability/insurance payments, or, conversely, incurring restrictions such as quarantine, compulsory admission for treatment, or suspension of the recognition of decision-making competence in certain areas. It defines and circumscribes fields of professional involvement, dictating which practitioners can justifiably intervene, and how. As a corollary and extension of this point, it can act as a site for political struggles, as there may be differences in opinion over whether and how a diagnosis should be applied and what the implications may be. More broadly, recognition of a diagnosis 'provides a cultural expression of what society is prepared to accept as normal and what it feels should be treated' (Jutel 2009, 279). These are among the important consequences of the decision to give HD official status.

Ian Hacking's work offers a useful structure for understanding how mental health conditions may move in and out of history. Hacking posited that many of the widespread forms that mental disorder takes are brought into being by the particular conditions obtaining in a given historical moment (the disorder's 'ecological niche'), and—if those conditions should change—the disorder may disappear or shift form again. He suggested four 'vectors' that may be at work in creating such a disorder's ecological niche: 1) medical taxonomy, a wider framework within which a putatively 'psychiatric' phenomenon can be classified; 2) cultural polarity, that the phenomenon should mediate two contradictory elements of the wider culture, one valued and one stigmatized or feared; 3) observability, that there must be a way for the phenomenon to be noticed as a contravention of norms; and 4) release, that the phenomenon should offer some form of release to the 'sufferer' even if it simultaneously causes difficulty or pain. As I will go on to show, attention to hoarding's modern history shows all four vectors plainly in action. Exploring the historical context that produced the *Divine Comedy*, however, casts considerably more doubt on whether they could be found so clearly at that time.

Historical Developments in the Creation of a Hoarding Diagnosis

Penzel credits psychologist William James as the first person to make an explicit link between hoarding behaviour and mental derangement. James wrote in 1893 that excessive hoarding was the consequence of 'insane [...] instincts' (James, cited in Penzel 12). Hoarding was discussed further, though briefly, by the psychoanalysts Sigmund Freud and Erich Fromm. What Freud and Fromm were describing does not fully correspond to the presentation of what we understand by hoarding today; for example, they emphasized the excessive orderliness of the hoarding type, in stark contrast to the disorder that typifies hoarding today (Lepselter 944; Herring 22). Yet it provided a conceptual framework that clinicians and others would use to make sense of such behaviours in psychopathological terms.

Despite sporadic case examples in the mental health literature and occasional flurries of media attention, most notably in the case of the Collyer Brothers of Harlem (Moran), hoarding generally remained of only minor interest to researchers into mental illness until the 1990s (Maier 328–30). Then, psychologist Randy Frost and his collaborators sparked a new focus on hoarding. They defined it for research purposes as 'the acquisition of, and failure to discard, possessions which appear to be useless or of limited value' (Frost and Gross 367), developed and refined a cognitive-behavioural model to account for hoarding behaviours (Frost and Hartl; Steketee and Frost 2003), and conducted a number of trials assessing the effectiveness of interventions with hoarding (see Steketee 2014 for a summary).

Frost and colleagues' pioneering efforts in the field were key to the eventual constitution of HD as a diagnosis in its own right with DSM-5. In fact, hoarding had already had a presence in the manual prior to this edition, but only as an aspect of both Obsessive-Compulsive Personality Disorder (OCPD) and Obsessive-Compulsive Disorder (OCD). The first of these, OCPD, appeared as 'Obsessive-Compulsive Personality' or 'anankastic personality' in DSM-II, and derived directly from the anal character type described by Freud. It was only in DSM-III-R that the criteria describing lack of generosity and inability to discard worthless items were added to the descriptors for OCPD (Fineberg et al. 2014).[2] Through DSM-IV, DSM-IV-TR and DSM-5, the diagnostic criteria have included 'unable to discard worn-out or worthless objects even when they have no sentimental value',[3] and 'adopts a miserly spending style toward both self and others; money is viewed as something to be hoarded for future catastrophes' (APA 2000, 726, 729); these two form part of a list of eight, four of which must be present in order for OCPD to be diagnosed. The true diagnostic utility of hoarding and miserliness within this set of criteria has been questioned, and it is significant that the *International Classification of Diseases 10th Edition* (ICD-10, the World Health Organization's international set of diagnostic codes) departs from the DSM approach: hoarding and miserliness do not appear among the criteria used in ICD-10 to diagnose anankastic personality disorder.

As several researchers pointed out, neither diagnostic option—OCPD or OCD—adequately described many cases presenting in clinical practice (Mataix-Cols et al.). The need to meet at least four of the criteria for OCPD presented challenges in applying the diagnosis to all hoarding profiles,[4] while the differences hoarding showed with other forms of OCD complicated its inclusion under that category also. Treatment guidelines for the overarching diagnosis were found to be less effective for those who hoarded. Because of these discrepancies, a distinct diagnosis of HD was proposed, assessed in field trials, and finally accepted for use in DSM-5 as an 'Obsessive-Compulsive Related Disorder' (OCRD) separate from the other two. Consequently, in the DSM-5:

> compulsive hoarding is simultaneously defined as an OCPD trait, an OCD symptom, and a stand-alone OCRD. (Fineberg et al. S44)

This is far from the only instance in psychiatry where such overlaps, co-morbid presentations, and potential confounding occur, and for the most part clinicians are well used to picking their way through this confusing territory with the aid of diagnostic guidelines. Equally, there is evidence to suggest that hoarding can come about for differing reasons and in different ways, so a single unitary classification may not be desirable (Pertusa et al. 375). Perhaps more significant is what it means for the research literature into hoarding, which has long been bedevilled by inconsistent measures and sampling criteria (Steketee and Frost 2014). Certainly few studies on hoarding carried out before 2013 adopted the precise criteria now used to define HD, but they nevertheless constitute the bulk of the evidence base cited in relation to the condition. Following DSM-5, this situation is slowly changing. Of note is that miserliness did not feature in HD, an observation which will become significant as this chapter unfolds.

Many commentators welcomed HD's entry into DSM-5 as a move heralding increased public and professional awareness of the difficulties that hoarding caused those who practised it. They reasoned that the existence of the new category would lead to more awareness and availability of treatments, and increase the likelihood of relevant authorities, such as housing officers, social services, or environmental health, taking an understanding rather than punitive approach (Mataix-Cols and Pertusa; Weiss and Khan). A minority of concerned social care practitioners and scholars within the critical humanities and social sciences questioned these assumptions, and some explicitly doubted whether introducing the label of a new mental disorder was the best path to take. Their critiques centred on: the potential stigma that the classification might evoke around those labelled; that it sweepingly disqualified as 'irrational' ways of relating to objects that might in some cases be creative or constructive aspects of individuals' worldview or well-being; and the risks that well-meaning human services practitioners might be encouraged by the new profile of hoarding to overreact to signs of clutter and disorder, resulting in unwarranted paternalistic interventions (Eddy; Herring; Lepselter; Orr, Preston-Shoot, and Braye). The influence of this group over formal diagnostic developments has been limited, but their reservations stand as potentially valuable cautions informing the work of professionals working with these issues and the reflections of academics researching the field.

Dante, Hoarding, and History

Though the implications of granting hoarding independent status as a diagnosis may be debated, the historical account of clinical developments is broadly accepted. However, the attempts to push accounts of hoarding back beyond the twentieth century, the era in which it became an object for clinical discussions, are more contested. These chart a distant prehistory, where some claim to detect the disorder's murky traces in literary sources that purportedly stand in for its absence in more empirical aspects of the historical record. Not only of interest to the small coterie of academics writing about and debating the history of hoarding, this view has achieved much wider currency, as this vignette from my own experience illustrates:

> 'Dante was writing about hoarding way back in his time!' This triumphant declaration came from Kim, a personal organiser in her early thirties, in the course of a friendly but animated discussion between us. We had found ourselves deep in conversation on the fringes of a national conference in the autumn of 2016, having made separate presentations on different aspects of hoarding. The immediate topic of debate was whether hoarding should be considered problematic behaviour that can be found transculturally and transhistorically (her position), or whether it is in many respects particularly characteristic of industrial and capitalist society, and becomes either more

or less problematic according to different social, cultural, and material conditions of life (my position). For Kim, this statement clearly trumped my position: how could hoarding be culturally contingent if it could be detected as a constant throughout the vagaries of history, down from fourteenth-century Florence to the contemporary world?

Kim is not the only individual to have pressed this point to me in such conversations. A number of others, their ranks drawn from among people who hoard, their relatives, clinical practitioners, and personal organisers, have conscripted Dante into the service of hoarding's claims to transhistoricity. They frequently cite Gail Steketee, the significance of whose research on hoarding with Randy Frost was noted above. She has often made the genealogical link between HD and Dante, most prominently in the publicly available web resource hosted by the International OCD Foundation, *From Dante to DSM-V* [*sic*]: *A Short History of Hoarding*. There she refers to Canto VII of the *Divine Comedy* as 'the earliest reference to hoarding' (Steketee 2013), before tracing a direct line to contemporary hoarding. Similar claims are made by other authors, such as depth-psychologist Renee Winters and clinical psychologist Fred Penzel. Penzel is unusual in this company in qualifying the statement with acknowledgement that 'although the historical record has some limited references to hoarding, not all types of hoarding are the same, nor has hoarding meant the same thing across different cultures and epochs' (Penzel 6).

The observation that the hoarding of which Dante writes is not the same as the hoarding described in DSM-5 has been made in passing before (Herring 21), but it is worth analysing more closely this passage of the *Divine Comedy* to clarify just how wide the gap is. As Virgil guides the narrating author on their tour through Hell, they reach the fourth circle. Here 'hoarders' and 'wasters' are punished together in two groups. 'To the sound of their own screams, / straining their chests, they rolled enormous weights' (Dante 1996 [1320?], Canto VII, ll. 26–27), perpetually crashing into each other before retreating and in turn being crashed into; Dante compares the ceaseless movement first one way, then another, around the circle, to the waves of the sea pounding the shore. The poem describes how:

> when they met and clashed against each other
> they turned to push the other way, one side
> screaming, 'Why hoard?' the other side, 'Why waste?' (ll. 28–30)

It is explained that many of the tormented crowd were priests, popes, and cardinals, 'in whom / avarice is most likely to prevail' (ll. 47–48), and here is the first clue that what Dante is discussing not only does not correspond to modern psychiatric and psychological conceptions of hoarding, but is diametrically opposed to them.

The DSM-5 definition of HD specifies that difficulty discarding items should be 'regardless of their actual value' (APA 2013, 247). 'Avarice', by contrast, focuses explicitly on things of worldly value. Throughout his works, Dante constantly condemned avarice, particularly among men of the Church. In this he was heavily influenced by theological discussions in preceding decades over whether avarice, rather than pride, might be the greatest of the capital sins; though Dante followed tradition in leaving pride in first place, he, like others whose concern arose partly from the growth of the merchant economy, was greatly exercised by the significance of avarice (Little 1971). In the *Convivio*, he distinguished between the *primo bene* (the first good—that is, God) and the *secondi beni* (secondary goods—that is, worldly things which, though as part of God's creation not objectionable in themselves, become vile when they lead humans away from God). In his later work on politics, the *De Monarchia*, Dante expanded on the reasons for his particular hatred of avarice among the capital sins: he saw how it had corrupted the Church of his time, leading the clergy and pope into the sin of simony (the selling of positions within the Church) and the misuse of Church wealth and power, and thereby leaving the people without a reliable source of moral guidance from the very institution that was divinely charged with providing it. The jealously guarded wealth of the Church could have provided justice if put to better use in providing for the needs of others; avarice therefore is opposed to the virtue of justice. What else, he wondered, drawing connections between moral and political theory, could cause so much destruction as riches, usually obtained illicitly, not conferring happiness, and leading to conflict when possessed? Dante agreed with Thomas Aquinas that among the fruits of avarice were inhumanity, violence, fraud, and treachery (Boyde 159–68).

If more proof were needed that Dante is targeting the *avari* ('avaricious') in this canto, rather than hoarders who fail to recognize agreed-upon value, it is that they are opposed to the other group who 'had such myopic minds they could not judge / with moderation when it came to spending' ('*fuor guerci / sì de la mente in la vita primaia, / che con misura nullo spendi ferci*'; ll. 40–42).

The present-day hoarders who best fit this description are those with the DSM-5 'excessive acquisition' specifier, whose 'spending' might be considered 'grandiose'; ironically, Dante saw this group as 'wasters'—the opposite to what the translation calls those who 'hoard'. Those who 'hoard', meanwhile, might more closely suit the 'miserly' disposition described in the OCPD diagnostic criteria, but show limited resemblance to the HD profile.

The description is followed by Virgil's excursus into criticism of both groups for trying to bring worldly Fortune under their control. This passage subtly evokes the medieval conception of the Wheel of Fortune, which in its turns was said to bring the noble into poverty and the poor man into wealth according to its own designs. Virgil states that neither building up wealth nor spending freely can enable humans to change what the divine plan has in store for them. Characteristically, the punishment Dante gives these sinners reflects their crime: for seeking to hold the wheel back from turning, they are themselves condemned to rush willy-nilly forwards and backwards around a circle, neither resting nor completing a full turn (Berk 145). Again, the emphasis is on the power or security, or else the opportunities for self-indulgence, conferred by riches, not on any disproportionate distress experienced when contemplating discarding seemingly worthless possessions.

The question is not only what Dante meant by 'hoard', but indeed *whether* he meant 'hoard'. The medieval Italian verb used was *'tenere'*, which has multiple translations including 'to have, hold, keep, possess, occupy a space' (Niccoli 555–59). It appears twice in this translation as 'hoard': the first time as *'perche tieni?'* (l. 30), glossed as 'Why do you hoard?', and the second time as *'mal tener'* (l. 58), glossed as 'hoarding'. The need to add the qualifier *'mal'*, meaning 'bad', to the second instance suggests that *'tener'* is not fully commensurable with 'hoarding', a word which has inherently negative semantic connotations in itself and would therefore render the adjective *'mal'* superfluous. Some English versions of the *Comedy* use alternative translations: '"Miser!" they shout' (Dante 1994, l. 30), '"Why do you hold?"' (Dante 1996, l. 30) and '"You miser!" Why?' (Dante 2006, l. 30) have been used to render *'perche tieni?'*; and 'ill keeping' (Dante 1939, l. 30; Dante 1980, l. 30) is a common translation for *'mal tener'*. As a poetic rendering, 'hoard' is a perfectly permissible gloss; however, it is doubtful whether it matches Dante's meaning as precisely as Steketee seems to have assumed. This forces us to consider whether this supposed historical evidence for hoarding might not be in part an illusion introduced in translation.

Steketee's *Short History* passes seamlessly from fourteenth-century Florence to the nineteenth-century novelists, Dickens, Balzac, Conan Doyle, and Gogol. Something comparable to modern-day hoarding is certainly more recognizable in the descriptions in these writers' works than in Dante's. Of Krook, from Dickens's 1852 work *Bleak House*, it is said that

> his whole stock from beginning to end, may easily be the waste paper he bought it as, for anything I can say. It's a monomania with him, to think he is possessed of documents. He has been going to learn to read them this last quarter of a century. (Dickens 14)

Key characteristics of HD are in evidence in these three lines: obsession with possessions without apparent value; the constant deferral of putting these items to use; even the association with mental derangement ('monomania'). Of Gogol's character Plyushkin, in the 1842 novel *Dead Souls*, the narrator comments:

> What need, one might ask, did Plyushkin have for such a mass of these artifacts? Never in all his life could they have been used even on two such estates as his—but to him it still seemed too little. […] whatever he came across—an old shoe sole, a woman's rag, an iron nail, a potsherd—he carried off and added to the pile that Chichikov had noticed in the corner of the room. (Gogol 132)

The full descriptions of Plyushkin's estate, with its disordered profusion, decay, and dust, again resonate with modern-day accounts of HD; even today, hoarding in Russia is commonly referred to as Plyushkin syndrome.

The gap of half a millennium between 'hoarding' in Dante and hoarding in these authors' books is left unremarked by Steketee, with the apparent implication that there was continuity even if it is either not attested to in the historical written record or she has not identified those instances where it is. Yet even a brief perusal of histories of material culture makes plain how unlikely it was that hoarding of objects regardless of their value had been seen as a problem, or even noticed at all, in the intervening period. By way of example, illustrations drawn from Cockayne's vivid depictions of the sensory environment in seventeenth- and eighteenth-century England drive home the point. Who would have registered the fire and hygiene risks of hoarding in an era when discharges from tanners, tallow chandlers, animal keeping, and slaughtering were largely unregulated; when blocking up of windows to avoid the Window Tax prevented light and air from penetrating dwellings; when building materials were highly combustible and candles were used for light; when houses themselves were hard to keep clean, rarely structurally sound, and their surrounding areas steeped in human, animal, and domestic waste (Cockayne 134–55)? The tenement overcrowding that was the reality of urban living for many could see dozens of people to a house: hoarding of people was thus much more common than hoarding of things, leaving little room for the accumulation of items few could anyway afford (Cockayne 149). Until waste collection became widespread in the twentieth century, it was standard in North America and Europe to simply throw waste out of the door (Strasser 8); such piles were a ubiquitous aspect of human habitation, rather than an anomaly. Essential practices of re-use, in pre-industrial societies like the one Dante lived in and that persisted for centuries after him, made the notion of hoarding items 'regardless of their value' largely meaningless; Strasser comments that it was only in the twentieth century that the circulation of objects in most households in the United States transitioned from a closed to an open system (Strasser 14). This is echoed in Britain, where Isabella Beeton's runaway Victorian bestseller *Book of Household Management*, though it extensively discussed both cleanliness and practices of re-use, did not so much as mention rubbish (Lucas 6). It is estimated that as late as the end of the nineteenth century, some 80% of household waste consisted simply of ashes from the fire (Lucas 13); there seems little scope amidst such material for hoarders to appropriate quantities of items that should rightly have been disposed of. Hoarding as a practice only comes to make sense against a cultural background where disposability is valued, and such a context only came into existence, in fits and starts and spread unevenly through society, relatively recently.

Reviewing this history in the light of Hacking's vectors illustrates the point. His first, 'medical taxonomy', was not readily available to Dante, yet hoarding could have been recognized within a moral-theological taxonomy of fault, had it been in evidence. The second, 'cultural polarity', was present in the form of frugality versus spendthriftiness, two opposing qualities that confronted each other in the fourth circle, but there is limited evidence to support the existence of a meaningful polarity between keeping and disposing. The third, 'observability', was likely absent in Dante's time and subsequent centuries; the forms of use, re-use and waste simply would not have allowed the problems posed by current forms of hoarding to become noticeable. As for the fourth, 'release', I can only speculate whether the opportunity to accumulate a massive 'hoard' of items in which only the owner can see worth might have afforded release to that individual in the fourteenth and subsequent centuries. In the industrial age brought on by the nineteenth century and continuing to the present day, the opportunities and social pressures brought by mass production to amass and retain possessions do seem to have afforded a form of 'release' for the person who hoards. It seems likely, therefore, that the five-century gap in the history of hoarding is more than coincidence, and that HD has a rather shorter history than has been claimed.

Discussion

So does any of this matter? Amidst the mobilization of narratives of suffering, brain scans, research papers and trials, severity rating scales, estimates of the disorder's economic cost to society, and all the other paraphernalia that modern mental health science calls on to consolidate a disorder's facticity and acceptability, are historical genealogies of the disorder any more than scholastic trivia? The *Divine Comedy* was undergirded by a comprehensive philosophical system working out right and wrong, 'correct' and 'pathological' behaviour, at least as encompassing as the DSM in its scope and internal logics of classification. The fact that this system occupied a moral-religious frame rather than a medical one only reflects the mindset of the time, which saw the two as intimately connected. But since few people today would turn to Dante for ethical, still less medical, guidance, does this historical inaccuracy merit any more than a footnote?

Perhaps. I might have thought little of the claim, had it not become apparent that it has become such common currency in the world of hoarding, among service users as well as researchers and clinicians. A proliferation of television shows and self-help books have solidified hoarding's place in the mind of the general public (Lepselter; Eddy) and the link between clutter and pathology has become well established. The more taken for granted the diagnosis becomes, the more likely hoarding is to be located as a pathology within the individual mind, and the less likely it is that questions are asked of the social arrangements that facilitate or encourage it (Smail)—after all, it has been unchanged for seven hundred years, hasn't it? It is not only critical scholars who have reservations about the ease with which a diagnosis of hoarding can lead to drastic effects on an individual's life; Rob Mitchell's blog post on the consequences of a lack of reflexivity over what was identified as a case of hoarding struck a chord with many, including the Chief Social Worker (England), Lyn Romeo (Mitchell).

Vikram Patel lists 'historical validity' among four types of validity which can support the value of a diagnosis in the absence of 'gold standard' (bio)markers (Patel 781). In producing such validity, the messiness of hoarding's heritage has been smoothed over and an unproblematized pathway plotted from the fourth circle of Dante's Hell to the 'Obsessive-Compulsive and Related Disorders' section of the 2013 DSM-5. Certainly, when Hoarding Disorder was newly named in DSM-5 as an officially recognized diagnostic classification, it was the crowning clinical stamp of authenticity for a 'problem' that had been confronting landlords and housing agencies, social workers, environmental health agencies, and fire and rescue for some time already (though not as long as Steketee made out). It was not a foregone conclusion that psychiatry's engagement with hoarding would further its medicalization; while entry of a diagnosis into the DSM may often promote the expansion of the clinical gaze into areas of human behaviour it did not previously concern itself with, it can also sometimes place limits on medicalization. This occurs when the new diagnostic category, by more tightly specifying the criteria for behaviours either to count as disorder or not, has the effect of restricting to defined limits a previously loosely defined grey area of medical intervention (Bryant). Yet the growth in hoarding categories, between OCPD, OCD, and now HD, suggests that this is not the direction of travel.

Implications and Conclusion

In this chapter, I have attempted to demonstrate that use of the *Divine Comedy* to make ontological claims about the historical existence of something akin to HD is misplaced. When considering the philosophical insights of Hacking and the material histories of Cockayne and Lucas, we cannot help but ask why the early modern historical record of hoarding is so scanty and Steketee is forced to fall back on literary illustrations. This unproblematized and ahistorical reading of Dante's work perhaps tells us more about contemporary needs to establish a clear genealogy for disorders than it does about pathological behaviours in the fourteenth century.

This is not to argue that literary portrayals have no role to play in the understanding of historical forms of 'madness' or mental distress. They can indeed make a valuable contribution, but this must be treated critically, with awareness of the dangers of basing ontological claims on decontextualized readings of literary works considered in isolation from their socio-cultural and linguistic hinterland. Even in relation to modern literature, straightforwardly deducing conclusions about diagnoses from literature can be a hazardous enterprise without knowledge of the background to the text; literature's primary concern is with the content of experience rather than the form it takes, whereas psychiatric diagnosis generally prioritizes form over content (Crawford et al. 50). Literature has many insights to offer into both subjective experience and the different ways in which unusual thoughts and behaviours may be perceived by others—which might indeed supply the details to allow readers to make inferences about hoarding and its reception in a particular time and place, Dickens and Gogol being cases in point. Yet the desire to find signs of a contemporary condition in past writings should not blind readers to the need for careful historicization if such analysis is to be meaningful.

Seen in the light of literature's contribution to understanding other worldviews, Dante's work does indeed shed light on a longer, and perhaps more intriguing, story of how humanity assessed its relationship with material possessions at different times and in different places. Underpinning Dante's representation of the fourth circle of Hell, and much else throughout the *Comedy* and his other works, is a framework offering a coherent account of what the 'good life' might be and the proper role of material possessions within it. This same thread runs through much subsequent literature, the abovementioned Gogol's *Dead Souls* being one outstanding example in its satirical treatment of how the ownership of human lives, deaths, and material things become interchangeable within the worldview the novel sought to critique. Approaching the literature in this way prevents critics from taking psychological pathology within individual characters for granted—though equally it does not preclude exploring this possibility within the character studies of fictional protagonists—and invites the reader to ask questions of how the social and historical circumstances within which the narrative is set might contribute to the experiences of individuals within the text.

The challenges of hoarding are not invented, and the DSM's effects depend on how practitioners use it; it can be used to support good care, or it can lend itself to 'hypo-narrativity' (Flanagan 867), where the only story anyone needs to know is seen to lie in the criteria listed in DSM-5 entry '300.3. Hoarding Disorder'. In this perhaps it is like Dante, who is poorly served by having his work reduced simply to a historical marker for evidence of the existence of Hoarding Disorder in medieval Florence. The richness of his narrative engagement with the ethical, political, and social issues of his day is something that contemporary mental health scholarship can learn from, in ensuring that the deeper, more humanistic dimensions of hoarding experience do not become lost in the wake of its encapsulation in the DSM.

Notes

1. See Muramoto (2014) for a discussion of the ontological, epistemic and ethical issues in this practice.
2. This revised version of the third edition was published in 1987.
3. The entry went on to add the following details:

    Often these individuals will admit to being 'pack rats'. They regard discarding objects as wasteful because 'you never know when you might need something' and will become upset if anyone tries to get rid of the things they have saved. Their spouses or roommates may complain about the amount of space taken up by old parts, magazines, broken appliances, and so on. (APA 2000, 726).

4. Some of the other criteria might fit relatively well with common hoarding presentations, e.g. 'perfectionism that interferes with task completion' (it is noted in the literature that perfectionist thinking prevents many people who hoard from making a start on clearing up if they cannot achieve it all within a short time [Burgess et al.]). However, others seem less compatible: the criterion 'is preoccupied with details, rules, lists, order, organisation, or schedules' does not fit well with the *dis*order so characteristic of HD and the observation that it often arises in part due to an inability to organize; 'adopts a miserly spending style' cannot be reconciled with the 'excessive acquisition' behaviour displayed by the majority of, albeit not all, people who hoard.

References

American Psychiatric Association, *Diagnostic and Statistical Manual of Mental Disorders, 4th Edition, Text Revision* (Washington, DC: American Psychiatric Association, 2000).

American Psychiatric Association, *Diagnostic and Statistical Manual of Mental Disorders, 5th Edition* (Washington, DC: American Psychiatric Association, 2013). https://doi.org/10.1176/appi.books.9780890425596

Berk, Philip R., 'Canto VII: The Weal of Fortune' in Allen Mandelbaum, Anthony Oldcorn, and Charles Ross (eds), *Lectura Dantis: Inferno* (Berkeley: University of California Press, 1999). https://doi.org/10.1525/9780520315808-008

Boyde, Patrick, *Human Vices and Human Worth in Dante's Comedy* (New York: Cambridge University Press, 2000).

Brumberg, Joan, *Fasting Girls: The Emergence of Anorexia Nervosa as a Modern Disease* (Cambridge, MA: Harvard University Press, 1988).

Bryant, Karl, 'Diagnosis and Medicalization' in P.J. McGann and David Hutson (eds), *Sociology of Diagnosis* (Bingley: Emerald, 2011). https://doi.org/10.1108/S1057-6290(2011)0000012007

Burgess, Alexandra, Randy O. Frost, Cheyenne Marani and Isabella Gabrielson, 'Imperfection, Indecision, and Hoarding', *Current Psychology* 37 (2018): 445–53. https://doi.org/10.1007/s12144-017-9695-4

Cockayne, Emily, *Hubbub: Filth, Noise & Stench in England* (New Haven: Yale University Press, 2007).

Crawford, Paul, Brian Brown, Charley Baker, Victoria Tischler, and Brian Abrams, *Health Humanities* (London: Palgrave Macmillan, 2015). https://doi.org/10.1057/9781137282613

Dante Alighieri, *Inferno: Dante Alighieri's Divine Comedy, Vol. 1*, trans. by Mark Musa (Bloomington: Indiana University Press, 1996 [1320?]).

Dante Alighieri, *Inferno*, trans. by John Dickson Sinclair (Oxford: Oxford University Press, 1939).

Dante Alighieri, *Inferno*, trans. by Allen Mandelbaum (New York: Bantam, 1980).

Dante Alighieri, *Inferno*, trans. by Steve Ellis (London: Chatto & Windus, 1994).

Dante Alighieri, *Inferno*, trans. by Robert Durling (Oxford: Oxford University Press, 1996).

Dante Alighieri, *Inferno*, trans. by Robin Kirkpatrick (London: Penguin, 2006).

Dickens, Charles, *Bleak House* (Oxford: Oxford University Press, 1996).

Easter, Michele, 'Interpreting Genetics in the Context of Eating Disorders: Evidence of Disease, Not Diversity', *Sociology of Health and Illness* 36.6 (2014): 840–55. https://doi.org/10.1111/1467-9566.12108

Eddy, Charmaine, 'Trash and Aesthetics in the Hoard', *Nanocrit* 7 (2015), https://nanocrit.com/issues/issue7/trash-and-aesthetics-hoard, accessed 20 April 2022.

Fineberg, Naomi, Samar Reghunandanan, Sangeetha Kolli, and Murad Atmaca, 'Obsessive-Compulsive (Anankastic) Personality Disorder: Toward the ICD-11

Classification', *Revista Brasileira de Psiquiatria* 36 (2014): S40–50. https://doi.org/10.1590/1516-4446-2013-1282

Flanagan, Owen, 'Identity and Addiction: What Alcoholic Memoirs Teach' in K.W.M. Fulford, Martin Davies, Richard G. Gipps, George Graham, John Sadler, Giovanni Stanghellini, and Tim Thornton (eds), *Oxford Handbook of Philosophy and Psychiatry* (Oxford: Oxford University Press, 2013). https://doi.org/10.1093/oxfordhb/9780199579563.013.0051

Frost, Randy, and Rachel Gross, 'The Hoarding of Possessions', *Behaviour Research and Therapy* 31.4 (1993): 367–81. https://doi.org/10.1016/0005-7967(93)90094-B

Frost, Randy, and Tamara Hartl, 'A Cognitive-Behavioural Model of Compulsive Hoarding' *Behaviour Research and Therapy* 34.4 (1996): 341–50. https://doi.org/10.1016/0005-7967(95)00071-2

Gogol, Nikolai, *Dead Souls* (London: Everyman's Library, 1996).

Hacking, Ian, *Mad Travelers: Reflections on the Reality of Transient Mental Illness* (Cambridge, MA: Harvard University Press, 1998).

Herring, Scott, *The Hoarders: Material Deviance in Modern American Culture* (Chicago: University of Chicago Press, 2014). https://doi.org/10.7208/chicago/9780226171852.001.0001

Jutel, Annemarie, 'Sociology of Diagnosis: A Preliminary Review', *Sociology of Health & Illness* 31.2 (2009): 278–99. https://doi.org/10.1111/j.1467-9566.2008.01152.x

Jutel, Annemarie, *Putting a Name to It: Diagnosis in Contemporary Society* (Baltimore: Johns Hopkins University Press, 2011).

Lepselter, Susan, 'The Disorder of Things: Hoarding Narratives in Popular Media', *Anthropological Quarterly* 84.4 (2011): 919–47. https://doi.org/10.1353/anq.2011.0053

Little, Lester K., 'Pride Goes Before Avarice: Social Change and Vices in Latin Christendom', *American Historical Review* 76.1 (1971): 16–49. https://doi.org/10.2307/1869775

Lucas, Gavin, 'Disposability and Dispossession in the Twentieth Century', *Journal of Material Culture* 7.1 (2002): 5–22. https://doi.org/10.1177/1359183502007001303

Maier, Thomas, 'On Phenomenology and Classification of Hoarding: A Review', *Acta Psychiatrica Scandinavica* 110 (2004): 323–37. https://doi.org/10.1111/j.1600-0447.2004.00402.x

Mataix-Cols, David, and Alberto Pertusa, 'Hoarding Disorder—Potential Benefits and Pitfalls of a New Mental Disorder', *Journal of Child Psychology and Psychiatry* 53.5 (2012): 608–18. https://doi.org/10.1111/j.1469-7610.2011.02464.x

Mataix-Cols, David, Randy Frost, Alberto Pertusa, Anna Lee Clark, Sanjaya Saxena, James Leckman, Dan Stein, Hisato Matsunaga, and Sabine Wilhelm, 'Hoarding

Disorder: A New Diagnosis for DSM-V?', *Depression and Anxiety* 27 (2010): 556–72. https://doi.org/10.1002/da.20693

McGann, P.J., and David Hutson (eds), *Sociology of Diagnosis* (Bingley: Emerald, 2011). https://doi.org/10.1108/S1057-6290(2011)12

McNally, Richard J., 'Is PTSD a Transhistorical Phenomenon?' in Devon E. Hinton and Byron J. Good (eds), *Culture and PTSD: Trauma in Global and Historical Perspective* (Philadelphia: University of Pennsylvania Press, 2016). https://doi.org/10.9783/9780812291469-003

Mitchell, Rob, 'Someone to Safeguard', 2016, https://lastquangoinhalifax.wordpress.com/2016/09/24/someone-to-safeguard/; https://adultpswnetwork.files.wordpress.com/2017/03/reflections-at-the-heart-of-social-work.pdf, accessed 28 January 2019.

Moran, Patrick, 'The Collyer Brothers and the Fictional Lives of Hoarders', *Modern Fiction Studies* 62.2 (2016): 272–91. https://doi.org/10.1353/mfs.2016.0033

Muramoto, Osamu, 'Retrospective Diagnosis of a Famous Historical Figure: Ontological, Epistemic, and Ethical Considerations', *Philosophy, Ethics, and Humanities in Medicine* 9 (2014): article 10. https://doi.org/10.1186/1747-5341-9-10

Niccoli, Alessandro, 'Tenere' in Umberto Bosco (ed.), *Enciclopedia Dantesca* (Rome: Istituto della Enciclopedia Italiana, 1976).

Orr, David M.R., Michael Preston-Shoot, and Suzy Braye, 'Meaning in Hoarding: Perspectives of People Who Hoard on Clutter, Culture and Agency', *Anthropology & Medicine* 26.3 (2017): 263–79. https://doi.org/10.1080/13648470.2017.1391171

Patel, Vikram, 'Why Mental Health Matters to Global Health', *Transcultural Psychiatry* 51.6 (2014): 777–89. https://doi.org/10.1177/1363461514524473

Penzel, Fred, 'Hoarding in History' in Randy Frost and Gail Steketee (eds), *Oxford Handbook of Hoarding and Acquiring* (Oxford: Oxford University Press, 2014). https://doi.org/10.1093/oxfordhb/9780199937783.013.001

Pertusa, Alberto, Randy Frost, Miguel Fullana, Jack Samuels, Gail Steketee, David Tolin, Sanjaya Saxena, James Leckman, and David Mataix-Cols, 'Refining the Diagnostic Boundaries of Compulsive Hoarding: A Critical Review', *Clinical Psychology Review* 30 (2010): 371–86. https://doi.org/10.1016/j.cpr.2010.01.007

Smail, Daniel, 'Neurohistory in Action: Hoarding and the Human Past', *Isis* 105.1 (2014): 110–22. https://doi.org/10.1086/675553

Steketee, Gail, *From Dante to DSM-V: A Short History of Hoarding* (2013), http://208.88.128.33/hoarding/hoarding.aspx?id=686&terms=a%20short%20history, downloaded 16 September 2017.

Steketee, Gail, 'Individual Cognitive and Behavioral Treatment for Hoarding' in Randy Frost and Gail Steketee (eds), *Oxford Handbook of Hoarding and Acquiring* (Oxford:

Oxford University Press, 2014). https://doi.org/10.1093/oxfordhb/9780199937783.013.018

Steketee, Gail, and Randy Frost, 'Compulsive Hoarding: Current Status of the Research', *Clinical Psychology Review* 23.7 (2003): 905–27. https://doi.org/10.1016/j.cpr.2003.08.002

Steketee, Gail, and Randy Frost, 'Phenomenology of Hoarding' in Randy Frost and Gail Steketee (eds), *Oxford Handbook of Hoarding and Acquiring* (Oxford: Oxford University Press, 2014). https://doi.org/10.1093/oxfordhb/9780199937783.013.008

Strasser, Susan, *Waste and Want: A Social History of Trash* (New York: Metropolitan Books, 1999).

Weiss, Kenneth, and Aneela Khan, 'Hoarding, Housing, and DSM-5', *Journal of the American Academy of Psychiatry and the Law* 43.4 (2015): 492–98.

Winters, Renee M., *The Hoarding Impulse: Suffocation of the Soul* (New York: Routledge, 2015). https://doi.org/10.4324/9781315730653

Young, Allan, *The Harmony of Illusions: Inventing Post-Traumatic Stress Disorder* (Princeton: Princeton University Press, 1995). https://doi.org/10.1515/9781400821938

14

Opening Up the Discourse of Male Eating Disorders: Personal Experience in German and English Narratives

Heike Bartel

Fictional and non-fictional writing about men's difficult personal experiences with food and food consumption in modern societies is still relatively rare compared to writing about women's experiences. Particularly at the extreme end of the spectrum of food consumption—the field of eating disorders (EDs)—reflections on the topic in art and literature focus predominantly on girls and women. This is in keeping with the focus in medical research and practice, which is largely driven by the fact that the majority of people with EDs—but crucially not all—are female.[1] Successive waves of feminist analysis of the changing social roles of girls and women have contributed to the understanding of the interconnectedness of the female body and food, weight and shape. Numerous studies in the field of women's writing (e.g. Bagley, Calamita, and Robson) highlight the links between the perception of women's bodies and female EDs. They explore the socio-cultural, economic, political, and aesthetic contexts that describe and prescribe women's roles in Western societies in various literary genres, including prose, poetry, drama, and notably autobiographical writing and self-help narratives. French feminist criticism has even coined the term 'écriture faminine', echoing the concept of *écriture féminine*, for writing 'rooted in or connected to anorexia' (Meuret 2008, 81). Susie Orbach, one of the leading feminist critics in the field, understands the significance of EDs as going beyond difficult relationships with food and the pressure to conform to female body stereotypes. She sees EDs as 'an expression of a woman's confusion about how much space she may take up in the world' (Orbach 1993, xii).

EDs—anorexia nervosa, bulimia nervosa, binge eating disorder, and other specified feeding and eating disorders—are serious and complex psychiatric disorders that can range from mild to severe, with anorexia nervosa showing 'the highest mortality of all mental health conditions' (Thompson 9).[2] The focus on female EDs is understandable and necessary given the prevalence and seriousness of the illness amongst girls and women, but this focus has also led to a 'glaring gender disparity' (Delderfield 2): the neglect of EDs in males and proper comparative study of EDs in different populations.[3]

It is a fact that men get eating disorders too.[4] In the Western world the number of boys and men affected by EDs is constantly rising (Colin and Lemberg 195) with figures in the UK estimated between 10% and 25% (Sweeting et al.). Any attempt to give accurate numbers 'is both difficult and self-defeating [...] difficult because baseline data on men are very hard to come by (existing measurers and diagnostic criteria are still highly feminised), and self-defeating because so often men will not report difficulties with eating' (Bryant-Jefferies vi). As a consequence, data may underestimate the problem and low figures circulated in the media may 'affect evaluations of [males'] personal susceptibility and hence help-seeking behaviour' (Sweeting et al.).

'Eating disorder symptomatology has been found to be quite similar in males and females' (Fichter and Krem 370) and the number of clinical studies on male EDs is slowly growing.[5] However, approaches so far have been largely framed through the discourse of female EDs and there is as yet no comprehensive socio-cultural approach towards understanding men and boys' experience of EDs. Jones and Morgan stress that 'the lack of equivalent discourse [compared to feminist theory] addressing male gender identity has left our knowledge of eating disorders in men aetiolated' (Jones and Morgan 29). Although Orbach's seminal title *Fat is a Feminist Issue* (1978) is often rephrased as 'Fat is a Man's Issue' in both medical and cultural studies (Andersen, Cohn, and Holbrook xiii; Gilman 1), this indicates that men's problems with food, weight, shape, and appearance tend to be researched not on their own terms. This chapter will show that there is room for a fruitful dialogue between feminist theory and the evolving critical approach to male EDs. However, it will also consider that the use of a 'female-centric lens' (Murray, Griffiths, and Mond 414–15) to view male EDs can reinforce a prevailing gender dichotomy which, in turn, is making it difficult for men and boys to articulate, communicate, and understand their health issues despite being 'Hungry for Words'.[6]

Method and Material

Drawing upon a small, as yet under-researched literary corpus of male-authored texts, this chapter aims to open up a discourse around male EDs and raise issues that can add both to the clinical and the socio-cultural exploration of the topic. I will focus on narratives by three authors: Michael Krasnow's 1996 *My Life as a Male Anorexic*, one of the first autobiographies by a man about his ED; Dave Chawner's 2018 *Weight Expectations: One Man's Recovery from Anorexia*, which charts Chawner's personal experiences and draws upon his own stand-up comedy material; and Benjamin von Stuckrad-Barre's 2016 *Panikherz* [Panic-Heart],[7] which reconstructs the author's personal experience with anorexia nervosa and bulimia nervosa and stylistically echoes his numerous publications in the genre of New German Pop Literature. The three texts, by men born in three different decades (Krasnow: 1969; Stuckrad-Barre: 1975; Chawner: 1989) and from three different geographic and socio-cultural spaces (North America, Germany, and the UK), vary considerably in style, context, and the authors' experiences of illness. What unites them, however, is that they are accounts of EDs experienced by heterosexual white men in Western society.[8]

The back cover of Krasnow's *My Life as a Male Anorexic* proposes that the author 'simply tells readers what his life is like and how anorexia has affected—even controlled—it'. Exploring the question of how a text, even one that promotes itself as an autobiography, can 'simply tell' the reader what an individual's 'life is like' is one aim of this chapter, especially when the narrative in this case is further complicated by a mental illness and its effects on the body. I will analyse all three texts within the broad theoretical frame of the genre of autobiography (Wagner-Egelhaaf; Smith and Watson; Lejeune) and its subgenre of 'illness autobiography', showing how these texts straddle, especially in the case of Chawner, the perceived divide between narratives of illness and recovery, and self-help books.[9] The intricate process of constructing and reconstructing experiences inherent in autobiographical writing reveals itself as even more complex in these three writings of a self affected by an ED. This self is, for example, inhibited by the gendered nature of EDs, affected by drug-induced memory loss, dominated by practitioners' opinions, and adverse to linear concepts of rehabilitation. It may use self-destruction as a coping mechanism or be empowered by models of recovery. I will also compare shifts and differences within and between the narratives, and will conclude with an evaluation of what they may contribute individually and collectively to an understanding—in both clinical and socio-cultural contexts—of male EDs and of recovery from such disorders.

The topic of male EDs involves consideration of a wide range of disciplines including medicine, psychology, sociology, gender studies, art, and literature. The extensive critical engagement with texts on contemporary female EDs has shown that a literary-analytic approach is highly suitable for dealing with this interconnectedness of areas and disciplines (Meuret 2007, 64). Applying such an interdisciplinary literary approach, this chapter asks what critical close readings of narrative texts can add to the understanding of lived experiences of illness. Aided and directed by the tools provided by literary scholarship, I will situate the narratives in the broad field that is now framed by the growing discipline of health humanities.

Krasnow, *My Life as A Male Anorexic*

Krasnow's 1996 text is often referred to as the first modern autobiography about a man's personal experience of an ED (Thapliyal, Mitchison, and Hay 112). According to the publisher's summary on the back cover, *My Life as a Male Anorexic* aims to 'begin to shed light on the little-known or discussed problem of male anorexia nervosa', which had been explored even less at the time of publication than today.

Krasnow was born in 1969 in Rochester, New York, and this was his first and only publication. He died in October 1997 aged twenty-eight and severely underweight.[10] The text puts a strong focus on Krasnow's experiences of treatment as an in- and outpatient in several hospitals and psychiatric units, and contains hardly any emotional disclosures. In its bleakness it is very powerful; it is described by one critic as 'terrifyingly spare and blunt' (Osgood 120).

Krasnow is at once author, protagonist, and first-person narrator. He remembers his eleven-year-old self proclaiming to his Jewish-American family that he feels 'fat' (Krasnow 3). He reconstructs the final moments he has as a nineteen-year-old with his dying father via the account provided by his mother, because electroshock therapy to treat his severe depression caused him temporary memory loss. He describes several attempts to run away from hospitals to starve himself to death and his efforts to lead an independent life, symbolized powerfully by his desire to own his own fridge, giving him control over his food consumption (27–30). In addition to the eleven short chapters authored by Krasnow, the book contains passages not written by him. Krasnow's publisher Harrington Park Press followed a trend particularly prominent in the 1970s and 1980s for narratives of personal experience of mental illness to 'contain editing or commentaries by mental health professionals' (Foster 42). A two-page preface by his doctor and a two-part appendix of fifty-three pages were added to Krasnow's eighty-four pages.[11] The appendix contains 'A Psychiatrist's Comments' by Stephen R. Wiener, who treated Krasnow, as well as three substantial discharge summaries from two different hospitals. These diverse sources invite us to query the notion of autobiography as 'simply telling' the reader what the subject's life is like. Moreover, they shift the focus onto a close analysis of the '*Konstruktcharakter*' [constructedness] of autobiographical writing (Wagner-Egelhaaf 61) and illness autobiographies in particular: the reconstruction of past events, especially when memory loss has occurred; and the contrast between personal and other accounts, particularly when these are affected by power structures inherent in patient–doctor or parent–child relationships. It is only by reading these elements together that the personal story unfolds in its complexity.

The medical documents inserted into the text create an implicit narrative of the individual's life and raise important questions.[12] As in other narratives of mental illness, these official notes and assessments by medical professionals can be seen as a way, here driven by the publisher, 'of lending to the story an authority and credibility it might otherwise be seen as lacking' (Foster 42). However, changing the perspective from patient to medical practitioner considerably affects the autarky of the subject's personal story: 'I felt that each item added to my story by somebody else […] would take away from it being my book', comments Krasnow in the epilogue (Krasnow 88). Moreover, the medical notes introduce a potent twofold dynamic to the text. This is particularly apparent regarding a hospital episode in which a severely undernourished protagonist is restrained and force-fed and resists violently. Here, the individual is described from two perspectives, in the clinical report and through the personal narrative. He is both the 'crazy' patient literally and metaphorically restrained and silenced by the feeding tubes, and he is the 'sane' narrating 'I' who coherently voices what he perceives as an abusive breach of trust. Echoing theoretical approaches that emphasize the importance and scope of patients' perspectives (e.g. Charon; Hawkins; Frank), Krasnow's personal narrative can be read here as a critique of 'dehumanizing treatment accorded by institutions to vulnerable people' and as empowering him as a patient to '"talk [...] back" to the authority of medical doctors' (Smith and Watson 146–47). Such dual-perspective narratives have the potential to 'hold [...] two socially constructed categories—normalcy and abnormalcy—in tension' (Smith and Watson 146). Acknowledging this tension may lead the reader to query the polarized understandings of 'healthy' versus 'ill', 'mad' versus 'sane'. Whilst in other narratives about personal experiences of mental illness the author may be able to reconcile these positions, in Krasnow's story they remain irreconcilable and contribute to the alienation of the subject from his surrounding world in general, and from medical practitioners in particular.

Rita Charon introduces *Narrative Medicine* as a way to strengthen in health practitioners, through the use of illness narrative, 'those cognitive and imaginative abilities that are required for one person to take in and appreciate the representation—and therefore reality—of another' (Charon 113). Correspondingly, Krasnow explicitly voices the intention of his book to 'lead to a greater awareness not only of anorexia, but male anorexia', hoping that this may help male sufferers and allow doctors to reach 'a better understanding of what goes through an anorexic's mind and be able to offer more help to a patient' (Krasnow 83). However, Krasnow's illness narrative is also a powerful and tragic testimony to the possible conflict between the standpoint of the suffering individual and medical advice. This conflict causes great pain and suffering for both sides, patient and carers/family, and ends in the subject of this story being unable to accept any help, in isolation and self-starvation.

A clinical study using autobiographical writings as case vignettes highlights that when compared to five other texts by men about their EDs, *My Life as a Male Anorexic* is the only story that does not end in recovery (Thapliyal, Mitchison, and Hay 113).[13] Nearly all personal narratives on the topic published between 2004 and 2018, whilst acknowledging difficulties and setbacks, emphasize recovery. This is expressed in titles such as: *A Young Man's Battle and Triumph over Anorexia* (Grahl) or *One Man's Recovery from Anorexia* (Chawner). Krasnow's 1996 narrative, not taking his sad demise less than a year after its publication into account, bucks this trend. It culminates in an overwhelming resistance to accepting any medical treatment aimed at increasing his weight. In the last chapter he describes moving away, living on his own and no longer seeking medical care. Despite a very desolate outlook on his life—'I don't care if I live or die' (Krasnow 83)—a sense of personal triumph and self-affirmation becomes apparent regarding his ability to function whilst maintaining a body weight deemed life-endangeringly low by health professionals.

Grasping the deep concerns of doctors and family, the protagonist in Krasnow's text nevertheless asserts: 'I'm holding on to anorexia and don't want to let go. The anorexia is my shield protecting me from something' (Krasnow 82). This statement gives the ED a function that is perceived as important for protecting and preserving a sense of self. However, clinically, this is termed 'self-destructive behaviour as coping mechanism' (Bräutigam and Herberhold 12). The protagonist's perception of his severe anorexia as positive and stabilizing, a 'win' and 'triumph' of the individual against medical intervention, is also reflected in the rhetoric. Experiences of feeling '"all-powerful" and in control' and decisions 'to run my life' (Krasnow 74, 79) are voiced almost exclusively in connection with a severe restriction of food and the maintenance of a dangerously low body weight. For the protagonist his anorexia is an integral part of his psychological self-formation, not self-destruction, although the destructive effects on his body are clear to the clinician, his family, and the reader.[14]

Other narratives about male anorexia echo this dynamic. 'No wonder I hadn't wanted to give it up—anorexia distracted, stabilised and explained me. [...] [A]norexia had been one of the only stable things I'd got' (Chawner 163, 165). However, whilst Chawner's recognition initiates for him the difficult process of recovery, Krasnow's illness narrative concludes with a desire to hold onto anorexia indefinitely.

Chawner, *Weight Expectations: One Man's Recovery from Anorexia*

In the epilogue to *My Life as a Male Anorexic*, Krasnow explains why he has refused to include a list of ED organizations in his book, as his publisher had suggested: 'You see, I don't believe in these places' (Krasnow 88). In stark contrast, Chawner in *Weight Expectations* not only emphatically recommends a number of charities and helplines (Chawner 187–88) but the author also actively supports several of them.[15] This is indicative of Chawner's positive treatment experience, in which these organizations played an important role, and also emphasizes that they have come a long way since the 1980s and 1990s and are now striving to offer help to all affected by EDs regardless of gender, age, or background.

Chawner describes receiving a clinical diagnosis after five years of not being able to communicate what had been affecting him: 'I didn't have the vocab to explain anorexia' (Chawner 97). In his narrative he retrospectively finds the words to explain and analyse his experience of developing anorexia as a late-teen and how it affected him at university and as he sought to establish a career. Interspersed with information outlining five stages of recovery, from 'Precontemplation' via 'Preparation' and 'Action' to 'Maintenance' and 'Relapse' (14), the text combines traits of self-help and personal illness and recovery narrative. Separate short texts inserted into the narrative, resembling post-it notes stuck onto the pages, link events in his life to these stages, for example: '"Precontemplation": Being unaware you have an eating disorder' (19). There are also 'notes' with 'Tips to help at this stage' and an extensive 'Maintenance' section (172–88). Playlists suggesting songs present another coping mechanism. At several points the text even abandons the narrative form and draws the ups and downs of particular periods of his life literally onto a graph (102, 108).

The back cover of Chawner's book advertises it as '[p]art memoir, part self-help guide', and the text indeed shows the close link between the two genres. Personal life stories, insofar as they are concerned with the individual overcoming crises and difficulties and moving on to recovery, have a long tradition of incorporating 'self-help' elements (Crowley 505–07). Whilst Krasnow's protagonist constructs his position in resistance to therapeutic approaches, Chawner's reconstructs his experiences of illness by closely following a step-by-step model of recovery, albeit one that also has room for relapses. This framework enables the author to retrospectively make sense of the development of his own illness, integrating important changes, such as his first love and heartbreak and his father's life-threatening heart attack, but also a large number of seemingly mundane life events that nevertheless impacted on his illness. Chawner structures his story with reflective insight, shifting the emphasis from illness to recovery narrative, and autobiography to self-help book. The book enables the reader to make sense of the illness and shows the way to possible recovery.

Authored by a man who articulates his struggle with an ED, Chawner's book not only challenges the stereotype of anorexia as 'female-only'; he also makes the self-help genre for which women are currently the 'main producers and consumers' (Crowley 506) more inclusive.

What makes this book stand out from other ED-recovery narratives is that it employs humour as a way to address male EDs and mental health. Chawner is a stand-up comedian and his shows 'Mental' (2018) and 'Over It—Death, Anorexia and Other Funny Things' (2015) draw on his personal experiences of illness. *Weight Expectations*, the title a comical echo of Dickens' *Great Expectations*, not only describes the ups and downs of his pathway into stand-up comedy as a career, but also echoes his comedy shows. It adapts some of his stand-up material and addresses the reader in a disarmingly direct and casual way that is very similar to Chawner's engagement with live audiences. The book emphasizes the importance of humour when dealing with the stigma and ignorance surrounding male EDs and mental health. 'Stand Up For Mental Health', a course that teaches individuals with mental illness to 'write, edit and perform stand-up comedy about their mental illnesses and the experiences surrounding them' (Maxwell, Lampshire, and Tse 88), stresses the important role humour can play in raising awareness of mental illness and in changing attitudes towards it. The programme emphasizes the potential of personal accounts of illness combined with comedy to 'unearth prejudices, offer information and challenge deeply entrenched perceptions', and to start new conversations (Maxwell, Lampshire, and Tse 90). Chawner too unlocks some of this power in a way that is, in his own words, 'fun, funny and helpful (or at least it's meant to be)' (Chawner 10). His book addresses general prejudices that anorexia is about 'wanting to look skinny and sexy, or a vanity project gone wrong' (61), or only represented by extremely thin individuals whose skeletal images in voyeuristic media 'get people watching or clicking links' (10–11). He also deals with gendered preconceptions including the deeply ingrained association of EDs with women and girls and, more recently, with gay men. Chawner addresses this with comical bluntness: 'If I had tooth decay, people wouldn't be interested if I'm male or female' (12). The comparison of EDs with tooth decay humorously underplays and normalizes EDs, portrays them as illnesses that can affect anybody regardless of gender, age, ethnicity, or background. It brings the discourse closer to home and destabilizes the (highly questionable) status of anorexia 'classically […] viewed as occurring primarily in young

White women, perhaps particularly in those of high socioeconomic status' (Crow 397). Open references to the sex life of a heterosexual anorectic man challenge gendered perceptions further. Chawner describes the loss and recovery of his libido, physiologically linked to his anorexia, and uses this to question definitions of masculinity: 'Therapy sparked a big change—I'd always been the anorexic camp guy with no sex drive. Now I was getting my masculinity and libido back, and it made me think, "Who *even* am I?"' (Chawner 167). This and other passages (e.g. 59–61) describe the male subject in what Carole Jones calls a state of 'unstable and paradoxical male identity' in reaction to the phenomenon that 'masculinity itself [is] a category obviously in flux' (Jones 13–14). Chawner's text opens up the possibility of using male EDs to ask much broader questions about what masculinity means in contemporary society.

Stuckrad-Barre, *Panikherz*

Stuckrad-Barre is one of the most prominent authors working in the genre of New German Pop Literature. In the 1990s, he and several other German-language writers continued to subvert the traditional distinction between 'High and Low Culture' as part of a literary trend that drew on earlier international twentieth-century pop art and literature.[16] These young, mainly male German writers drove the pop trajectory faster and more aggressively into the twenty-first century than their pop art predecessors. They steered their writing towards a seemingly wilful superficiality with a strong penchant for popular culture, media consumption, advertising, and fashion, combined with a deliberate avoidance of political, historical, or moral topics. Critics of this new type of pop literature, with its seeming emphasis on superficial consumerist values, on shopping, fun, drug use, and hedonism, excoriated it at the time. It was criticized as one-dimensional and shallow, limited to 'straightforward inventories of the present moment' that deflected attention from 'big meaning' (McCarthy 8). However, current scholarship recognizes that some of these texts are highly innovative in their approaches to literary aesthetics, the role of culture, and in particular the struggle of the (mostly male) individual in a superficial and consumerist society where media and popular lifestyle dictate looks, and money is the only marker of success. Scholars increasingly see in the seemingly detached and uncritical inventory of modern urban life a critical power, akin to the one Jones finds in Irvine Welsh's 1993 novel *Trainspotting*, to 'reflect the dominant culture' and distort its values (Jones 73). This aesthetic and cultural background to Stuckrad-Barre's work is more than a frame for the text. It is an important component of his engagement with EDs.

The first-person narrator of *Panikherz* struggles to get through modern urban life with its trademark ingredients of pop culture: 'love, misery, grief, alienation, existential crises initiated by drug experiences, sexuality and violence' (Mehrfort, cited in McCarthy 9). Stuckrad-Barre pushes the boundaries of this catalogue to the extreme by adding anorexia and bulimia to the list. The protagonist's anorexia develops into bulimia when he turns, halfway through this 564-page book, to self-induced vomiting to counteract the binge-eating behaviour spurred by his food restriction (Stuckrad-Barre 223). Stuckrad-Barre is at once author, protagonist, and first-person narrator. As in Chawner's book, pop music plays an important role in Stuckrad-Barre's text, which chronicles his life as a music journalist, working for a record label, as a writer for a successful German talk show, and as an acclaimed author and literary 'pop-star'. It also outlines in detail his cocaine and alcohol addiction, and his ED. *Panikherz* interconnects ED and addiction by describing anorexia and bulimia as integral to a brutal step-by-step self-destruction, where cocaine and alcohol are part of complex addictive and anorectic/bulimic behaviour patterns and are also used to stifle or satisfy hunger. Compared to Chawner's emphasis on the everyday normalcy of EDs, *Panikherz* presents a sufferer with an extreme lifestyle without any rhythm or boundaries, epitomized by the place where the I-narrator lives and writes *Panikherz*: the infamous Chateau Marmont hotel on Los Angeles' Sunset Boulevard, place of frequent encounters with subversive art and artists, including the author of the controversial novel *American Psycho* (1991), Bret Easton Ellis. In this environment it is not only female size zero that is promoted; expectations of a particular body shape and size bear on males as well. Here, representations of extreme male thinness and emaciated 'heroin chic' push at the boundaries of what is perceived as a traditional masculine physique, particularly in the creative sector—for example in the protagonist's idol David Bowie.[17] Other names of male disordered eaters in the entertainment industry also scratch at the gendered image of EDs: John Lennon, Elvis Presley, and Elton John, all known for having a problematic relationship with food, are named as the protagonist's *'Brüder im Geiste'* [brothers in spirit] (225–26). The protagonist receives the diagnosis of his own ED very late after onset and pins his hopes on a German ED clinic where he has to face his

'Albtraum' [nightmare] of having to achieve a healthy *'NORMALGEWICHT'* [NORMAL WEIGHT] (244; emphasis in original). Here he finds himself to be the only male patient amongst teenage girls, and responds to the gendered codification of the illness with a term that ironically belittles his own fraught experience and the severity of the illness itself: *'Mädchenkrankheit'* [girls' illness] (244). However, deluding himself and deliberately deceiving the therapists throughout, the protagonist-turned-rebellious-patient makes a deliberate mockery of this therapy attempt. His eventual pick-up by a taxi-driving drug dealer is described in a way that takes any notion that this discharge means he is *'GEHEILT'* [HEALED] (251; emphasis in original) *ad absurdum*.

The narrative structure of *Panikherz* disrupts any linearity of illness, treatment, and recovery/healing. Passages describing youth and childhood are interrupted by passages narrated from a present-day perspective. The style follows a spiralling and associative logic that mirrors the uncontrolled pattern of periods of serious drug abuse, and extreme food restriction followed by food binges, followed by purging. The crisis of the unhinged protagonist is reflected in a deliberately unhinged narrative expressed both through content and form. One example would be the numerous words throughout the text that are printed seemingly at random in capital letters, making them part of normal sentence structures but at the same time interrupting the flow of reading—such as the abovementioned *'GEHEILT'* and *'NORMALGEWICHT'*. These words can be read as ironic commentaries highlighting empty phrases: 'JUNIOR PRODUCTMANAGER PROGRESSIVE' (164), or as flashing advertisements or neon signs: 'DIET COKE' (481). Sometimes they seem only to follow the rambling logic of an erratic narrative: *'EINEN'* [ONE] (127); in other passages they clearly signal distress, as in *'NORMALGEWICHT'* [NORMAL WEIGHT] (244). However, the interpretations are interchangeable: a word like *'NORMALGEWICHT'* can be read simultaneously as an advert, an empty phrase, a distress signal, or a random word, subverting any singular reading. This practice signals the unreliability of fixed references and an overlapping of discourses, in particular words related to the central topics of food consumption, therapy, and addiction, so indicating a total lack of orientation. Such deliberately disorientating language mirrors the protagonist's mind in freefall and thus inscribes the pathological into the text. The final image leaves it unclear whether the subject has recovered or self-destructed, whether this is the end or the beginning of his story, or in fact another intertextual element, here alluding to the famous opening of Billy Wilder's 1950s film *Sunset Boulevard*: '*Der Tote im Pool erzählt seine Geschichte*' [The dead man in the pool tells his story] (564). However, the emphasis on '*erzählen*' [to narrate] and the fact that *Panikherz* containing this 'story' exists, highlights the potential of writing itself as aiding survival, self-affirmation, and even recovery.

The youthful risk-taking behaviour in Stuckrad-Barre's previous fictional texts reaches with this very personal account in *Panikherz* an utterly unglamorous climax. Describing himself as reduced to a whimpering wreck collapsed in front of the toilet bowl by the dictate of endless repetitions of eating and vomiting, interrupted only by secret and ashamed food shopping excesses (224), Stuckrad-Barre shatters any illusion of rockstar-cool. He destroys the myth of a carefree and culturally celebrated ideal of youth and also his own '*Popstarmaske*' [popstar-mask] (Kauer 141). Stuckrad-Barre's *Panikherz* can be read as an autobiographical narrative that emphatically rejects the notion of the life story as a successful *Bildungsroman* or recovery narrative that ultimately leads the protagonist to overcome various crises and become integrated into a meaningful and wholesome life and society (Wagner-Egelhaaf 181–83). Authoritative figures or institutions—for example parents, doctors, or clinics—that are traditionally seen as facilitating progress and personal betterment are represented as ignorant at best and damaging at worst (Wagner-Egelhaaf 189–94). *Panikherz* presents an autobiographical illness narrative that questions traditional notions of recovery, and challenges on a personal and a cultural level the concept of the self as a body and mind that can be restored, saved, and healed. By weaving anorexia and bulimia into a scathing inventory of postmodern life, Stuckrad-Barre's text emphasizes a subject in deep crisis, fragmented and radically distanced from its environment, combining personal story and '*Zeitgeistanalyse*' [analysis of the zeitgeist] (Siebrasse). For German art historian Florian Illies, *Panikherz* is the final self-destructive push of New German Pop Literature that burns itself out alongside its protagonist (Illies).

Conclusion and Relevance for Healthcare

The close readings of the above three texts have aimed to open up a discourse of male EDs and highlight the need for further engagement with the topic. Moreover, given the disparate styles and contents of the texts, it is not surprising that we cannot extrapolate a single unified 'message' regarding male EDs.

The parallels and points of comparison this literary analysis has identified can, however, be used to delineate a field of enquiry and make recommendations for future research.

Part of opening this discourse lies in unlocking the interdisciplinary potential of literary texts to inform and influence clinical treatment of male EDs. All three texts raise in their individual ways points that healthcare providers should attend to, especially insofar as they also correspond to findings by clinical research (referenced in parentheses). All three authors relate ignorant or negative attitudes of medical professionals, often represented by the local doctor as first port of call, who are ill-prepared to engage openly with the male individual and consider an ED diagnosis. Combined with an initial lack of awareness of their illness, as voiced by all three protagonists, this is a dangerous combination, adversely affecting, delaying, or hindering diagnosis and treatment (Thapliyal, Mitchison, and Hay; Bannatyne and Stapleton 2015).[18] Given the emphasis on early intervention as vital for successful recovery (Andersen 137; Stanford and Lemberg; Räisänen and Hunt), a clear need emerges for more specialized medical training in relation to EDs (Thapliyal, Mitchison, and Hay), but also for better-informed teachers, sports and drama coaches, and other professionals. That all three protagonists express a feeling of standing out during group therapy sessions at ED clinics where teenage girls are in the majority highlights the need to explore specialized male-orientated therapy options (Brown, Griffiths, and Murray; Bannatyne and Stapleton). This is especially important in light of the male-specific issues described particularly by Chawner and Stuckrad-Barre—for example the effects of anorexia on sexual dysfunction and libido (Brown, Griffiths, and Murray). Passages that describe personal experiences of inpatient treatment, e.g. by Krasnow, also throw light on problems that may particularly affect males. These include reactions to the authority of male or female practitioners; the loss or feared loss of the father (Krasnow and Chawner) or father figure (Stuckrad-Barre) through ill health (Thompson 10; Andersen 46); the role of sport and over-exercising from a male perspective—different from female over-exercising (Brown, Griffiths, and Murray); and patterns of drug and alcohol abuse, particularly in male peer groups (Bräutigam and Herberhold 91).

Viewed in a wider socio-cultural context, all three texts provide glimpses into how men relate to their bodies and especially how 'the' anorectic male body is viewed by themselves and by others. Building on existing studies engaging with representations of masculinity and of the male body in broader socio-cultural terms (e.g. Adams and Savran; Gardiner), examples from male ED narratives can add further insights to the field. Together the three texts discussed here chart, for example, how public perception of the extremely thin male body changes between 1996 and 2018 in different national and cultural contexts. Krasnow's text includes references to skeletal victims in Nazi concentration camps (Krasnow xi), comments such as 'You look as though you have AIDS' (81) and, in a newspaper, references to Franz Kafka's 1922 short story 'A Hunger Artist' (Norman). Stuckrad-Barre's text illustrates a specific cultural performance of not only female but also male thinness prominent in pop culture. Chawner's text alerts us to the public perception of anorectic men as gay. Clearly, as one expert in the field comments, '[f]or male eating disorders research to advance, diversification of approach is required' (Delderfield 2). The questions and perceptions in our three texts point to the need to broaden clinical approaches by taking full account of different historical, national, and socio-cultural backgrounds.

In *Writing Size Zero*, a study of female anorexia in literary texts, Isabelle Meuret, citing Antony Easthope's *Literary into Cultural Studies*, writes of 'a serious discourse of knowledge' (Meuret 2007, 60–61; Easthope 6). This chapter proposes that a literary-analytical approach to narratives of male EDs offers significant opportunities for establishing a discourse of knowledge (see Bartel). As Sandy Petrey argues, nuanced literary study 'doesn't exclude other disciplines, it allows us to use them while maintaining the integrity of our own' (Petrey 16). Literary studies bring together the many aspects inherent in textual representations of male EDs. Above all, this approach pays close attention to the language, form, and style used to articulate, communicate, and understand personal experience of illness and the vast surrounding experiences of life. Through this approach the three texts have revealed an array of insights into male EDs and associated issues: innovatively introducing the power of humour to break down stereotypes and normalize how we approach the illness (Chawner); powerfully linking the personal illness narrative with a much more expansive cultural critique (Stuckrad-Barre); or giving unique and urgent insights into an ultimately destructive route to self-affirmation through anorexia (Krasnow). Together with other texts—referenced here, or still to be discovered—they can help towards figuring a serious discourse of male EDs.

Notes

1. In the UK between 75% and 90% of the approximately 1.25 million people suffering from EDs are female. Figures from the UK's largest ED charity Beat with consideration of Sweeting et al. (2015). https://www.beateatingdisorders.org.uk/media-centre/eating-disorder-statistics, accessed 7 January 2019.
2. For a comprehensive account of the broad spectrum of EDs, see e.g. Treasure, Schmidt, and Furth 2003; Downs et al., 2022.
3. The importance of addressing 'atypical EDs' is starting to be recognized, e.g. in the *Clinical Handbook of Complex and Atypical Eating Disorders* (Andersen, Murray, and Kaye), where Arcelus et al. address EDs in the LGBTQ population (327–43), Ramirez et al. present EDs amongst ethnic minorities (344–62), and Runfola et al. address midlife-onset in ED (363–83).
4. Charities such as 'Male VoicED' and the now ceased 'Men Get Eating Disorders Too' as well as 'Beat Eating Disorders' and 'First Steps Eating Disorder' are leading successful campaigns raising awareness of male EDs.
5. For an overview of literature see Murray et al.
6. 'Hungry for Words' is an AHRC-funded project on male EDs that has inspired this research. Special thanks go to co-investigator Nadia Micali and to Huw Grange for their invaluable help and support. https://www.nottingham.ac.uk/research/groups/hungry-for-words/index.aspx.
7. All translations from *Panikherz* are my own.
8. Future research would benefit from focusing on the differences between treatment options and medical systems in these countries.
9. Einat Avrahami and others problematize illness autobiography as a 'subgenre' challenging 'accepted definitions' of autobiography (Avrahami 1–16). The term 'pathography', e.g. as defined by Hawkins (1999), adds further dimensions to the discussion. This emphasizes the need—addressed in this volume—to advance genre definitions in the field, show crossovers but also outline differences. For further discussion see also Carel; Jurecic; Smith and Watson.
10. His weight is given by the sensationalist *Broward Palm Beach New Times* as sixty-four pounds and his height as five foot ten (Norman).
11. The book also contains six pages of family photos depicting Krasnow in an increasingly emaciated state. These visual representations of the male anorectic body deserve closer critical analysis, e.g. via Wilson's research (2014).
12. Patient confidentiality would pose legal problems in disclosing such documents nowadays.
13. Titles analysed by Thapliyal, Mitchison, and Hay are: Bruni; Henning; McBride; Croteau; Grahl. Added to this list can be further single publications in English:

Simon; Saxen; Prager; Evans; Chawner; and in German: Frommert; Slim. For further titles see Delderfield's extensive bibliography (Delderfield 14; 28–38).
14. Bray and Colebrook emphasize theories of anorexia—particularly in women and girls in the context of patriarchal oppression—as an 'active event rather than [...] the negation of some ground' (Brasy and Colebrook 63).
15. Chawner is e.g. patron for First Steps Eating Disorders and partner in the 'Hungry for Words' project; see footnote 6. Special thanks to him for his support.
16. Leslie Fiedler provided the seminal essay for this concept in 1971.
17. European culture interlinks creative 'romantic agony' with very thin 'pallid, rachitic young men', e.g. linking stylized symptoms of tuberculosis with great creativity, as Susan Sontag highlights quoting Théophile Gautier (1811–1872): 'When I was young [...] I could not have accepted as a lyrical poet anyone weighing more than ninety-nine pounds' (Sontag 26). Many thanks to Lasse Raaby Gammelgaard for a valuable exchange of thoughts on this.
18. See also the project @ConsiderMaleEDs, aimed at GPs as part of 'Hungry for Words', University of Nottingham.

References

Adams, Rachel, and David Savran (eds), *The Masculinity Studies Reader* (Chichester: Wiley Blackwell, 2002).

Andersen, Arnold, *Males with Eating Disorders* (New York: Psychology Press, 1990).

Andersen, Arnold, Leigh Cohn, and Thomas Holbrook, *Making Weight: Men's Conflicts with Food, Weight, Shape and Appearance* (Carlsbad, CA: Gürze, 2000).

Anderson, Leslie K., Stuart B. Murray, and Walter H. Kaye (eds), *Clinical Handbook of Complex and Atypical Eating Disorders* (Oxford: Oxford University Press, 2018). https://doi.org/10.1093/med-psych/9780190630409.001.0001

Avrahami, Einat, *The Invaded Body: Reading Illness Autobiographies* (Charlottesville/London: University of Virginia Press, 2007).

Bagley, Petra, Francesca Calamita, and Kathryn Robson (eds), *Starvation, Food Obsession and Identity: Eating Disorders in Contemporary Women's Writing* (Oxford: Peter Lang, 2018). https://doi.org/10.3726/b10998

Bartel, Heike, *Men Writing Eating Disorders. Autobiographical Writing and Illness Experience in English and German Narratives* (Bingley: Emerald, 2020). https://doi.org/10.1108/9781839099205

Bannatyne, Amy, and Peta Stapleton, 'Educating Medical Students about Anorexia Nervosa: A Potential Method for Reducing the Volitional Stigma Associated with the Disorder', *Eating Disorders* 23.2 (2015): 115–33. https://doi.org/10.1080/10640266.2014.976102

Bräutigam, H., and M. Herberhold, '"I Couldn't Find the Food I Liked": Anorexia in Boys: Three Case Reports' in Pamela I. Swain (ed.), *Anorexia Nervosa and Bulimia Nervosa: New Research* (New York: Nova Science, 2006), 91–104.

Bray, Abigail, and Claire Colebrook, 'The Haunted Flesh: Corporeal Feminism and the Politics of (Dis)Embodiment', *Signs* 24.1 (1998): 35–67. https://doi.org/10.1086/495317

Brown, Tiffany A., Scott Griffiths, and Stuart B. Murray, 'Eating Disorders in Males' in Leslie K. Anderson, Stuart B. Murray, and Walter H. Kaye (eds), *Clinical Handbook of Complex and Atypical Eating Disorders* (Oxford: Oxford University Press, 2018), 309–26. https://doi.org/10.1093/med-psych/9780190630409.003.0018

Bruni, Frank, *Born Round: The Secret History of a Full-Time Eater* (Waterville, ME: Thorndike Press, 2010).

Bryant-Jefferies, Richard, *Counselling for Eating Disorders in Men: Person-Centred Dialogues* (Oxford/Seattle: Radcliffe, 2005).

Carel, Havi, *Illness: The Cry of the Flesh* (Abingdon: Routledge, 2013).

Charon, Rita, *Narrative Medicine: Honoring the Stories of Illness* (Oxford: Oxford University Press, 2006).

Chawner, Dave, *Weight Expectations: One Man's Recovery from Anorexia* (London/Philadelphia: Jessica Kingsley, 2018).

Colin, Leigh, and Raymond Lemberg, *Current Findings on Males with Eating Disorders* (London/New York: Routledge, 2014).

Croteau, Jean Derek, *My Thinning Years: Starving the Gay Within* (Center City, MN: Hazelden, 2014).

Crow, Scott J., 'Eating Disorders in Young Adults' in John E. Grant and Marc N. Potenza (eds), *Young Adult Mental Health* (Oxford: Oxford University Press, 2010), 397–405. https://doi.org/10.1093/med:psych/9780195332711.003.0024

Crowley, Karlyn, 'Self-Help Narrative' in Victoria Boynton and Jo Malin (eds), *Encyclopedia of Women's Autobiography, Vol. 1* (Westport, CN/London: Greenwood, 2005), 505–07.

Delderfield, Russell, *Male Eating Disorders: Experiences of Food, Body and Self* (Basingstoke: Palgrave Macmillan, 2018). https://doi.org/10.1007/978-3-030-02535-9

Downs, James, Mark Hopfenbeck, Hannah Lewis, Isla Parker and Nicole Schnackenberg (eds), *The Practical Handbook of Eating Difficulties. A Comprehensive Guide from Personal and Professional Perspectives* (Shoreham-by-Sea: Pavilio, 2022).

Easthope, Antony, *Literary into Cultural Studies* (London: Routledge, 1991).

Evans, John, *Becoming John: Anorexia's Not Just for Girls* (Didcot: Xlibris, 2011).

Fichter, Manfred, and H. Krem, 'Eating Disorders in Males' in Janet Treasure, Ulrike Schmidt, and Eric van Furth (eds), *Handbook of Eating Disorders* (Chichester: Wiley, 2003), 369–84. https://doi.org/10.1002/0470013443.ch23

Fiedler, Leslie, *Cross the Border—Close the Gap* (New York: Stein & Day, 1971).

Foster, Juliet L.H., *Journeys Through Mental Illness: Client Experiences and Understanding of Mental Distress* (Basingstoke: Palgrave Macmillan, 2007). https://doi.org/10.1007/978-1-137-05545-3

Frank, Arthur, *The Wounded Storyteller: Body, Illness and Ethics* (Chicago: University of Chicago Press, 1995). https://doi.org/10.7208/chicago/9780226260037.001.0001

Frommert, Christian, *"Dann iss halt was!"* (Munich: Mosaik, 2013).

Gardiner, Judith Kegan (ed.), *Masculinity Studies and Feminist Theory* (New York: Columbia University Press, 2002).

Gilman, Sander, *Fat Boys: A Slim Book* (London/Lincoln: The University of Nebraska Press, 2004).

Grahl, Gary A., *Skinny Boy: A Young Man's Battle and Triumph over Anorexia* (Clearfield, UT: American Legacy Media, 2007).

Hawkins, Anne Hunsaker, *Reconstructing Illness: Studies in Pathography* (West Lafayette, IN: Purdue University Press, 1999).

Henning, Dennis, *Hiding Under the Table* (Albuquerque, NM: Americana Publishing, 2004).

Illies, Florian, '"Panikherz": Der verlorene Sohn', *Zeit*, 31 March 2016, https://www.zeit.de/2016/13/panikherz-benjamin-von-stuckrad-barre-roman, accessed 7 January 2019.

Jones, Carole, *Disappearing Men: Gender Disorientation in Scottish Fiction* (Amsterdam/New York: Rodopi 2009). https://doi.org/10.1163/9789042026995

Jones, William, and John Morgan, 'Eating Disorders in Men: A Review of the Literature', *Journal of Public Mental Health* 9.2 (2010): 23–31. https://doi.org/10.5042/jpmh.2010.0326

Jurecic, Ann, *Illness as Narrative* (Pittsburgh, PA: University of Pittsburgh Press, 2012).

Kauer, Katja, 'Der Zauber männlicher Verletzlichkeit oder *das Mannsein stehe ich dann also mal im Wortsinn nicht durch*' in Katja Kauer (ed.), *Pop und Männlichkeit: Zwei Phänomene in prekärer Wechselwirkung* (Berlin: Frank & Timme, 2009), 119–48.

Krasnow, Michael, *My Life as a Male Anorexic* (New York/London: Harrington Park Press, 1996).

Lejeune, Philippe, *Le Pacte autographique, Vol I* (Paris: Éditions du Seuil, 1975).

Maxwell, Victoria, Debra Lampshire, and Samson Tse, 'Public Relations and Communication' in Chris Lloyd, Robert King, Frank Deane, and Kevin Gournay (eds), *Clinical Management in Mental Health Services* (Chichester: Wiley Blackwell, 2009), 80–93.

McBride, Gregg, *Weightless: My Life as a Fat Man and How I Escaped* (Las Vegas, NV: Central Recovery Press, 2014).

McCarthy, Margaret (ed.), *German Pop Literature: A Companion* (Berlin: de Gruyter, 2015). https://doi.org/10.1515/9783110275766

Meuret, Isabelle, *Writing Size Zero: Figuring Anorexia in Contemporary World Literatures* (Amsterdam/New York etc: Peter Lang, 2007).

Meuret, Isabelle, 'Writing Size Zero: Figuring Anorexia in Contemporary World Literatures' in Peter L. Twohig and Vera Kalitzkus (eds), *Social Studies of Health, Illness and Disease: Perspectives from the Social Sciences and Humanities* (Amsterdam/New York: Peter Lang, 2008), 75–94. https://doi.org/10.1163/9789401205917_006

Murray, Stuart B., Scott Griffiths, and Jonathan M. Mond, 'Evolving Eating Disorder Psychology: Conceptualising Muscular-Orientated Disordered Eating', *British Medical Journal of Psychiatry* 208.5 (2016): 414–15. https://doi.org/10.1192/bjp.bp.115.168427

Murray, Stuart B., Jason M. Nagata, Scott Griffiths, Jerel P. Calzo, Tiffany A. Brown, Deborah Mitchison, Aaron J. Blashill, and Jonathan M. Mond, 'The Enigma of Male Eating Disorders: A Critical Review and Synthesis', *Clinical Psychology Review* 57 (2017): 1–11. https://doi.org/10.1016/j.cpr.2017.08.001

Norman, Bob, 'The Hunger Artist', *Brodwark Palm Beach New Times*, 19 April 1998, https://www.browardpalmbeach.com/news/the-hunger-artist-6332189, accessed 7 January 2019.

Orbach, Susie, *Fat is a Feminist Issue: The Anti-Diet Guide to Permanent Weight Loss* (New York: Paddington, 1978).

Orbach, Susie, *Hunger Strike: The Anorectic's Struggle as a Metaphor for our Age* (London: Penguin, 1993).

Osgood, Kelsey, *How to Disappear Completely: On Modern Anorexia* (New York: Overlook, 2013).

Petrey, Sandy, 'When Did Literature Stop Being Cultural?', *Diacritics* 28 (1998): 12–22. https://doi.org/10.1353/dia.1998.0024

Prager, Michael, *Fat Boy Thin Man* (Los Gatos, CA: Smashwords, 2010).

Räisänen, Ulla, and Kate Hunt, 'The Role of Gendered Constructions of Eating Disorders in Delayed Help-Seeking in Men: A Qualitative Interview Study', *British Medical Journal Open* 4 (2014). https://doi.org/10.1136/bmjopen-2013-004342

Saxen, Ron, *The Good Eater: The True Story of One Man's Struggle with Binge Eating Disorder* (Oakland, CA: New Harbinger, 2007).

Siebrasse, Brigitte, 'Panikherz', *Psychosoziale Rundschau*, 29 March 2017, https://www .psychiatrie.de/buecher/sucht/stuckrad-barre-panikherz.html, accessed 7 January 2019.

Simon, Scott, *Male Bulimia: My Dark Demon* (Lincoln, NE: iUniverse, 2006).

Slim, Jim, *Auferstanden aus der Magersucht* (Wroclaw: Create Space Independent Publishing Platform, 2015).

Smith, Sidonie, and Julia Watson, *Reading Autobiography: A Guide for Interpreting Life Narratives* (Minneapolis, MS: University of Minnesota Press, 2010).

Sontag, Susan, *Illness as Metaphor and AIDS and its Metaphors* (London: Penguin, 2009 [1978]).

Stanford, Stevie C., and Raymond Lemberg, 'Measuring Eating Disorders in Men: The Development of the Eating Disorder Assessment for Men (EDAM)', *Eating Disorders* 20 (2012): 427–36. https://doi.org/10.1080/10640266.2012.715522

Stuckrad-Barre, Benjamin von, *Panikherz* (Cologne: Kiepenheuer & Witsch, 2016).

Sweeting, Helen, Laura Walker, Alice Maclean, Chris Patterson, Ulla Räisänen, and Kate Hunt, 'Prevalence of Eating Disorders in Males: A Review of Rates Reported in Academic Research and UK Mass Media', *International Journal of Men's Health* 14.2 (2015). : DOI: 10.3149/jmh.1402.86.

Thapliyal, Priyanka, Deborah Mitchison, and Phillipa Hay, 'Insights into the Experiences of Treatment for An Eating Disorder in Men: A Qualitative Study of Autobiographies' in Amanda Sainsbury and Felipe Q. da Luz (eds), *Advances in the Prevention and Management of Obesity and Eating Disorders: Special Issues Edition of Behavioural Sciences* (Basel: MDPI, 2018), 107–23. DOI:10.3390

Thompson, Dominique, 'Boys and Men Get Eating Disorders Too', *Trends in Urology and Men's Health* 8.2 (2017): 9–12. https://doi.org/10.1002/tre.568

Treasure, Janet, Ulrike Schmidt, and Eric van Furth (eds), *Handbook of Eating Disorders. Second Edition* (Chichester: Wiley, 2003). https://doi.org/10.1002/0470013443

Wagner-Egelhaaf, Monika, *Autobiographie* (Stuttgart/Weimar: Metzler, 2000). https://doi.org/10.1007/978-3-476-04037-4

Wilson, Susannah, 'The Iconography of Anorexia in the Long Nineteenth Century' in Ji Wong Chung, Francesca Scott, and Kate Scath (eds), *Picturing Women's Health* (London: Routledge, 2014), 77–104.

Afterword

Lasse Raaby Gammelgaard

This is not the first book to explore the interdisciplinary interrelations and discussions that the topic of literature and madness gives rise to, nor will it be the last. Literature and madness is an inexhaustible topic that will continue to develop and be relevant for both existential and societal reasons for as long as literature and minds exist. Furthermore, the aim to depict minds that function outside of what a society at a certain historical point in time perceives as constituting normalcy will likely continue to be tied with experimental literature, a literature that is playful and that pushes the limits of what is conventional and possible within literature's subsets of genres. Thus, this book is part of an ongoing tradition of research devoted to exploring literature and madness, with an equal interest in uncovering the possibilities of literature and various functions of the human mind.

This volume offers state-of-the-art research on questions related to literature and madness. The contributing scholars work at universities in North America, Western Europe (including the United Kingdom and Scandinavia), the Middle East, and Australia. The literature examined in the chapters is by authors from Persia, the Republic of Ireland, South Africa, the United Kingdom, New Zealand, Canada, the United States of America, Australia, the Netherlands, Italy, and Germany. Although most cases of literature represented historically in the volume are from either the twentieth or the twenty-first century, there is also a case of Arabic literature dating back to the seventh century, as well as literature by Dante from the late medieval period—both of which, by the way, are brought into a dialogue with contemporary clinical psychiatry. From the perspective of literary genres, the chapters of this volume examine novels, short prose, autobiographies, epic poetry, lyric poetry, graphic novels, and patient stories on blogs and in databases. Additionally, two chapters reflect on creative writing. The chapters discuss cases applicable to several different types of mental illnesses, and symptoms related to specific mental illnesses—for instance, melancholia, psychosis, schizophrenia, trauma, bipolar disorder, hoarding disorder, eating disorder, to name a few. The chapters furthermore reflect on topics like anti-psychiatry, Apartheid, and digital sexual assault. Finally, various types of literary theory are employed in the interpretations of the cases, like postcolonial theory, enactivist cognitive theory, narrative theory, genre theory, psychoanalysis, and theory of creative writing. Hence, the volume is marked by diversity on all levels.

Despite the diversity of the material, all contributing authors write about literature in relation to madness, investigating what literature can teach us about mental illness, and how knowledge of mental illness can inform how we approach and interpret specific literary texts and genres. The volume is divided into three parts, although, of course, there are thematic overlaps with two or all three parts in each chapter.

The book opened with literary history and socio-political perspectives. It is misleading to think that only literature of a somewhat distant past is historical. All literature, including contemporary literature, is historical. Nonetheless, and as evidenced by research on madness in relation to a history-of-medicine approach, there often is a gap in the historical knowledge about the perception of mental illness, and in those cases, examples drawn from literature will continue to illuminate the topic of the past. Simultaneously, new theoretical developments may be applied to readings of the literature of the past, yielding new insights from the texts. Literature always to some extent reflects the historical time of its creation, and therefore madness literature at any given time will reflect and comment—whether directly or indirectly—on socio-political perspectives of a society's value system in relation to mental health issues. Future research on historical and socio-political perspectives on mental illness should then continue to highlight the alternative inside perspective presented through literature, and additionally continue to act as watchdog, representing subjective, idiosyncratic views on issues such as coercion in psychiatry (whether through medicine, fixation, or otherwise).

AFTERWORD

The second and largest part of the volume, devoted to literary theory and the experience of mental illness, demonstrates that well-established theories like psychoanalysis and narrative theory are far from exhausted. New theoretical developments applied to traditional cases still shed new light on canonical texts. Furthermore, a lot of the work done within phenomenology and cognitive science as well as research into affect theory will make, I believe, an even bigger impact on research into madness literature within the near future. At the same time, authors invent new genres or combine existing genres in new ways to achieve their artistic goals. These literary experiments force theorists to reshape and rethink their concepts or even create new ones. For instance, the past forty-five years of experiments with blending fictive and autobiographical material in new ways has led to a revolution of theory production within the field of life writing. Another related example is the emergence of the graphic memoir, a genre that mixes comics with autobiographical writing/drawing. A significant portion of the production within both trends represents illnesses in general, among them mental illnesses.

The third part of the book is about literary instrumentality and clinical psychopathology. Although the entire book fits under the umbrella term of health humanities and literature and medicine, this part does so in the most direct way, since it suggests ways in which literature may influence and be influenced by clinical practice. One may roughly divide instrumental approaches into two categories: therapy and education.

On the one hand, literature can be applied as a kind of treatment that supplements other psychological approaches, for instance through reading and writing literature alone or in groups. Guided reading and shared reading as well as creative writing and therapeutic writing are increasingly being employed to produce psychologically healing effects to the person reading or writing. This is something that both patients and professionals within healthcare can do, since professionals working with mental illnesses are likely to experience traumatizing events as well during their career. Both reading and writing as therapy fall under the larger category of art therapy. Reading and writing for both patients and healthcare professionals are part of the revolution of narrative medicine, which I take to be a part of the health humanities in general. And, of course, the notion that literature may have a healing power is not new. To give just one salient example, the philosopher and politician John Stuart Mill claims in his autobiography from 1873 to have overcome a severe depression with suicidal ideation by reading the poetry of William Wordsworth.

On the other hand, literature has the potential to be put to use in educational contexts. As mentioned in the introduction, psychiatric nosology neglects a large part of the human experience and understanding of what it means to be in ill mental health. Students of psychiatry are learning the standardized symptoms and clusters of symptoms, and they learn to identify them in textbook case stories. Literary examples can be employed to problematize such generalizing simplifications of human suffering, but they can also further supplement psychiatric understandings. Literary texts can provide a fuller view into the minds of people, reflecting on causes and motivations, and attempt to explain mental illnesses (including experiences of psychosis) as meaningful experiences. Literature can also show an episode from different viewpoints; in addition to the patient's point of view, literary representations might represent the perspective of the doctor, of a next of kin, or the public viewing something from the outside. Future work on literary instrumentality would do good to further explore and validate literature employed in creative interventions and in the training of healthcare professionals.

This afterword is intended as a reflection on the volume and on which directions research on madness literature might take in future studies. Whatever lies ahead, I think it is safe to say that madness literature—and hopefully also research into literature and mental illness—will perform an important role as a necessary humanistic intervention in a field otherwise dominated by positivist epistemology, creating both dialogue and productive tension between literary and medicalized understandings of mental illness.

Index

Page numbers followed by 'n' refer to endnotes.

4E theories   13, 96–98, 106–7

Abbott, Porter   9–10, 93
Acker, Kathy   143, 158–60; female characters of   146–48; fragments and fragmentation of narratives   150–54; identity and   155–58; plagiarism   155, 157; 'Politics'   152–53; psychosis   144, 151, 154; sexual trauma in writing   145–50; split identity   156
Agnes's Jacket (Hornstein)   119
Albinali, Hajar Ahmed   27
Aldworth, Susan   124
Alighieri, Dante   240, 245, 251–54; "Hell"   246, 252, 253; hoarding and history   245–51
Aliyev, Rustam M.   26
Allan, Clare   78, 79, 81, 82, 87; *Poppy Shakespeare. See Poppy Shakespeare* (Allan)
altered experiential worlds   98–102
anankastic personality   243
anomalous self-experience, clinical evidence of   131–32
anti-psychiatric movement   4, 12, 41–43, 52
anti-psychiatry ethos   41, 42, 52
apartheid   13, 58; camp system   61–69; food in camp system   70–72; madness and   59–61
'Apartheid Thinking' (Coetzee)   59, 67
Attridge, Derek   61
Attwell, David   63

Atwood, Margaret   129; *Surfacing* (Atwood)   132, 135–38, 140
authenticity   128–30, 134, 139

Baker, Charley   140
Baldwin, James   77–78
Bateson, Gregory   121
Bateson, Mary Catherine   121
Beckett, Samuel   41, 42, 44, 45, 50, 53–56; free indirect discourse   43
Beeton, Isabella   250
Bennett, Jane   122; vibrant matter   120–21
Bennett, Jill   180, 181, 184, 190, 195; *Empathic Vision* (Bennett)   180, 184; traumatic memory   191
Beresford, Peter   4
Bernaerts, Lars   6
binge-eating behaviour   269
bipolar disorder   14, 15, 168, 178; 'Disorder' (Dawson)   172–75; 'Eclipse' (Bloch)   175–77; poems about   168–78; 'Returning from the Shopping Center to the Suburbs' (Cooley)   168–72; two moods of   176–77
blackness   78
Blanchot, Maurice   133
blended psychiatry   224–25
Bloch, Chana: 'Eclipse'   175–77
Blood and Guts in High School (Acker)   145
The Body Keeps the Score (Van der Kolk)   182–83
Bolton, Gillie   204

INDEX

Bourdieu's field theory   221–23
Bracken, Patrick   144
brain landscape   124
brain science   113
Bright Lights, Big City (McInerney)   138
Brink, André   59–60, 67
Britton, Celia M.   60, 68
Brooks, Peter   5
bulimia   269
Bürgel, Johann C.   25
Burke, Alban   64, 66
The Burning Bombing of America (Acker)   147–48, 151, 156
Burwick, Frederick   2
Butler, Judith   223, 235

Casey, R.J.   194
celestial language   112
Charon, Rita   10, 106, 264
Chawner, Dave   272, 273; *Weight Expectations: One Man's Recovery from Anorexia*   265–68
Chekhov, Anton   75
The Childlike Life of the Black Tarantula by The Black Tarantula (Acker)   156, 157
Christensen, Robert Zola   209, 214
Christianity   35–36
Chute, Hillary   183
Clarissa (Richardson)   133, 137
cluster   84–85
Coates, Kimberly Engdahl   165, 167, 178
Cockayne, Emily   249
Coetzee, J.M.   58, 59, 61, 63, 64, 69, 71–73; 'Apartheid Thinking'   59, 67; *Life & Times of Michael K*. See *Life & Times of Michael K* (Coetzee)
Cohn, Dorrit   5, 99
Collins, William   61
Collyer Brothers of Harlem   243
common memory   191
confirmation bias   51
confusion of self with not-self   129–32, 134, 135, 138–40
consciousness as vibrant materiality   120–22
contemptus mundi   35
Convivio (Dante Alighieri)   247
Cook, Emma   87
Cooke, Nathalie   136
Cooley, Peter: 'Returning from the Shopping Center to the Suburbs'   168–72
Crawford, Paul   10, 229, 235

creative writing   206, 207
creativity   122–25; and madness   7–8; and mental illness   7; and schizophrenia   8
cultural negotiation   221–24
cultural polarity   250

Dante Alighieri   16, 239–54
Dastan-ı Leyli vu Mecnun (Fuzuli)   28
data production: therapeutic reading   207, 208, 211, 213–16
Dawson, Erica: 'Disorder'   172–75
De Monarchia (Dante Alighieri)   247
Dead Souls (Gogol)   253
Deleuze, Gilles   181, 186–88; encountered sign   184, 195
delusional mood   99
De-Medicalizing Misery: Psychiatry, Psychology and the Human Condition (Rapley, Moncrieff, and Dillon)   164
demonic possession: in *Layla and Majnun*   29–32
depersonalization disorder (DPD)   132
detour   60–61, 68–69, 72
diagnosis: history of   240–42; of hoarding disorder (HD)   243–44
Diagnostic and Statistical Manual of Mental Disorders (DSM)   9, 164–66, 169, 172, 174, 175, 178, 240, 243, 244, 246–48, 251–54
diagnostic criteria   243
diagnostic typology   9
Dick, Leslie   146
Dickens, Charles   249, 253
Die Blechtrommel (Grass)   133, 134
digital sexual assault (DSA)   15, 201–2, 212–14; planning writing workshops for victims   206–10
Dillon, Jacqui   164
diminished selfhood, literary evidence of   132
'Disorder' (Dawson)   172–75
dissociation   182–84, 187, 189–91; art as   194–95
The Divided Self (Laing)   42, 47, 48, 54
divided selves   48, 53–56
Divine Comedy (Dante)   240, 246, 248, 251–53
djinn   31, 32
Dols, Michael   27, 33
Doppelganger   138
DPD. *See* depersonalization disorder (DPD)

INDEX

DSA. *See* digital sexual assault (DSA)
DSM. *See Diagnostic and Statistical Manual of Mental Disorders* (DSM)
Ḏulfaqāri, Ḥasan   25

eating disorders (EDs)   16, 259–60
'Eclipse' (Bloch)   175–77
'écriture faminine'   259
The Edible Woman (Atwood)   129, 136
EDs. *See* eating disorders (EDs)
embodied, enactive, embedded, and extended mind   96–98
Empathic Vision (Bennett)   180, 184
empathy   84; and the gaze   191–94
Empire of the Senseless (Acker)   147, 149, 159
encountered sign   184, 195
epistemic (in)justice   231–34
Equality Act of 2010   87
ethics in therapeutic writing   211–13
evil eye   32

failures of speech   115–19
Faulkner, William   6
Feder, Lillian   6
feeble-mindedness   59, 69, 70
Felman, Shoshana   4, 5
female eating disorders (EDs)   260
field theory   221–23
first-person narratives   128–31, 134
Flint, Kate   105
Fludernik, Monika   139
fou imaginant   6
Foucault, Michel   62, 65, 69, 140
Frame, Janet   111–15, 124–25; *Scented Gardens for the Blind*   111, 115–22
Frank, Arthur   6
Franssen, Gaston   221
'Freaks and the American Ideal of Manhood' (Baldwin)   78
Freud, Sigmund   4, 5, 242–43; psychoanalysis   113, 114; theory of the unconscious   117
Fricker, Miranda   232
Fromm, Erich   242–43
Frost, Randy   243, 246
Fuchs, Thomas   96
Fuzuli   28, 29, 33

Ganjavi, Nizami   23–24; *ghazal* poetry   24–26; *Leili o Majnun. See Leili o Majnun* (Ganjavi); mental illness   24; *Panj Ganj* or *Khamsa* (Quintet)   25
Garnham, Nicholas   222
Genette, Gérard   130
Geworfenheit   63–65, 67–69
ghazal poetry   24–26
ghuls   32
Gilman, Charlotte Perkins   133–34
Glissant, Édouard   58–61, 68, 72
Goffman, Erving   77
Gogol, Nikolai   249, 253
Goldsmith, Rachel E.   183, 184
Gordimer, Nadine   62, 68
Grass, Günter   133, 134

Al-Habeeb, Ahmad   35
habitus   223
Hacking, Ian   242, 250
Haines, Steve   182
hallucination   99
Hartman, Geoffrey H.   166, 170
Hayman Wilson, Hayman Wilson   34
HD. *See* hoarding disorder (HD)
health humanities   8–11
Health Humanities (Crawford)   10–11
'Hell' (Dante)   246, 252, 253
Hennion, Antoine   235
Herman, David   99, 106, 107n1
Herman, Luc   223–24
hermeneutical injustice   232–34
Hesmondhalgh, David   222
history of medicine   6–7
hoarding disorder (HD)   16, 239–40, 246–49, 251, 252; diagnosis of 243–44; DSM-5 definition of 247; historical developments in creation of 242; key characteristics of 249
Hoffmann, E.T.A.   4
Holten, Emma   201
homodiegetic narration   130
Hornstein, Gail A.   119
Hume, Katherine   157
hyperreflexivity   7, 8, 131

ICD-10. *See International Classification of Diseases 10th Edition* (ICD-10)
identity: confusion   129–32, 134, 135, 138–40; of madness   13, 78, 80, 82, 85–88
illness narratives   6, 222–24, 235; Dutch   231–34; and epistemic (in)justice   231–34; male EDs. *See* male eating disorders (EDs); manic

287

INDEX

depression. *See* manic depression narratives
Ilott, Sarah   72
imaginary body   117
Incandescent Alphabets (Rogers)   123
industrial therapy   66
Ingram, Allan   131
insanity   32, 36, 41, 49, 95, 104, 107, 155
International Classification of Diseases 10th Edition (ICD-10)   243–44
Involuntary Commitment Act of 1973   64, 65
ipseity disturbance   129, 131, 132
irreducible particularity   9, 10
al-Iṣbahānī, Abū Bakr Muḥammad ibn Dāwūd   27
Islam   36; madness in   37
Islamic psychology, modern: Nizami's poem and   36–37
Islamic psychotherapeutic models   36–37

Jaëck, Nathalie   8
James, William   242
Jāmī, Nur ad-Dīn Abd ar-Rahmān   33
Jamison, Kay Redfield   7
jann   30–31
Jaspers, Karl   154
al-Jawzi, Ibn   28
Jones, Carole   268
Jones, Tiffany Fawn   65, 71
Jones, William   34, 260
Joranger, Line   174–75
jouissance   118
al-junūn   30
al-Jurjani, Zayn al-Din Sayyed Isma'il ibn Husayn   29

Karkas (Schavemaker)   229–31, 233–35
Keitel, Evelyne   153, 231
Kent, Gerry   36–37
Khairallah, As'ad E.   35, 36
Kinsella, Elizabeth Anne   232, 233
Koelewijn, Rinskje   231
Kofoed, Jette   211
Kotowicz, Zbigniew   52
Krasnow, Michael   273; *My Life as a Male Anorexic*   262–65
Kronfol, Ziad   31

Lacan, Jacques: psychoanalysis   13–14, 112–14; theory of the unconscious   117, 118
Ladegaard, Nicolai   203

Laing, Ronald D.   41–44, 46–48, 53–56, 131; mental illness   55; Murphy and   48–52; schizoid   53; schizophrenia   42, 53, 54
larynx lips tongue   116
Le discours antillais (Glissant)   58, 60
Leader, Darian   129–30, 139, 144
LeBlanc, Stephanie   232, 233
Leili o Majnun (Ganjavi)   12, 23–25; madness and demonic possession in   29–32; modern Islamic psychology   36–37; physiological readings of, mythos   27–29; spiritualist and Sufi interpretations of   33–36; summary of the poem   26–27
Life & Times of Michael K (Coetzee)   58–61; apartheid camp system in   61–69; food in apartheid camp system   70–72; Michael's self-starvation   70–73
literature   3; and madness   3–8, 128, 132–37, 139, 140, 282, 283
Llambías, Pablo   203, 204, 208, 214
Lotringer, Sylvere   155, 156, 158
love madness: in Arabic and Persian literature   24–26
love-melancholia   27–29

McCloud, Scott   187, 192, 196
McGrath, Patrick   134–35
McInerney, Jay   138
McNichol, Kathleen   205, 206, 208, 210, 213–16
'Mad persons'   232–33
madness   2, 10, 44, 56, 65, 93, 99, 102; and apartheid   59–61; border   78, 85; creativity and   7–8; defined   58; function of   75–78; identity of   75, 78, 80, 82, 85–88; in Islam   37; Islamic conceptions of   23; in *Layla and Majnun*   29–32; *Life & Times of Michael K* (Coetzee)   61–69; literature of   3–8, 128, 132–37, 139, 140, 282, 283; love, in Arabic and Persian literature   24–26; Majnun's   33, 35; *versus* sanity   154; women's   147, 150
Madness and Modernism: Insanity in the Light of Modern Art, Literature, and Thought (Sass)   7–8
male anorexia. *See* male eating disorders (EDs)
male eating disorders (EDs)   260, 271–73; *My Life as a Male Anorexic*

INDEX

(Krasnow) 262–65; *Panikherz* 268–71; *Weight Expectations: One Man's Recovery from Anorexia* (Chawner) 265–68
manic depression 221
manic depression narratives 222–23; *Karkas* (Schavemaker) 229–31, 233–35; PsychoseNet case 227–29, 233–35; Story Bank for Psychiatry (*Verhalenbank Psychiatrie*) case 224–27, 233–35
Matzerath, Oskar 133, 134
medical taxonomy 250
medieval Christianity 35–36
melancholia 1, 7, 23, 27–29, 46, 61
mental disorders 97, 240, 242
mental distress 85, 95, 132
Mental Health Clustering Tool (MHCT) 84, 85
mental illness 2, 8–9, 24, 31, 42, 55, 95, 107, 113; creativity and 7, 123–24; Majnun's 28; poetry and 166–68, 178; and Woolf, Virginia 167–68, 175
mental institutions 49, 71
Metzl, Jonathan 77
Meuret, Isabelle 273
MHCT. *See* Mental Health Clustering Tool (MHCT)
mind: embodied, enactive, embedded, and extended 96–98; as matter 124
miserliness 243, 244
Mitchinson, Kevin 124
modern Islamic psychology 36–37
Moncrieff, Joanna 164
Morgan, John 260
Morgenthaler, Walter 124
Mrs Dalloway (Woolf) 93–95; altered experiential worlds of characters 98–102; connecting the characters 95, 96, 102–4, 106; critics of 94; embodied, enactive, embedded, and extended mind 96–98; reading in space and time 105–7
Munro, Martin 68–69
Murphy (Beckett) 41–44, 47, 48; divided selves 53–56; Murphy and Laing 48–52; Murphy's introduction to asylum life 44–46
My Life as a Male Anorexic (Krasnow) 262–65

nafs 33, 35

narratives: fiction 10; illness. *See* illness narratives; medicine 264; theory 5, 6
Neoplatonism 34–36
neuropsychiatry 114
NHS England 84–85
Noë, Alva 106
Nora van Middelaar (fictional narrator) 229–31
Nünning, Ansgar 130

Obsessive-Compulsive Disorder (OCD) 243, 244
Obsessive-Compulsive Personality Disorder (OCPD) 243, 244, 248
Obsessive-Compulsive Related Disorder (OCRD) 244, 252
On Being Ill (Woolf) 6, 165, 167–68, 170, 178
ontological anxiety 137
Orbach, Susie 259, 260
Ormston, Camille 124
other/otherness 62, 68, 70–72, 81, 206
Outsider Art: Visionary Worlds and Trauma (Wojcik) 123

Panikherz (Stuckrad-Barre) 268–71
Panj Ganj or *Khamsa* (Quintet) 25
Parnas, Josef 131
Parrish, Tommi 182; *Perfect Hair*. *See Perfect Hair* (Parrish); sensorial Figure 180, 186–88, 196; treatment of trauma 188
participatory research approach 207
Patel, Vikram 252
Penzel, Fred 242, 246
Perfect Hair (Parrish) 180, 181, 183, 184, 196–97; art as dissociation 194–95; contents of the body 186; empathy and the gaze 191–94; fact of the body 186–88; meaning of colour and the line 188–90; self-empathy 194; table of contents 184–85; violence of discourse 190–91
Petrey, Sandy 273
Pitchford, Nicola 146, 147
plagiarism 155, 157
Plyushkin syndrome 249
'Politics' (Acker) 152–53
Poppy Shakespeare (Allan) 75, 84, 85; identity of madness 75, 78, 80, 82, 85–88; normalizing madness 78–83
Porter, Roy 6, 130–31

INDEX

postcolonial fiction   183
postcolonial political rhetoric   36
postcoloniality   60
postmodern fiction   183
post-traumatic memory   180, 184
Prinzhorn, Hans   123
pronominal shift   14, 129–33, 136, 138, 140
psychiatric diagnosis   83–84
psychiatric nosology   284
psychiatric phenomenon   242
psychoanalysis   5; Freud, Sigmund   113, 114; Lacan, Jacques   13–14
psychoanalytic theory   113, 120
psychological trauma   182–84. *See also* dissociation
psychopathographic narratives   154
psychophysical misfit   137
PsychoseNet   227–29, 233–35
psychosis   14, 112–15, 117–19, 130, 143–44, 151–54, 158, 159
psychotic delusion   122
psychotics   54

Quayson, Ato   62

Radden, Jennifer   2, 7–9
Rapley, Mark   164
'Reading' (Woolf)   105
reading psychosis   153
'Returning from the Shopping Center to the Suburbs'(Cooley)   168–72
Richardson, Samuel   133, 137, 139
Rieger, Branimir   5
Rimmon-Kenan, Shlomith   166
Rip Off Red, Girl Detective (Acker)   148–49
Rogers, Annie G.   111–15, 117–20, 122–25; *Incandescent Alphabets*   123
Rogers, Sean   182

sane schizoid   53, 56
sanity   36, 41, 82, 95, 104, 107; madness *versus*   154. *See also* insanity
Sarabando, Andreia   121
Sass, Louis A.   7–8, 99, 129, 131, 138
Satterlee, Michelle   183, 184
Saussure, Ferdinand de   136
Scented Gardens for the Blind (Frame)   115–22; consciousness as vibrant materiality   120–22
Schavemaker, Femke: *Karkas*   221, 229–31, 233–35

Scheepers, Floortje   221, 224–25
schizophrenia   7–8, 12, 42, 44, 48, 50–56, 111–14, 124, 131, 132, 144, 155, 158
Schlichter, Annette   147, 156
Scott, Bonnie Kime   95
Scott, Ronnie   181
second-person narratives   138–39. *See also* first-person narratives
self and the world   99, 101, 102
self-empathy   194
self-harm   147–50
sensation   186–88
sense memory   191
sexual violence   145–50
Seyed-Gohrab, Ali-Asghar   33, 34
Short History (Steketee)   249
Showalter, Elaine   77
signe du miroir   138
Sina, Ibn   27–29, 31
Skott-Myhre, Hans A.   4
Smith, David L.   84
The Space of Literature (Blanchot)   133
Spider (McGrath)   134–35
split consciousness   43
spoiled identity   77, 85–88
Staunæs, Dorthe   211
Steenberg, Mette   203, 204, 206, 208, 214
Steketee, Gail   246, 248, 252
Story Bank for Psychiatry (*Verhalenbank Psychiatrie*)   224–27, 233–35
Strasser, Susan   250
Stuckrad-Barre, Benjamin von   272, 273; *Panikherz*   268–71
Sufi interpretations: of *Layla and Majnun*   33–36
Suhaila Ghuloum   31
Surfacing (Atwood)   132, 135–38, 140

tabi'   31
testimonial injustice   232, 233
therapeutic philosophy   47
therapeutic reading   203–5, 215–16, 283
therapeutic writing   202–6, 215–16, 283; as ethics   211–13; example of task   210–11; media ethics   211; practice   206–9; principles for progression of   208; and problem of data production   213–15; tasks   213–14; workshop for DSA victims   206–10
Thiher, Allen   6

INDEX

Thompson, Geoffrey 48
The Tin Drum. See Die Blechtrommel (Grass)
Todorov, Tzvetan 5
Touched with Fire: Manic-Depressive Illness and the Artistic Temperament (Jamison) 7
trauma: psychological 182–84
Trauma is Very Strange (Haines) 182
traumatic memory 191
'tunnelling process': Woolf, Virginia 13, 95, 96, 106

Udhrī poetry 24, 25
Udhrite love 25
UK National Institute for Health and Care Excellence (NICE) 144
Ussher, Jane M. 150

Van der Kolk, Bessel A. 182–83
veils 33, 34
Vervaeck, Bart 223–24
vibrant materiality: consciousness as 120–22
Vibrant Matter: A Political Ecology of Things (Bennett) 120–21
Virgil 246, 248

Wahass, Saheed 36–37

Weber, Alan S. 31
Weight Expectations: One Man's Recovery from Anorexia (Chawner) 265–68
'What Does It Mean to Be Mad? Diagnosis, Narrative, Science, and the DSM' (Abbott) 9–10, 93
Wheeler, Kathleen 154
willful blindness 51
Williams, Valeria 234
Winters, Renee 246
Wisdom, Madness and Folly (Laing) 42, 47
Wojahn, David 168
Wojcik, Daniel 123
Wolff, Janet 222–23
Wollen, Peter 146, 151
women's madness 147, 150
Woolf, Virginia 6, 93–96, 165; *On Being Ill* 165, 167–68, 170, 178; mental illness and 167–68, 175; *Mrs Dalloway. See Mrs Dalloway* (Woolf); tunneling process to connect the characters 13, 95, 96, 106; understanding of the mind 97–98
Writing Size Zero (Meuret) 273

The Yellow Wallpaper (Gilman) 133–34

Zaikowski, Carolyn 145

Lightning Source UK Ltd.
Milton Keynes UK
UKHW011226040922
408256UK00002B/13